Handbook of Gastrointestinal Drug Therapy

Handbook of Gastrointestinal Drug Therapy

Second Edition

Edited by
Michael M. Van Ness, M.D.
Associate Professor of Internal Medicine, Northeastern Ohio Universities College of Medicine, Rootstown; Attending Physician, Canton Affiliated Hospitals, Canton, Ohio

Michael S. Gurney, M.D.
Partner, West Hills Gastroenterology Associates P.C.; Attending Physician, St. Vincent Medical Center and Legacy Affiliated Hospitals, Portland, Oregon

D. Michael Jones, M.D.
Chief, Division of Gastroenterology, National Naval Medical Center, Bethesda, Maryland

Foreword by
Stanley B. Benjamin, M.D.
Chief, Division of Gastroenterology and Professor of Medicine, Georgetown University School of Medicine, Washington, D.C.

Little, Brown and Company
Boston New York Toronto London

Second Edition

Library of Congress Cataloging-in-Publication Data

Handbook of gastrointestinal drug therapy / edited by Michael M. Van Ness, Michael S. Gurney, D. Michael Jones ; foreword by Stanley B. Benjamin. — 2nd ed.
p. cm.
Includes bibliographical references and index.
ISBN 0-316-89731-0
1. Gastrointestinal agents—Handbooks, manuals, etc. I. Van Ness, Michael M. II. Gurney, Michael S. III. Jones, D. Michael (Dan Michael)
[DNLM: 1. Gastrointestinal Disease—drug therapy—handbooks. WI 39 H2355 1995]
RM355.H36 1995
616.3′3061—dc20
DNLM/DLC
for Library of Congress 95-8044
CIP

Printed in the United States of America

RRD-VA

Editorial: Nancy Megley and Richard L. Wilcox
Production Editor: Karen Feeney
Copyeditor: Libby Dabrowski
Indexer: Nancy Newman
Production Supervisor: Louis C. Bruno, Jr.
Cover Designer: Louis C. Bruno, Jr.

To

Hyman J. Zimmerman, M.D.,
Professor of Medicine, Georgetown Universit
School of Medicine, and Distinguished
Physician, Veterans Administration
Medical Center, Washington, D.C.

and

Frank Ruddle, Ph.D.,
Professor of Biology, Yale University,
New Haven, Connecticut

Their dedication to the art and science of clinical medicine and basic science research has been an inspiration to all who have been privileged to know and work with them.

Contents

V. MOTILITY DISORDER DRUGS

VI. GASTROENTEROLOGY PROCEDURE-RELATED DRUGS

Foreword

This application of pharmacologic principles to gastrointestinal drug therapy is required for the safe and effective treatment of diseases of the gastrointestinal tract. Given the ubiquitous nature of disorders of the gastrointestinal tract, all physicians, from the primary-care provider to the subspecialty consultant, need a complete and thorough understanding of available drugs. *Handbook of Gastrointestinal Drug Therapy,* Second Edition, not only provides a solid foundation for the family practitioner, internist, or general surgeon but also goes beyond a review of approved agents and indications and provides an up-to-date analysis of some promising experimental drugs. Last, the authors look at non–FDA-approved uses of currently available agents and examine the potential benefit of some nonapproved drug applications.

The editors, Drs. Michael M. Van Ness, Michael S. Gurney, and D. Michael Jones, are uniquely qualified to provide this type of analysis. They have worked in the rich environment of the National Naval Medical Center, have conducted their own research, and have benefitted from a referral system that places the Naval Medical Center at the focus of a worldwide medical network. The editors also have daily contact with colleagues at the National Institutes of Health, the National Cancer Institute, Georgetown University, and the Armed Forces Institute of Pathology.

They are to be congratulated for preparing a useful and informative text that provides physicians at all levels of practice with current and practical guidelines on gastrointestinal drug therapy.

Stanley B. Benjamin, M.D.

Preface

Handbook of Gastrointestinal Drug Therapy, Second Edition, was inspired by our participation in teaching conferences in the Gastroenterology Division of the Department of Internal Medicine at the National Naval Medical Center, Bethesda, Maryland and the Gastroenterology Fellowship Program at the Portsmouth Naval Hospital Norfolk, Virginia. The intellectual stimulation of young, aggressive and eager Fellows in gastroenterology caused us to review and update our knowledge of the medications useful in the treatment of gastrointestinal diseases.

Although many of the agents discussed in the book are well known to students and practicing physicians, the application of these drugs in a thoughtful and consistent manner to routine and not-so-routine situations demands a conscientious approach to the mechanism of action and pharmacodynamics of each agent.

We have not steered away from newer agents with narrow applications, nor have we avoided discussion of drugs with utility outside the Food and Drug Administration guidelines. Use of such drugs demands a thorough understanding of the risks and benefits inherent in the use of the drug in question. To keep as current as possible in this regard, we have focused considerable attention on the most recent literature available for review, as well as on our own experiences.

It is a testimony to the Gastroenterology Division at National Naval Medical Center, as well as the Department of Internal Medicine, that many of its members produced and refined this work while continuing to provide outstanding care, perform quality research, and support the needs of a large and growing beneficiary population.

The house officers and secretarial staff of the Department of Internal Medicine, Northeastern Ohio Universities College of Medicine, under the direction of Andrew Ognibene, Brigadier General, U.S. Army Medical Corps (ret.), at Aultman Hospital and Timken Mercy Medical Center, supported and advanced this effort enthusiastically.

Last, without the patience and love of our wives, Jean and Pamela, and our children, Emma, Claire, Elliott, Kaitlin, Emily, Evan, Tessa, and Travis, this book could not have been written.

M.M.V.N
M.S.G.
D.M.J.

Contributing Authors

Richard D. Baertlein, M.D.
Chief Resident in Medicine, St. Vincent Medical Center, Portland, Oregon

James A. Butler, M.D.
Assistant Professor of Medicine, Uniformed Services University of the Health Sciences, F. Edward Hébert School of Medicine; Staff Gastroenterologist and Internist, National Naval Medical Center, Bethesda, Maryland

Michael Carboni, M.D.

Brooks D. Cash, M.D.
Instructor in Medicine, Department of Internal Medicine, Uniformed Services University of the Health Sciences, F. Edward Hébert School of Medicine, Bethesda, Maryland

M.R. Chowdhury, M.D.
Teaching Fellow, Uniformed Services University of the Health Sciences, F. Edward Hébert School of Medicine, Bethesda, Maryland

Walter J. Coyle, M.D.
Clinical Fellow, National Naval Medical Center, Bethesda, Maryland

J. Thomas Dorsey III, M.D.
Clinical Assistant Professor of Medicine, West Virginia University School of Medicine, Morgantown; Staff, Ohio Valley Medical Center, Wheeling, West Virginia

Thomas A. Dowgin, M.D.
Assistant Professor, Uniformed Services University of the Health Sciences, F. Edward Hébert School of Medicine, Bethesda, Maryland; Staff Gastroenterologist and Internist, National Naval Medical Center, Bethesda, Maryland

Frank A. Hamilton, M.D., M.P.H.
Branch Chief, Digestive Diseases Branch, National Institutes of Health; Consultant, Division of Gastroenterology, National Naval Medical Center, Bethesda, Maryland

Barry E. Herman, M.D.
Assistant Professor of Internal Medicine, Uniformed Services University of the Health Sciences, F. Edward Hébert School of Medicine; Staff Gastroenterologist, National Naval Medical Center, Bethesda, Maryland

David A. Johnson, M.D.
Associate Professor of Medicine, Eastern Virginia School of Medicine, Norfolk, Virginia

Mark H. Johnston, M.D.
Clinical Fellow, Division of Gastroenterology, National Naval Medical Center, Bethesda, Maryland

George Koval, M.D.
Partner, West Hills Gastroenterology Associates P.C., Portland, Oregon

Thong P. Le, M.D.
Clinical Fellow, Division of Infectious Diseases, National Naval Medical Center, Bethesda, Maryland

C. Samuel Ledford, M.D.
Instructor in Medicine, Department of Internal Medicine, National Naval Medical Center, Bethesda, Maryland

Michael F. Lyons, M.D.
Staff, Department of Gastroenterology, Madigan Army Medical Center, Tacoma, Washington

John D. Malone, M.D.
Associate Professor, Uniformed Services University of the Health Sciences, F. Edward Hébert School of Medicine; Head, Division of Infectious Diseases, National Naval Medical Center, Bethesda, Maryland

David J. Roberts, M.D.
Assistant Professor of Medicine, Uniformed Services University of the Health Sciences, F. Edward Hébert School of Medicine; Staff, Division of Gastroenterology, National Naval Medical Center, Bethesda, Maryland

Rodger A. Sleven, M.D.
Partner, West Hills Gastroenterology Associates P.C., Portland, Oregon

Amy M. Tsuchida, M.D.
Chief, Department of Gastroenterology, Madigan Army Medical Center, Tacoma, Washington

John J. Vargo, M.D.
Staff Gastroenterologist, Cleveland Clinic, Cleveland, Ohio

Margaret Andrea Wise, R.N., C.G.C.
Certified Gastroenterology Registered Nurse, North Canton, Ohio

Notice

The indications and dosages of all drugs in this book have been recommended in the medical literature and conform to the practices of the general medical community. The medications described do not necessarily have specific approval by the Food and Drug Administration for use in the diseases and dosages for which they are recommended. The package insert for each drug should be consulted for use and dosage as approved by the FDA. Because standards for usage change, it is advisable to keep abreast of revised recommendations, particularly those concerning new drugs.

Anti-Ulcer and Antigastroesophageal Reflux Disease Drugs

Treatment of Acid-Peptic Disease

Over the past two decades, the treatment of peptic ulcer and gastroesophageal reflux disease has been revolutionized by the development of effective drugs for suppression of acid secretion, the widespread use of endoscopic instruments that give precise diagnostic information, the acceptance of newer invasive methods such as esophageal manometry and 24-hour pH probe monitoring, and our increasing understanding of the role of *Helicobacter pylori.* With these advances, new challenges arise, such as how to treat early recurrence of peptic ulcer disease, how best to give prophylaxis of stress mucosal ulceration and bleeding, what to do with the patient who has refractory acid-peptic disease, and how best to eradicate *H. pylori.*

Historical Perspective

Until the introduction of competitive H_2-receptor antagonists in 1978, medical therapy of peptic ulcer disease was limited to antacid therapy with dietary and life-style regulation. In 1915, Sippy introduced a powder consisting of calcium carbonate, sodium bicarbonate, magnesium oxide, and bismuth subcarbonate. Approximately 60 percent of ulcers healed on his "Sippy diet," but serious life-style disruptions and occasional complications of the alkaline diet such as the milk-alkali syndrome occurred in up to one-third of patients. Severe metabolic alkalosis, azotemia, and hypercalcemia caused death in rare (<5%) cases.

As late as 1974, Menguy stated that the ulcer patient needed to "lead a stereotyped existence" so as not to stimulate the sensitive "ulcer-prone" stomach.

The problems of recurrent and recalcitrant ulcers and complications such as bleeding, perforation, and gastric outlet obstruction provided surgeons with the impetus to develop innovative procedures to deal with these problems. In 1881, Woffler performed the first gastrojejunostomy for an obstructing carcinoma of the stomach, and in the same year Billroth accomplished the first successful gastric resection by performing a gastroduodenostomy for a pyloric carcinoma.

The incidence of dumping in the 2- to 5-year period after surgery ranges from 27 percent for selective vagotomy and drainage to 4 percent for parietal cell vagotomy. Diarrhea is reported in 17 percent of the patients who had total vagotomy and drainage, compared to only 3 percent of the patients who underwent parietal cell vagotomy. Ulcer recurrence is seen in 16 percent of the parietal cell vagoto patients, 14.9 percent of the selective vagotomy and drainage patients, and 9.6 percent of the total vagotomy and drainage patients.

Uncontrollable bleeding, perforation, and refractory gastric outlet obstruction remain clear and compelling reasons for surgical intervention. The costs and consequences of surgical intervention remain strong incentives for use of effective medical therapy.

Currently, H_2-receptor antagonists as a class are the "gold standard" by which to measure agents that are effective in the treatment of acid-peptic disease. To review, acid secretion results from parietal cell receptor stimulation by one or more secretagogues: histamine, acetylcholine, or gastrin. Agents that block interaction of these agonists with the H_2-histamine receptor, the M_1-cholinergic receptor, and the gastrin receptor decrease the acidity and volume of gastric secretions. At present, four H_2-receptor antagonists are approved by the Food and Drug Administration for treatment of duodenal ulcer disease: cimetidine (introduced in 1977), ranitidine (introduced in 1982), famotidine (introduced in 1987), and nizatidine (introduced in 1988). The agents differ in chemical structure, potency, and dosage. All are remarkably safe and effective. The use of one or all of these agents can be justified in a number of other conditions, including gastroesophageal reflux disease, prophylaxis against and treatment of acute allergic drug reactions, stress mucosal ulceration prophylaxis, acute acetaminophen overdose, and pill-induced esophagitis. It can also be used as an adjunct in the treatment of acute upper gastrointestinal hemorrhage and to facilitate eradication of *H. pylori*.

The most powerful suppressor of acid secretion currently available is the substituted benzimidazole omeprazole. It inhibits the action of the hydrogen ion/potassium (H+/K+)–adenosine triphosphatase (ATPase) present on the luminal portion of the parietal cell membrane, thereby markedly decreasing basal and pentagastrin-stimulated acid secretion. Although not approved by the Food and Drug Administration for peptic ulcer disease, omeprazole heals duodenal ulcers more rapidly and with prompter pain relief than do the H_2-receptor antagonists. In one trial omeprazole healed 100 percent of peptic ulcers that were refractory to treatment with H_2-receptor antagonists, colloidal bismuth, or sucralfate alone and in combination. Omeprazole is known to cause enterochromaffinlike cell hyperplasia and carcinoid tumors in rats. Bacterial overgrowth of the stomach and proximal duodenum with oral flora is commonly seen as a *Candida albicans* esophagitis, most likely a consequence of prolonged acid suppression.

Agents that enhance mucosal defenses are also available. Sucralfate, a basic aluminum salt of sucrose octasulfate, becomes viscous and adhesive at a pH less than 4 and binds to ulcerated mucosa. It protects gastric mucosa by an increase in intramucosal prostaglandin E_2, by inhibition of pepsin, and by absorption of bile acids. It accelerates healing of mucosal lesions compared to placebo therapy and is approved for the short-term treatment of acute duodenal ulcer. Like the H_2-receptor antagonists, its use can be justified from evidence in the medical literature for a number of other conditions, such as prophylaxis against stress-induced mucosal ulceration, bile reflux gastritis, refractory peptic ulcer disease, and drug-induced gastritis (from aspirin, other nonsteroidal anti-inflammatory agents, and alcohol).

Another class of compounds that enhance mucosal defenses are the prostaglandins, derivatives of arachidonic acid, that are found in most mammalian tissues and have many biologic properties. In the gastric mucosa, the endogenous prostaglandins E_2 and I_2 decrease gastric acid secretion and accelerate ulcer healing. Exogenous prostaglandinlike drugs appear to act by a "cytoprotective" mechanism at low doses and an antisecretory mechanism at higher doses. Although controversy exists as to the components of cytoprotection (thickened gastric mucus, decreased epithelial cell exfoliation, maintenance of gastric blood flow, or restoration of the hydrophobic nonwettable surface of the gastric mucosa), use of these agents (misoprostol, enprostil) in doses that suppress acid secretion is effective in the treatment of peptic ulcer.

Renewed interest in the infectious component to the pathogenesis and early recurrence of peptic ulcer disease has sparked interest in the anti-ulcer effects of bismuth. The organism *H. pylori* is associated with acute and chronic gastritis, a susceptibility to antral ulceration, and a possible association with gastric lymphoma. This organism is most effectively eradicated by a combination of bismuth and antimicrobial agents. The utility of bismuth alone or in combination with antimicrobial agents for treatment of duodenal ulcers has been shown. Eradication of the organism was associated with recurrence of ulcers in fewer than 20 percent of cases, compared to ulcer recurrence in nearly 50 percent of cases treated with acid suppression alone. The role of bismuth remains to be clearly defined, but its potential uses are generating considerable interest and excitement. The risks of bismuth therapy and toxicity are being elucidated.

Suggested Readings

Bayerdorffer E, et al. Double-blind treatment of early gastric MALT-lymphoma patients by *Helicobacter pylori* eradication. Gastroenterology 1994; 106:A370.
The favorable response to Helicobacter pylori *eradication leads this group to suggest that primary gastric MALT-lymphoma may be directly related to* H. pylori *gastritis.*

Behar J, et al. Efficacy of sucralfate in the prevention of recurrence of duodenal ulcer (abstr). Gastroenterology 1986; 90:1343.
Sucralfate, 1 gm after meals twice a day, was found to decrease the duodenal ulcer relapse rate (35%, N=30) at 1 year compared to placebo (81%, N=31).

Christiansen J, et al. Prospective controlled vagotomy trial for duodenal ulcer. Ann Surg 1981; 193:49–55.
A prospective evaluation of the effectiveness, morbidity, mortality, and ulcer recurrence rate after parietal cell vagotomy, truncal vagotomy and drainage, and selective gastric vagotomy and drainage. Complications were fewest but ulcer recurrences highest in the parietal cell vagotomy group.

Fried M, et al. Duodenal bacterial overgrowth during treatment in outpatients with omeprazole. Gut 1994; 35:23–26.
Duodenal bacterial overgrowth is common in omeprazole patients. Malabsorption of fat has not been studied.

Hamilton I, et al. Healing and recurrence of duodenal ulcer after

treatment with tripotassium dicitrato bismuthate (TDB) tablets or cimetidine. Gut 1986; 27:106–110.
The patient cohort treated with TDB had a recurrence rate of 25 percent at 12 months, compared to a recurrence rate of 68 percent in the cimetidine-treated group.

Hasan M, Sircus V. The factors determining success or failure of cimetidine treatment of peptic ulcer. J Clin Gastroenterol 1981; 3:225–229.
Drinking up to 5 pints of beer a day did not interfere with duodenal ulcer healing in British patients.

Lam S-K, et al. Prostaglandin E_1 (misoprostol) overcomes the adverse effect of chronic cigarette smoking on duodenal ulcer healing. Dig Dis Sci 1986; 31 (Feb suppl):68S–74S.
Misoprostol overcame the adverse effects of cigarette smoking on duodenal ulcer healing.

Marcuard SP, et al. Omeprazole therapy causes malabsorption of cyanocobalamin (vitamin B_{12}). Ann Intern Med 1994; 120: 211–215.
Significant reductions in vitamin B_{12} are seen in patients who take omeprazole, 20 mg. Absorption decreased from 2.3 percent before therapy to 0.9 percent after treatment.

Marshall BJ, Warren JR. Unidentified curved bacilli in the stomach of patients with gastritis and peptic ulceration. Lancet 1984; i:1311–1315.
The authors noted curved, gram-negative rods in the stomach of patients with gastritis and were motivated to fulfill Koch's postulates in a subsequent report. A new and provocative line of research was initiated based on these observations and may explain the cause of refractory ulcer disease in a subset of chronically achlorhydric patients.

Menguy RB. Stomach. In SI Schwartz (ed), *Principles of Surgery.* New York: McGraw-Hill, 1974.
A comprehensive review of the state-of-the-art treatment of peptic ulcer disease immediately before the introduction of H_2-receptor antagonists into clinical practice.

Muller AF, et al. Primary gastric lymphoma in Nottinghamshire, U.K. Gastroenterology 1994; 106:A419.

Parsonnet J, et al. *Helicobacter pylori* infection and gastric lymphoma. N Engl J Med 1994; 770:1267–1271.
Non-Hodgkin's lymphoma affecting the stomach is associated with previous H. pylori *infection. A cause-and-effect role remains to be proved.*

Simko V, Michael S. Retrospective analysis of toxicity of oral bismuth. Gastroenterology 1994; 106:A181.
Bismuth toxicity is seen with serum levels of 50 to 100 mg/liter and is manifested by confusion, dysarthria, myoclonus, lethargy, and coma.

Sontag S, et al. Cimetidine, cigarette smoking, and recurrence of duodenal ulcer. N Engl J Med 1984; 311:689–693.
Continued cigarette smoking during the time of treatment to prevent recurrent ulcer negated the benefits of cimetidine therapy. Optimal prophylaxis against ulcer recurrence requires cessation of smoking.

Walan A, et al. Effect of omeprazole and ranitidine on ulcer healing and relapse rates in patients with benign gastric ulcer. N Engl J Med 1989; 320:69–75.

In a study of 602 patients with benign gastric ulcer, healing rates at 4 weeks were 80 percent in the 40-mg omeprazole group and 59 percent in the ranitidine group. In a subgroup of 68 patients taking concurrent nonsteroidal anti-inflammatory agents, the healing rates were 81 percent in the 40-mg omeprazole group and 32 percent in the ranitidine group.

Antacids

Michael M. Van Ness

Even with the widespread availability of H_2-receptor antagonists, sucralfate, and other effective agents, antacids still have a place in the treatment of acid-peptic disease. Antacids work by neutralizing gastric acid. The neutralizing capacity, sodium content, monthly cost of therapy, and number of tablets containing 140 mEq of acid-neutralizing capacity vary widely (Table 1-1). Unlike sodium bicarbonate (baking soda), none of the acid-neutralizing compounds listed in Table 1-1 is absorbed into the systemic circulation.

The different agents—aluminum hydroxide, magnesium hydroxide, calcium carbonate, and aluminum phosphate—have several distinguishing features. The aluminum-containing compounds (aluminum hydroxide and aluminum phosphate) tend to be constipating and hence are frequently combined with agents that tend to produce diarrhea, such as magnesium hydroxide. Fordtran and Barreras have shown that calcium carbonate, a very effective acid-neutralizing drug, when taken in 4- to 8-gm/day dosages, causes a nearly 50 percent increase in acid output (4–7 mEq/hr), with a fall in gastric pH from a baseline of 1.7 to 1.2. This acid rebound is believed to be secondary to contact of the small-bowel mucosa with calcium, not antral alkalinization or elevated serum total calcium levels, despite an average rise of serum calcium levels of 0.7 mg/dl.

Brody and Bachrach have advanced the idea that the rapid acid-neutralizing capacity of liquid antacids (<15 minutes) makes them superior to the slower acid-neutralizing antacid tablets.

INDICATIONS

Antacids are indicated in the treatment of common heartburn (pyrosis), symptomatic hiatal hernia and peptic esophagitis (gastroesophageal reflux disease), gastritis, and peptic ulcer.

Peterson and associates showed that 30 ml of a Mylanta-like antacid (capable of neutralizing 154 mEq acid), given 7 times a day (1 and 3 hours postcibal and at bedtime), resulted in a duodenal ulcer healing rate of 78 percent after 4 weeks of therapy, compared to a 45 percent healing rate in patients treated with placebo. The daily acid-neutralizing action of the dosages used in the study was 1078 mEq.

Fordtran has reinforced the notion that adequate quantities of liquid antacids must be taken to optimize duodenal ulcer healing rates and that failure to heal duodenal ulcers with antacids may result simply from inadequate dosing. Other authors disagree. In a study from Norway, Berstad and associates found that two antacid tablets 7 times a day for 4 weeks resulted in a healing of peptic ulcers in 81 percent of patients (N=78) despite only 280 mEq daily acid-neutralizing capacity. Interestingly, Berstad's group found that the anticholinergic drug pirenzepine, an M_1-muscarinic receptor antagonist, in combination with a low dose of antacids, was equivalent to a double dose of antacid in the healing of duodenal ulcers. They believe that this combination may improve patient compliance compared to high-dose antacids alone.

Table 1-1. Comparison of liquid and tablet antacids

	Acid-neutralizing capacity (mEq/ml)	Volume containing 140 mEq (ml)	Sodium content (mg/5 ml)	Monthly cost of therapy ($)
Antacids (liquid)				
Aluminum hydroxide, magnesium hydroxide				
Maalox TC	4.2	33	1.2	44
Delcid	4.1	34	1.5	57
Aluminum hydroxide, magnesium hydroxide, simethicone				
Maalox Plus	2.3	61	2.5	68
Mylanta-II	3.6	39	1.1	63
Gelusil	2.2	64	0.7	80
Gelusil II	3.0	47	1.3	74
Riopan Plus	1.8	78	0.7	78
Calcium carbonate, glycine				
Titralac	4.2	33	11.0	35

	Acid-neutralizing capacity (mEq/tablet)	Volume containing 140 mEq (tablets)	Sodium content (mg/tablet)	Monthly cost of therapy ($)
Antacids (tablets)				
Aluminum hydroxide, magnesium hydroxide				
Camalox	16.7	8	1.5	54
Aluminum hydroxide, magnesium hydroxide, simethicone				
Maalox Plus	5.7	25	1.4	106
Mylanta-II	11.0	39	1.1	63
Gelusil II	8.2	17	2.1	107
Riopan Plus	10.0	14	0.3	76
Calcium carbonate				
Tums	10.5	13	2.7	56
Alka-2	10.5	13	2.0	58
Calcium carbonate, glycine				
Titralac	9.5	15	0.3	57
Aluminum carbonate				
Rolaids	6.9	20	53.0	86
Aluminum hydroxide				
Amphojel	2.0	70	7.0	360

Priebe and associates have demonstrated the utility of an intensive antacid regimen in the prevention of stress mucosal ulceration and acute gastrointestinal bleeding. Mylanta-II, at an initial dose of 30 ml/hour via nasogastric (NG) tube, was compared to a cimetidine regimen, at an initial dose of 300 mg intravenously every 6 hours. Both regimens were titrated to a gastric pH greater than 3.5. The highest hourly quantity of antacid given was 120 ml. The most intensive cimetidine regimen was 400 mg every 4 hours. Upper gastrointestinal bleeding was defined by the presence of frank blood on NG aspirate or a series of three positive guaiac tests. In the 37 patients treated with antacids, no bleeding was noted. Of the 38 patients treated with cimetidine, 7 bled. Four of the antacid patients developed diarrhea, one exhibited hypermagnesemia, and one experienced persistent metabolic alkalosis (6 of 37, or a 16% complication rate). Cost, patient comfort, and staff hours for drug administration were not commented on in the report. Although this remains a landmark study, more recent data on continuous infusion H_2-receptor antagonist therapy for prevention of stress mucosal ulceration and bleeding suggest certain advantages to this form of therapy compared to antacids.

One study, performed by Rydning and associates, has shown a positive benefit of low-dose antacids, one tablet with 30 mEq acid-neutralizing capacity, on healing of gastric ulcers. A total of 67 percent of 42 gastric ulcers were healed at 4 weeks, compared to 25 percent of 44 gastric ulcers in patients given placebo.

Simethicone is often added to antacid formulations. It has trivial acid-neutralizing capability and is included only for its so-called antigas characteristics. Simethicone works better on Madison Avenue than in the gastrointestinal tract.

Antacids are particularly useful in treatment of patients with chronic renal failure. Blood loss as high as 6 ml/day can occur from the gastrointestinal tract of uremic patients. Gastritis and duodenitis are present in 60 to 80 percent of patients with chronic renal failure. Postdialysis gastric acid hypersecretion is common (15–20% of patients). Aluminum hydroxide not only neutralizes gastric acid but blocks absorption of phosphate. Hyperphosphatemia commonly occurs when serum creatinine approaches 3 mg/dl and is best prevented by the administration of aluminum-containing antacids. Once serum phosphate levels are demonstrated to be normal, calcium-containing antacids such as calcium carbonate can be added to maintain serum calcium levels and to minimize osteomalacia. Constipation can occur with aluminum hydroxide.

Magnesium-containing antacids can precipitate hypermagnesemia in patients with chronic renal failure and are to be avoided in these individuals.

CONTRAINDICATIONS

There are few contraindications to the use of antacids. As emphasized in the previous discussion, adequate dosing to ensure ulcer healing requires a high degree of patient compliance. Magnesium-containing antacids should be avoided in patients with chronic renal failure as central nervous system depression, skin irritation, and, rarely, muscle paralysis with respiratory failure can occur.

Concurrent use of antacids and tetracycline is contraindicated. Calcium binds and prevents absorption of tetracycline. Although on[e] might think that aluminum- or magnesium-based antacids wou[ld] useful in this situation, these ions chelate tetracycline as efficiently as calcium. Furthermore, by raising gastric pH, these agents ionize tetracycline, thereby further impairing its absorption.

Antacids are well recognized for their ability to decrease the absorption of iron and cimetidine.

ADMINISTRATION

For treatment of acute peptic ulcer disease, it is recommended that 30 ml of a single-strength antacid (e.g., Maalox or Mylanta) or 15 ml of a double-strength antacid (e.g., Maalox Plus or Mylanta II) be administered 1 and 3 hours after meals and at bedtime for a total of 4 weeks. Despite Berstad's data from Norway, this amount of antacid is probably required to ensure optimal healing of duodenal ulcer.

For treatment of other acid-related conditions such as gastroesophageal reflux disease, symptomatic hiatal hernia, and heartburn, administration of antacid is on an as-needed basis, not to exceed four to six doses a day.

In the patient with chronic renal failure, dosages must be adjusted on an individual basis. For control of hyperphosphatemia, 30 ml with each meal is an appropriate starting dose.

PEARLS AND PITFALLS

1. Magnesium-containing antacids are contraindicated in patients with chronic renal failure.
2. Adequate acid-neutralizing capacity (as much as 1000 mEq) is required to ensure optimal duodenal ulcer healing.
3. Absorption of tetracycline, iron, and all H_2-receptor antagonist agents is inhibited by aluminum-, magnesium-, and calcium-containing antacids.
4. Simethicone is virtually useless in the treatment of acid-peptic disease.
5. Aluminum-containing antacids tend to be constipating. Magnesium-containing antacids tend to be laxatives.
6. In patients with chronic renal failure, aluminum-containing antacids for phosphate binding are best administered at mealtime.

Suggested Reading

Barreras RF. Acid secretion after calcium carbonate in patients with duodenal ulcer. N Engl J Med 1970; 282:1402–1405.
Excessive rebound of acid output is seen after calcium carbonate ingestion. In the third hour after calcium carbonate ingestion, the mean acid output in a cohort of 20 men was 11.4 mEq/hour (basal acid output 5.3 mEq/hr).

Berstad A, et al. Controlled clinical trial of duodenal ulcer healing with antacid tablets. Scand J Gastroenterol 1982; 17:953–959.
A provocative study indicating that a low-dose antacid regimen may be efficacious in the treatment of duodenal ulcer disease.

Berstad A, Weberg R. Antacids in the treatment of gastroduodenal ulcer. Scand J Gastroenterol 1986; 21:385–391.
A comprehensive review of the clinical trials involving antacids in the treatment of peptic ulcer disease.

Brody M, Bachrach WH. Antacids I. Comparative biochemical and economic considerations. Am J Dig Dis 1959; 4:435–458.

These authors demonstrated the superiority of liquid antacids ove tablets in terms of capacity to rapidly neutralize gastric acid.

Chobanian MC, Chobanian SJ. Hollow Organ and Liver Disease ir the Chronic Dialysis and Transplant Patient. In SJ Chobanian and MM Van Ness (eds), *Manual of Clinical Problems in Gastroenterology*. Boston: Little, Brown, 1993.

An up-to-date review of the use of antacids in patients with chronic renal failure.

Fordtran JS. Acid rebound. N Engl J Med 1968; 279:900–905.

Calcium carbonate, both 4- and 8-gm doses, induces gastric acid hypersecretion.

Fordtran JS, Morawski SG, Richardson CT. In vivo and in vitro evaluation of liquid antacids. N Engl J Med 1973; 288:923–928.

As shown in Table 1-1, different antacids vary markedly in their in vivo and in vitro acid-neutralizing capacity.

Peterson WL, et al. Healing of duodenal ulcer with an antacid regimen. N Engl J Med 1977; 297:341–345.

The first clear demonstration of efficacy of a large-dose antacid regimen in the healing of duodenal ulcer. After 4 weeks of therapy with 30 ml antacid 7 times a day (1080 mEq acid-neutralizing capacity), ulcers were healed completely in 28 of the 36 antacid-treated patients, compared to 17 of the 38 placebo-treated patients. This article remains the standard against which other antacid trials must be compared.

Priebe HJ, et al. Antacid versus cimetidine in preventing acute gastrointestinal bleeding. N Engl J Med 1980; 302:426–430.

A landmark study demonstrating that an intensive antacid regimen can decrease the incidence of upper gastrointestinal bleeding in an intensive care unit. In comparison to a regimen of intermittent cimetidine therapy, less upper gastrointestinal tract bleeding was noted in the antacid group. Complications occurred in 16 percent of the antacid-treated cohort. No side effects from cimetidine were noted even though it was used in doses as high as 400 mg intravenously every 4 hours.

Rydning A, et al. Healing of benign gastric ulcer with low-dose antacids and fiber diet. Gastroenterology 1986; 91:56–61.

A 6-week, low-dose, aluminum-magnesium antacid regimen, 120 mEq/day, in combination with low- and high-fiber diets was associated with a 67 percent gastric ulcer healing rate (28 of 42 patients), compared to a 25 percent healing rate (11 of 44 patients) in those treated with placebo. The amount of fiber did not correlate with ulcer healing.

2 H₂-Antagonists

Margaret Andrea Wise and Michael M. Van Ness

Cimetidine

Cimetidine, the first histamine type 2–receptor antagonist, has had a marked impact on the practice of gastrointestinal medicine. Medical and surgical approaches to duodenal ulcer disease, gastric ulcer disease, gastric acid hypersecretory states, and other conditions related to the secretion of gastric acid, such as gastroesophageal reflux disease and stress-related mucosal bleeding, are dramatically different since the introduction of cimetidine in 1977 as the pioneer in this new class of agents.

MECHANISM OF ACTION

Cimetidine is a structural analogue of histamine with an aliphatic side chain attached to an imidazole ring (Fig. 2-1). It binds reversibly with the H_2-receptor, thereby inhibiting the accumulation of intracellular cyclic AMP. Although H_2-receptors have been identified in the uterus, the cardiac atria, and the cutaneous vascular bed, and on T-suppressor cells, the primary locus of cimetidine action is in the stomach, where parietal cell acid secretion is suppressed.

Cimetidine is a moderately potent inhibitor of parietal cell acid secretion. Basal acid output is decreased 90 percent for the 6 hours after a 300-mg dose. Nocturnal acid output is reduced by 67 percent. Pepsin concentration in gastric secretions is not reduced by cimetidine. However, by decreasing the total volume of gastric secretion, total pepsin secretion is likewise reduced. Furthermore, as depicted in Table 2-1, elevations in gastric pH decrease the activity of pepsin, a useful fact in the treatment of acid-peptic diseases.

The pharmacokinetic properties of cimetidine are outlined in Table 2-2. Cimetidine is a weak imidazole base that is well absorbed from the small intestine, with peak blood levels reached 60 to 90 minutes after ingestion. The drug's half-life is about 2 hours. Because 50 to 70 percent of an oral dose is excreted unchanged by the kidneys, renal failure markedly prolongs the half-life of cimetidine to 3.5 hours and dosage reductions are appropriate.

Cimetidine absorption is modestly inhibited by concurrent antacid dosing. Antacids (Mylanta-II, Maalox, ALternaGEL, or milk of magnesia) decrease peak serum concentrations and total cimetidine absorption by one-third. A more sustained rise in nocturnal intragastric pH is achieved by cimetidine administration alone at bedtime as compared to cimetidine and antacids together. Likewise concurrent iron administration appears to decrease cimetidine uptake and acid suppression.

INDICATIONS

Cimetidine is indicated for the short-term treatment of active duodenal ulcer disease, for the short-term maintenance against recurrence of duodenal ulcer disease, for the short-term treatment of active benign gastric ulcer disease, and for the treatment of pathologic hypersecretory conditions such as Zollinger-Ellison syndrome.

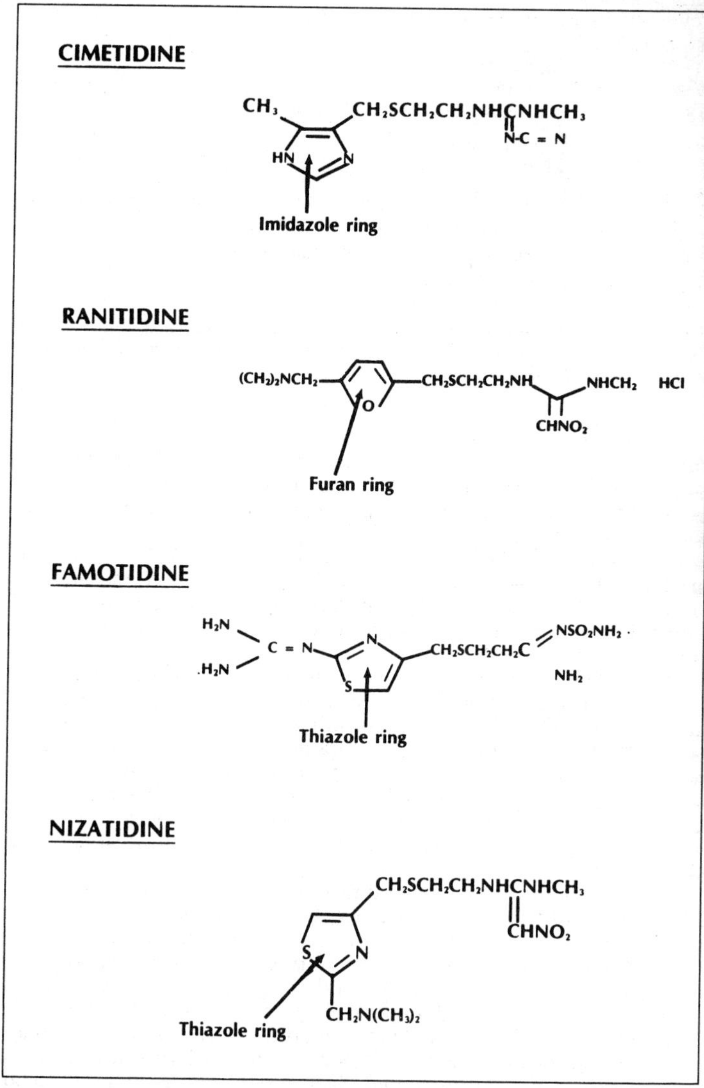

CIMETIDINE

CH_3 $CH_2SCH_2CH_2NHCNHCH_3$
N-C ≡ N
HN N
Imidazole ring

RANITIDINE

$(CH_3)_2NCH_2$ O $CH_2SCH_2CH_2NH$ $NHCH_3$ HCl
$CHNO_2$
Furan ring

FAMOTIDINE

H_2N
C = N N $CH_2SCH_2CH_2C$ NSO_2NH_2
H_2N S NH_2
Thiazole ring

NIZATIDINE

$CH_2SCH_2CH_2NHCNHCH_3$
$CHNO_2$
S N
$CH_2N(CH_3)_2$
Thiazole ring

Fig. 2-1. Structure and formula of available H_2-receptor antagonists.

Table 2-1. Significance of intragastric pH values

pH	Significance
>3.5	Decreased frequency of bleeding
>4.5	Pepsin inactivated
5	99.9% of acid neutralized
<5–7	Abnormalities in coagulation time, platelet aggregation, polymerization of fibrinogen
>7	Decreased frequency of rebleeding
>8	Pepsin destroyed

Source: From DA Peura, Recognizing, setting therapeutic goals, and selecting therapy for the prevention and treatment of stress-related mucosal damage. Pharmacology 1987; 7:95S–103S.

Cimetidine is the most widely studied H_2-receptor antagonist in the treatment of active duodenal ulcer disease. It is clearly superior to placebo in the treatment of duodenal ulcer disease. Cimetidine is equivalent to intensive antacid regimens in terms of duodenal ulcer healing rates.

In trial after trial, the duodenal ulcer healing rate by endoscopic criteria after 4 weeks of therapy with cimetidine, 300 mg orally 4 times a day, has been over 70 percent. Pain relief and decreased antacid consumption are clearly achieved as early as 5 to 7 days into therapy.

In an effort to increase patient compliance, simplified dosing regimens have been studied. Based on studies of nocturnal acid output, Capurso and his colleagues, performing a prospective, double-blind study of 187 patients with acute duodenal ulcer in seven medical centers, compared the ulcer healing rates of cimetidine, 400 mg twice a day and 800 mg at bedtime. After 4 weeks of therapy, 65 of the 96 patients (68%) receiving 400 mg cimetidine twice a day and 76 of the 91 patients (84%) receiving 800 mg cimetidine at bedtime were healed.

Not all patients with duodenal ulcer disease heal with cimetidine. The factors that determine the success or failure of cimetidine were examined by Hasan and Sircus in 1981. They found that early age of onset of the disease, smoking cigarettes, continued use of nonsteroidal anti-inflammatory agents, and heavy alcohol intake (>5 pt of beer per day) correlated independently with treatment failure.

Cimetidine is effective in decreasing the recurrence rate of duodenal ulcer disease. Sontag and associates have shown that, whereas the recurrence rate for duodenal ulcer in patients receiving placebo is approximately 48 percent at 6 months and 50 percent at 12 months, the recurrence rate for patients receiving cimetidine, 400 mg at bedtime, is 17 percent at 6 months and 28 percent at 12 months.

Cimetidine also benefits those patients who have suffered a perforated duodenal ulcer. Simpson and associates evaluated the postoperative course of 60 patients with perforated duodenal ulcer treated by simple closure with an omental patch and cimetidine. Re-operation, rebleeding, and recurrent peptic symptoms were significantly lower in the cimetidine-treated group than in the control group.

Cigarette smoking negates the benefit of cimetidine prophylaxis against recurrent duodenal ulcer disease. Among nonsmokers re-

Table 2-2. Pharmacokinetic properties of intravenous H_2-receptor antagonists in patients with normal renal function

	Cimetidine	Ranitidine	Famotidine	Nizatidine
Volume of distribution (liters/kg)	0.8–2.1	1.2–1.9	1.1–1.4	0.8–1.5
Plasma protein binding (%)	13–25	15	15–20	35
Elimination half-life (hr)	1.6–2.1	1.6–2.1	2.5–3.5	1.0–2.0
Renal clearance (ml/min)	293–486	489–512	304	500
Plasma clearance (ml/min)	442–702	568–709	412	666–1000

Adapted and reproduced with permission from MJ Ostro. Pharmacodynamics and pharmacokinetics of parenteral histamine (H_2)-receptor antagonists. Am J Med 1987; 83 (suppl 6A):15–20.

ceiving cimetidine prophylaxis, the recurrence rate of symptomatic duodenal ulcer after 1 year of observation was 4 percent. Among nonsmokers receiving placebo the recurrence rate of symptomatic duodenal ulcer was 13 percent, compared to a recurrence rate of 22 percent for smokers receiving cimetidine. The duodenal ulcer recurrence rate for smokers receiving placebo was 51 percent.

Cimetidine is effective in the treatment of benign gastric ulcer. Hentschel and associates studied the effect of cimetidine in a double-blind, multicenter trial. Of 130 patients who completed the initial 8 weeks of cimetidine therapy, 200 mg 3 times a day with 400 mg at bedtime, 112 (86%) healed. Of these 112, 84 then remained in the trial for one year. They received either cimetidine, 400 mg, or placebo at bedtime. On maintenance therapy, 72 of the 84 (86%) remained healed after one year, compared to only 45 percent on placebo.

Cimetidine is effective in the treatment of Zollinger-Ellison syndrome and other hypersecretory states (short-bowel syndrome, systemic mastocytosis, and endogenous hyperhistaminemia from basophilic leukemia). Cimetidine provided the first medical treatment alternative to total gastrectomy. In the initial series of patients with Zollinger-Ellison syndrome, reported in 1978, 40 of 61 patients had relief of symptoms with cimetidine, 300 mg 4 times a day. Daily doses were increased in the other 21 patients as necessary to control symptoms and ranged as high as 600 mg 4 times a day. Symptoms of pain, nausea, vomiting, and diarrhea were either completely or markedly improved in all patients. Patients in this study received the drug for as long as 18 months. No patient rejected the drug although six of them developed gynecomastia. Tumor progression was not affected by cimetidine. Saeed and associates have demonstrated a clear correlation between the total daily oral dose of cimetidine and the continuous intravenous dose required to decrease basal acid output to less than 10 mEq/hour. In 47 Zollinger-Ellison syndrome patients undergoing operation, this degree of acid suppression allowed an uncomplicated perioperative course.

The benefits of continuous infusion cimetidine in the treatment of patients with upper gastrointestinal hemorrhage include less rebleeding and lower mortality. Rather than intermittent bolus injections of cimetidine, continuous infusion therapy is recommended. Ostro and associates have shown that continuous infusion administration achieves a gastric pH above 6 in 80 percent of patients, with little fluctuation in serum concentration. Siepler and Trudeau found that 50 mg cimetidine every hour intravenously combined with 30 ml antacid every 2 hours decreased rebleeding and mortality in an indigent population admitted to an intensive care unit.

Because (1) stress-related mucosal damage occurs in patients with trauma, burns, and serious medical illness (Table 2-3); (2) stress reduces duodenal bicarbonate secretion (Fig. 2-2); and (3) gastric acid is essential for the development of stress-related mucosal damage, prophylaxis of stress-related mucosal ulcerations was sought. In one of the first studies, Halloran and associates found that only 2 of 26 cimetidine-treated patients suffering severe head injury experienced upper gastrointestinal bleeding that was serious enough to require blood transfusion, whereas 8 of 24 placebo-treated patients did require blood transfusion for stress-related mucosal bleeding.

Continuous infusion cimetidine therapy is superior to intermittent cimetidine or antacid therapy for the prevention of stress-related mucosal injury and bleeding (Fig. 2-3). Cimetidine therapy is also

Table 2-3. Natural history of stress-related mucosal damage

Author(s), year	Population	Number of patients	Percent with lesions	Percent bleeding
Lucas, 1971	Trauma	42	100	21
Czaja, 1974	Burns	32	86	22
LeGall, 1976	ICU			
	sepsis	14	100	21
	no sepsis	16	48	0
Kamada, 1977	Head injury		75	17
Peura, 1985	ICU	18	83	39
Poleski, 1986	MICU		60	

Source: Adapted from DA Peura, Stress-related mucosal damage. Am J Med 1987; 83 (suppl 6A):4–11.

Fig. 2-2. Schematic representation of the various factors thought to be responsible for the pathogenesis of stress-related mucosal damage. (From TA Miller, Stress Erosive Gastritis. In FG Moody (ed). *Surgical Treatment of Digestive Disease.* Chicago: Year Book, 1986. Pp 203–215.)

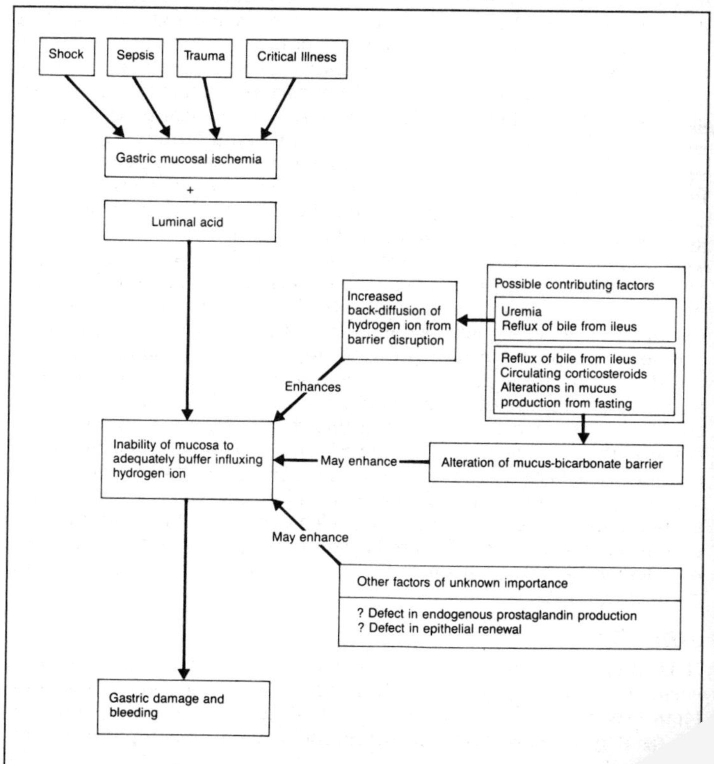

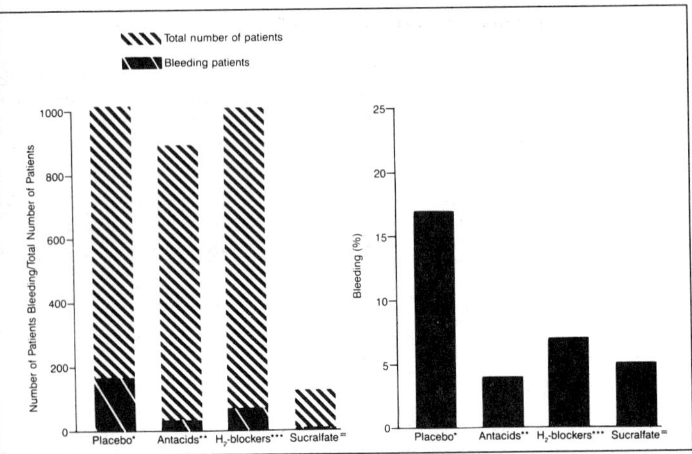

Fig. 2-3. Comparison of bleeding rates in 21 prospective studies of prophylaxis against stress ulcer bleeding in medical and surgical patients. (From GR Zuckerman, R Shuman. Therapeutic goals and treatment options for prevention of stress ulcer syndrome. Am J Med 1987; 83 (suppl 6A):33.)

of benefit to patients in whom stress-related mucosal bleeding develops. As shown by Peura and Johnson, endoscopic signs of bleeding cleared or did not develop in 20 of 21 patients treated with cimetidine. To facilitate continuous administration to critically ill patients, cimetidine can be added to hyperalimentation solutions. The delivery of 37.5 to 50.0 mg/hour results in steady-state concentrations of 0.6 to 1.0 μg/ml cimetidine in patients without renal failure. The failure of either intensive antacid therapy or cimetidine to control gastric pH should alert the practitioner to the possibility of sepsis.

Cimetidine has been evaluated for the treatment of gastroesophageal reflux disease. Although the drug has no effect on either the lower esophageal sphincter, clearance of acid from the esophagus, or gastric emptying, it decreases both symptoms of reflux and the need for antacids compared to placebo. Even in patients with scleroderma and severe gastroesophageal reflux symptoms, cimetidine promotes healing of esophagitis. Cimetidine also promotes healing of other complications of gastroesophageal reflux disease such as esophageal stenoses. In patients with Barrett's esophagus, use of cimetidine decreases gastrin-stimulated acid secretion and the number of reflux episodes per 24 hours. Interestingly, Lieberman has demonstrated that intensive short-term therapy (300 mg cimetidine 4 times a day and 10 mg metoclopramide 4 times a day) for gastroesophageal disease not associated with decreased lower esophageal sphincter pressure (< 5 mm Hg) may suffice to allow for gradual tapering and ultimate discontinuation of cimetidine and metoclopramide.

SIDE EFFECTS

It is likely that no drug in use today in gastroenterology has been scrutinized as closely as cimetidine for the development of side effects. Given the drug's astonishingly widespread use and the number of organ systems with H_2-receptors, the frequency of hepatic, central nervous system, renal, cardiovascular, and endocrine side effects is surprisingly low.

Hepatotoxicity was one of the first side effects noted after introduction of cimetidine. Villeneuve and Warner published a case report of an 83-year-old woman in whom a hypersensitivity-type reaction to cimetidine developed. She had begun cimetidine, 300 mg orally 4 times a day, in October 1977 for iron-deficiency anemia associated with Barrett's esophagus. In February 1978, her liver-associated enzymes showed a serum glutamic oxaloacetic transaminase (SGOT) of 935 units/liter, an alkaline phosphatase of 160 units/liter, and a bilirubin of 15 mg/dl. Cimetidine was discontinued, and the liver-associated enzymes were normalized. This type of reaction is rare. In a retrospective analysis of 1189 recipients of cimetidine, Porter and associates found only one possible case of cimetidine-induced hepatitis (Table 2-4).

Low levels of transaminase elevation are not uncommon with intravenous cimetidine. Cohen and Fabre prospectively evaluated 100 normal volunteers who received intravenous bolus injection and infusion of cimetidine and ranitidine 4 times a day for 7 to 10 days. Transaminase values less than 100 units/liter were noted in 19 percent of cimetidine and 24 percent of ranitidine recipients, typically after 5 to 7 days of therapy. No functional abnormalities were noted (i.e., elevation of prothrombin time, decreased albumin level, or elevation of serum bilirubin).

The incidence and severity of mental status changes associated with cimetidine are almost invariably increased in patients with renal or hepatic failure. Except in the patient with renal failure and

Table 2-4. Intravenous cimetidine use in 1189 hospitalized patients: Adverse reactions ranked by investigator's impression

Adverse reaction	Definite or probable	Possible	Total
Neuropsychiatric	11	8	19
Blood disorders	5	3	8
Rash	2	1	3
Increased creatinine	2	1	3
Drug fever	1	2	3
Drowsiness		1	1
Nausea		1	1
Convulsions	1		1
Abnormal coagulation	1		1
Altered liver tests		1	1
Totals (%)	23(1.9%)	18(1.5%)	41(3.5%)

Reproduced with permission from JB Porter et al, Intensive hospital monitoring study of intravenous cimetidine. Arch Intern Med 1986; 146: 2237–2239.

liver failure, serum trough concentrations of cimetidine greater than 1.25 μg/ml are rarely associated with central nervous system abnormalities. To minimize the possibility of these untoward side effects, cimetidine dosages should be reduced in these patients.

Renal disease is rare as a consequence of cimetidine therapy. Rudnick and associates have described two cases of acute, partially reversible interstitial nephritis from cimetidine use. Symptoms of fatigue, fever, and anorexia developed 1 month after initiation of therapy. Serum creatinine levels of 6.7 and 8.1 mg/dl were seen in conjunction with moderately severe azotemia (blood urea nitrogen of 32 and 88 mg/dl). Cellular invasion of the interstitium with preserved glomerular and vascular architecture were seen on kidney biopsy. Near normalization of renal function occurred within 1 month of cessation of therapy.

Cimetidine and ranitidine have been associated with the development of sinus bradycardia after oral and intravenous administration. At the time of Tanner's 1988 report, about 144 million prescriptions for cimetidine (1.6 cases of bradycardia per 10 million prescriptions), 41.5 million prescriptions for ranitidine (3.6 cases of bradycardia per 10 million prescriptions), and 1.5 million prescriptions for famotidine (no reports received) had been written with a total of 39 spontaneous reports to the Food and Drug Administration (FDA).

The antiandrogenic effects of cimetidine were published as early as 1979, when decreased rat and dog seminal vesicles and prostate weights were noted. Jensen reported antiandrogenic effects in Zollinger-Ellison patients. A total of 50 percent of the 22 men with Zollinger-Ellison syndrome and gastric hypersecretion who took a mean daily cimetidine dose of 5.3 gm experienced either impotence, tender gynecomastia, or both. Gynecomastia is not observed more frequently in patients receiving cimetidine than in those given placebo who are not treated for Zollinger-Ellison. With discontinuation of cimetidine, the impotence and tenderness disappeared over a month. Resolution of gynecomastia took as long as 3 months.

A potential benefit of the antiandrogenic activity of cimetidine is the fact that, as observed by Terruzzi and associates, high-density lipoprotein (HDL) levels increase an average of 14 percent with cimetidine, 800 mg/day (Table 2-5). The clinical applicability of this observation remains unknown.

Table 2-5. Factors affecting HDL cholesterol

Increased levels	Decreased levels
Female sex	Male sex
Physical activity	Smoking
Lean body	Obesity
Estrogens	Androgens
Nicotinic acid	Hypertriglyceridemia
Alcohol	High-carbohydrate diet
Heparin	Diabetes
Familial hyperalphalipoproteinemia	Tangier disease

Reproduced with permission from SM Sabesin and SW Weidman, Histamine H_2-receptor antagonists and high-density lipoproteins. Pharmacology 1987; 7: 116S–

Drug interactions of significance are known to occur with cimetidine. Feely and associates have shown in normal volunteers that acute and chronic cimetidine use reduces hepatic blood flow 25 to 33 percent. Cimetidine is known to bind reversibly the cytochrome P-450 system and to alter levels of drugs metabolized by this system. Theophylline, warfarin, diazepam, and phenytoin (Dilantin) serum concentrations are increased approximately 30 percent by concurrent cimetidine therapy (Fig. 2-4). Increases in theophylline levels can be minimized by nocturnal cimetidine administration.

Although the addition of cimetidine to the drug regimen of a patient taking warfarin increases serum warfarin levels, little change is noted in serum prothrombin time. The reason is that the R(−) enantiomer of warfarin is the more potent anticoagulant but only the R(+) enantiomer serum concentration is increased by cimetidine.

Cimetidine's affinity for the cytochrome P-450 system is potentially beneficial in acetaminophen overdose. Mitchell and colleagues have shown that pre- and post-treatment with cimetidine of rats given toxic doses of acetaminophen decrease both the magnitude of the rise and mortality. As depicted in Fig. 2-5, the benefit from cimetidine occurs by inhibition of production of the postulated acetaminophen toxic metabolite (*N*-acetyl-*p*-benzoquinone imine). Ci-

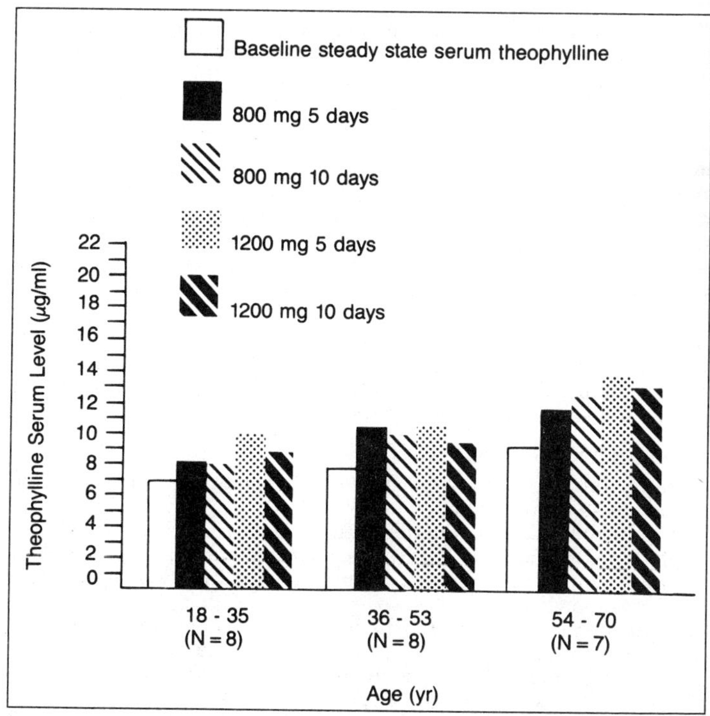

Fig. 2-4. Effect of age and cimetidine dose on theophylline level. (From C De Angelis et al. Effect of low-dose cimetidine on theophylline metabolism. Clin Pharmacol 1983; 2:563–567.)

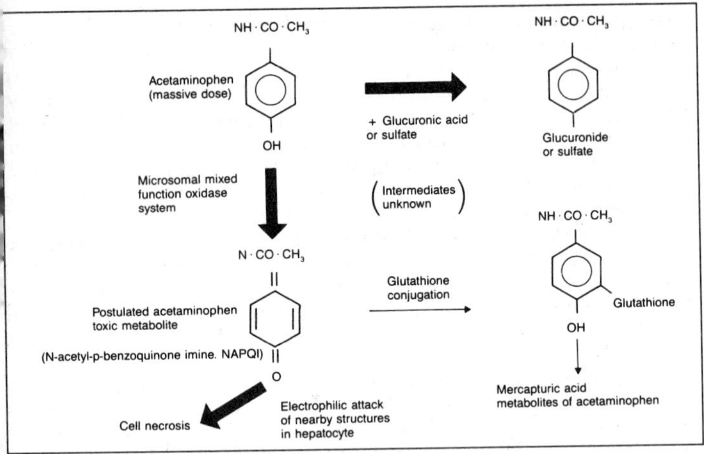

Fig. 2-5. Pathways of acetaminophen metabolism following ingestion of massive quantities of the drug. (From M Black. Hepatotoxic and hepatoprotective potential of histamine (H_2)-receptor antagonists. Am J Med. 83 (suppl 6A):71.)

metidine, 37.5 mg/hour intravenously, serves only as an adjunct to the primary medical therapy of *N*-acetylcysteine (Mucomyst, 140 mg/kg loading dose orally as soon as possible after the ingestion of acetaminophen, then 70 mg/kg orally every 4 hours for 17 doses).

ADMINISTRATION

The oral and parenteral doses and dosage intervals are presented in Table 2-6. Chronic renal failure patients with creatinine clearances of less than 20 to 35 ml/minute should be dosed every 12 hours instead of every 6 hours.

Continuous infusions of cimetidine should be given as a primed infusion with a 150-mg loading dose followed by a constant infusion. The infusion solution is made by adding 900 mg cimetidine to 250 ml of 5% dextrose in water (final cimetidine concentration 3.6 mg/ml 5% D/W). The initial infusion rate is 10 ml/hour (36 mg/h). If gastric pH by nasogastric aspirate is less than 4, the infusion rate can be increased to 14 ml/hour (50 mg/h).

PEARLS AND PITFALLS

1. Rapid intravenous administration of cimetidine and ranitidine can cause bradycardia.
2. The introduction of cimetidine to patients receiving either theophylline, warfarin, Dilantin, diazepam, lidocaine, propranolol, or procainamide may require downward adjustment of the dosages of these medications.
3. Antacids modestly inhibit the oral absorption of cimetidine.
4. Failure to neutralize the gastric pH of a seriously ill patient receiving cimetidine for prophylaxis against stress-related mucosal bleeding should raise the possibility of sepsis.
5. Gynecomastia from high-dose cimetidine therapy may require 3 months to resolve.

Table 2-6. Indications and dosage for H_2-receptor antagonists

Drug	Indications	Dosage	
		Oral	Parenteral
Cimetidine	Duodenal ulcer		
	• active	800 mg qhs, 300 mg qid, or 400 mg bid	300 mg q6–8h
	• maintenance	400 mg qhs	
	Gastric ulcer		
	• active	300 mg qid	300 mg q6–8h
	Zollinger-Ellison	300 mg qid	300 mg qid
		with dosage adjustment as necessary	
Ranitidine	Duodenal ulcer		
	• active	150 mg bid, or 300 mg qhs	50 mg q6–8h
	• maintenance	150 mg qhs	
	Gastric ulcer		
	• active	150 mg bid	50 mg q6–8h
	GERD*	150 mg bid	
	Zollinger-Ellison	150 mg bid	150 mg bid
		with dosage adjustment as necessary	
Famotidine	Duodenal ulcer		
	• active	20 mg bid, or 40 mg qhs	20 mg q12h
	• maintenance	20 mg qhs	
	Zollinger-Ellison	20 mg bid	20 mg q12h
		with dosage adjustment as necessary	
Nizatidine	Duodenal ulcer		
	• active	150 mg bid, or 300 mg qhs	
	• maintenance	150 mg qhs	

*GERD = gastroesophageal reflux disease.

Ranitidine

Ranitidine was introduced into clinical practice in July 1983. Potent, effective, and safe, it has broadened the utility of H_2-receptor antagonists in the treatment of acid-peptic diseases.

MECHANISM OF ACTION

Ranitidine is a potent competitive inhibitor of the binding of histamine to parietal cell H_2-receptors. As depicted in Fig. 2-1, it has a furan ring instead of the imidazole ring of cimetidine. Ranitidine binds minimally to androgen receptors, the cytochrome P-450 system, and peripheral lymphocytes. It is about 12 times more potent at inhibiting pentagastrin-stimulated acid output in humans than is cimetidine. As with cimetidine, pepsin secretion is reduced by virtue of the overall decrease in gastric acid secretion, although the concentration of pepsin is not substantially reduced.

PHARMACOKINETICS

Absorption of an oral dose of ranitidine, 150 mg, is rapid, occurs in the upper digestive tract, and is not inhibited by food. Although peak drug levels occur about 2 hours after ingestion, significant inhibition of acid secretion continues for 8 to 10 hours. Peak serum concentration after a 150-mg dose ranges from 200 to 600 μg/ml and correlates with the percent reduction in acid output. The mean inhibition of 24-hour acid secretion in patients with duodenal ulcer who are receiving 150 mg ranitidine twice a day is 70 percent.

Chronic liver disease can alter ranitidine pharmacokinetics. In normal patients and patients with compensated cirrhosis (albumin > 3 gm/dl, no ascites), bioavailability of ranitidine is approximately 50 percent, half-life is about 2.5 hours, and the volume of distribution is 1.2 liters. However, in cirrhotic patients with prolonged prothrombin times (twice normal), ranitidine serum concentrations and bioavailability both tend to be higher, and half-life is longer, effects believed to be secondary to decreased hepatic metabolism and a slight decrease in glomerular filtration rate. Only in patients with severe renal and hepatic disease is dose reduction necessary.

The pharmacokinetic properties of intravenous ranitidine are presented in Table 2-2.

INDICATIONS

As outlined in Table 2-6, ranitidine is indicated for treatment of active duodenal ulcer disease, short-term maintenance against recurrence of duodenal ulcer disease, active gastric ulcer disease, gastroesophageal reflux disease, and Zollinger-Ellison syndrome and other gastric acid hypersecretory states.

Numerous studies have demonstrated the effectiveness of ranitidine in the short-term treatment of uncomplicated duodenal ulcer disease. Ulcer healing by endoscopic criteria has been documented in about 70 percent of patients after 4 weeks of ranitidine therapy, 150 mg twice a day, and in about 90 percent after a total of 8 weeks of drug. These figures are comparable to those seen in published studies of the effectiveness of cimetidine in the short-term therapy of duodenal ulcer disease.

Nocturnal administration of ranitidine, 300 mg, was studied in an effort to improve patient compliance. Colin-Jones and associates reported the results of a trial of 102 patients treated with either 150 mg ranitidine twice a day or 300 mg ranitidine at bedtime. Healing rates for the patients receiving ranitidine twice a day were 84 percent (48 of 57), compared to 96 percent (43 of 45) for the patients receiving the single bedtime dose. Pain relief was comparable between the two treatment groups. Untoward side effects were rare (one patient receiving ranitidine, 150 mg twice a day, developed cholestatic jaundice that resolved and did not necessitate drug withdrawal).

Maintenance of remission of duodenal ulcer disease is a desired effect of any treatment regimen. The cumulative remission rate for symptomatic recurrences in 367 patients with duodenal ulcer treated with ranitidine and reported by Penston and Wormsley was 95 percent at 1 year, 88 percent at 3 years, and 86 percent at 5 years. Significantly, recurrent duodenal ulcer bleeding was rare (1.1%) in patients receiving continuous therapy.

Ranitidine is effective in the treatment of acute gastric ulcers. At a dosage of 150 mg twice a day, it healed 58 percent of benign gastric ulcers after 4 weeks. After 8 weeks of continued therapy, 77 percent of the gastric ulcers were healed. These results are similar to those of Bardham and associates, who found that 68 to 85 gastric ulcers healed after 8 weeks of ranitidine therapy (150 mg orally twice a day). Cessation of smoking, long duration of therapy (up to 12 weeks), and cessation of agents injurious to the gastric mucosa appear to be factors that correlate with successful healing of gastric ulcers.

Ranitidine is useful in the treatment of patients with gastroesophageal reflux disease. Compared to placebo, ranitidine clearly improves symptoms of heartburn. In addition, in a trial reported by Zimmerman and associates of 64 patients (older than 60 years) with gastroesophageal reflux disease treated with either ranitidine, 150 mg twice a day, or placebo, endoscopic evidence of healing was observed in 52 percent of the ranitidine patients, compared to only 33 percent of the placebo patients.

Patients with severe gastroesophageal reflux disease complicated by nonallergic asthma or cough may also benefit from ranitidine therapy. The best predictor of benefit in this situation was found by di Stefano and associates to be a positive pulmonary aspiration test (egg labeled with 4.5 μCi technetium [Tc] 99m–DTPA).

Like cimetidine, ranitidine is approved for use in patients with Zollinger-Ellison syndrome and other gastric acid hypersecretory states. Patients need sufficient ranitidine to suppress basal acid secretion to less than 10 mEq/hour. While the patient is receiving therapy, peptic ulcers should not develop according to endoscopic criteria. The follow-up period is at least 6 months long. Unlike cimetidine, ranitidine has no apparent adverse effects such as impotence or tender gynecomastia.

Like cimetidine, ranitidine is used in several clinical situations in which suppression of gastric acid is desirable. Dawson and Cockel studied 158 consecutive patients with acute upper gastrointestinal hemorrhage, comparing ranitidine, 150 mg orally 3 times a day, to placebo in ability to decrease the incidence of recurrent hemorrhage. Among patients with duodenal ulcer as the etiology of their upper gastrointestinal hemorrhage, the rate of rebleeding with ranitidine treatment, 3 of 27, was significantly lower than that seen among patients treated with placebo, 11 of 26 ($p < 0.05$).

Ranitidine is also effective in raising gastric pH in critically ill patients with respiratory failure. In a prospective evaluation, Rigaud and associates gave a 35-mg loading dose and 17.5 mg/hour by continuous intravenous infusion and found that 65 percent of the time gastric pH was maintained above 4.

Ranitidine can decrease the incidence of stress-related mucosal bleeding in critically ill patients. Reid and Baycliff found that only 2 of 33 patients in a group receiving a primed infusion of ranitidine (50-mg loading dose with 12.5 mg/hr) had clinical evidence of upper gastrointestinal hemorrhage. Siepler and associates found that ranitidine, 50-mg bolus with an 8-mg/hour infusion, was equivalent to cimetidine, 300-mg bolus with a 50-mg/hour infusion, in elevating gastric pH above 5, preventing upper gastrointestinal hemorrhage.

and decreasing transfusion requirements in 227 intensive care unit patients. Interestingly, Ruiz-Santana and colleagues found that total parenteral nutrition, sucralfate, and ranitidine were equally effective in decreasing stress gastritis and hemorrhage.

Ranitidine has proved effective in suppression of gastric acid hypersecretion resistant to cimetidine therapy. Three cases were reported by Danilewitz and associates in 1982. All three patients were treated with intravenous cimetidine (one received a total of 1.2 gm/day and two were given a total of 2.4 gm/day, all intravenously) and experienced persistent high-volume gastric outputs and basal acid secretion (pH of gastric aspirate 1, acid output 15 mEq/hr). With initiation of ranitidine, 300 mg/day in divided doses, acid secretion was controlled.

Ranitidine is effective in controlling the high acid outputs characteristic of many patients with Barrett's esophagus. Collen and associates found that the mean basal acid output (BAO) was 8.3 mEq/hour in the Barrett's patients, compared to a mean basal acid output of 3.2 mEq/hour in normal control subjects ($p = 0.001$). He also noted that ranitidine dosages correlated with the basal acid output in these patients. Using the formula, daily ranitidine dose equals 100 times the BAO minus 407, 15 of the Barrett's patients in the study required a mean of 890 mg/day for complete control of symptoms and healing of esophagitis. No untoward side effects were noted from use of these higher doses of ranitidine.

Ranitidine can also prevent the development of duodenal ulcers and gastric erosions in patients receiving nonsteroidal anti-inflammatory agents. Lanza and associates studied 119 patients receiving nonsteroidal anti-inflammatory agents for rheumatologic conditions and found that ranitidine, 150 mg orally twice a day, prevented the development of duodenal ulcers in 62 patients, compared to the development of duodenal ulcers in 4 of 57 patients receiving placebo ($p<0.01$).

Ranitidine utilized in combination with amoxicillin (750 mg po tid) and metronidazole (500 mg po tid) resulted in an 88 percent rate of eradication of *Helicobacter pylori.* More important, only 8 percent of these patients experienced ulcers in 12 months of follow-up.

SIDE EFFECTS

Ranitidine is a remarkably safe agent with rare side effects limited primarily to drug-induced hepatitis and headache. The incidence of drug-induced hepatitis from oral ranitidine was estimated by Dobbs and associates to be 0.06 to 0.08 percent.

Ranitidine is not known to possess antiandrogenic properties, is not known to change serum concentrations of high-density lipoproteins, and is not thought to be useful in the treatment of acetaminophen overdose. Ranitidine may compete with acetaminophen for available hepatic glutathione thereby inhibiting acetaminophen metabolism and potentiating toxicity.

The incidence of hepatitis has been reported sporadically but appears to be as high or higher with ranitidine than with cimetidine. In an analysis of the short- and long-term untoward effects of oral ranitidine, Simon and associates found some elevations in the liver-associated enzymes of ranitidine-treated patients. The elevations were small, of little clinical significance, and infrequent. The incidence of drug-induced hepatitis was estimated by Dobbs and associates to be 0.06 to 0.08 percent.

The incidence of drug-induced hepatitis is higher with intravenous administration. Cohen and Fabre conducted a prospective evaluation of 100 normal volunteers and found transaminase values of less than 100 units/liter in 9 percent of the subjects receiving 50 mg ranitidine every 6 hours for 5 days, and in 28 percent who received 100 mg ranitidine every 6 hours for 5 days.

Headache and other central nervous system effects may complicate ranitidine therapy (Table 2-7). In Cohen and Fabre's study, 4 of the 51 patients receiving ranitidine developed headache, compared to no headache in the 7 subjects who received saline injections and 3 in the group of 43 who received intravenous cimetidine.

As with cimetidine, bradycardia from both oral and intravenous ranitidine use is well described but rare (see Tanner letter).

A recent study showed that gastric emptying, as measured by nuclear medicine emptying times, is impaired in patients with duodenal ulcer who are treated with ranitidine.

Clinically significant interactions with theophylline have also been well documented. A study of hospitalized patients found the frequency of this interaction roughly comparable to the experience with cimetidine. Ranitidine also causes a slight decrease in warfarin clearance, but this has not been clinically significant.

ADMINISTRATION

The oral and parenteral doses and dosage intervals are presented in Table 2-6. The dosage of ranitidine should be reduced to 150 mg every 24 hours for patients with renal failure who have creatinine clearances of less than 50 ml/minute.

Continuous infusion ranitidine should be given as a primed infusion with a 50-mg loading dose followed by a constant infusion. The infusion solution is made by adding 300 mg ranitidine to 250 ml of 5% dextrose in water (final ranitidine concentration, 1.2 mg/ml 5% D/W). The initial infusion rate is 10 ml/hour (12 mg/hr).

PEARLS AND PITFALLS

1. Ranitidine is only one of several H_2-receptor antagonists currently approved by the Food and Drug Administration for treatment of gastroesophageal reflux disease.
2. Ranitidine contains a furan ring and has no known antiandrogenic activity.
3. Ranitidine is 5 to 10 times more potent on a molar basis than cimetidine.
4. Intravenous ranitidine is associated with rises in liver-associated enzymes (usually < 100 units/liter) without demonstrable changes in synthetic function (albumin, bilirubin, or coagulation parameters).
5. Ranitidine has no role in the treatment of acute acetaminophen overdose.
6. Ranitidine bioavailability is not changed in patients with chronic liver disease unless severe hepatic decompensation occurs.
7. Ranitidine given with amoxicillin, metronidazole, and bismuth can eradicate *H. pylori* in 85 percent of patients.

Table 2-7. Central nervous system toxicities following ranitidine administration: Case reports

Author, year	Number of patients	Symptom	Dose	Recurrence on rechallenge
Billings, 1986	3	Depression	150 mg bid	yes
Epstein, 1985	5	Headache	150 mg bid	yes
Silverstone, 1984	1	Confusion	150 mg bid	no
Hughes, 1983	1	Confusion	150 mg bid	no
Mandal, 1986	1	Confusion	150 mg bid	no
Mani, 1984	1	Confusion	150 mg bid	no
Price, 1985	1	Hallucinations	150 mg bid	yes
Sonnenblick, 1986	1	Hallucinations	150 mg bid	no

Reproduced with permission from JW Freston, Safety perspectives on parenteral H2-receptor antagonists. Am J Med 1987; 83 (suppl 6A): 60.

Famotidine

Famotidine is a newer, more potent, competitive histamine H_2-receptor antagonist that is effective in the treatment of duodenal ulcer disease, benign gastric ulcer, and Zollinger-Ellison syndrome. At this time, after careful study and intense scrutiny, famotidine appears to be relatively free of untoward side effects.

MECHANISM OF ACTION, PHARMACOKINETICS, AND PHARMACODYNAMICS

Famotidine is based on a thiazole ring, compared to an imidazole ring for cimetidine and a furan ring for ranitidine (see Fig. 2-1). Like these agents, it is a competitive antagonist for the histamine H_2-receptor. It is estimated to be 30 to 40 times more potent than cimetidine and 7 to 10 times more potent than ranitidine. Famotidine inhibits basal and pentagastrin-stimulated parietal cell acid output but has no effect on nonparietal cell (bicarbonate) gastric secretion. Reductions in pepsin output parallel reductions in volume of secretion, not changes in pepsin concentration. The half-life of famotidine is longer than that of cimetidine or ranitidine (see Table 2-2) such that significant inhibition of pentagastrin-stimulated acid secretion (50% of control) persists even 12 hours after a 20-mg oral dose.

Famotidine does not influence serum concentrations of medications metabolized by the cytochrome P-450 mixed-function oxidase system. Unlike cimetidine, an agent known to have the property of impairing hepatic microsomal drug-oxidizing capacity, famotidine does not increase serum concentrations of diazepam. The effect of famotidine administration on serum concentrations of other agents metabolized by this system—theophylline, warfarin, lidocaine, acetaminophen, azothymidine (AZT)—has not been studied but is likely to be similar.

The effect of famotidine on renal tubular secretory mechanisms was studied by Klotz and associates. Because renal clearance of famotidine exceeds the creatinine clearance, one can assume that famotidine, like many drugs, is secreted by the renal proximal tubule. With respect to procainamide, Klotz's group found that famotidine does not interfere with the clearance, half-life, or plasma concentration of procainamide or its metabolite *N*-acetyl procainamide.

INDICATIONS

As depicted in Table 2-6, famotidine is indicated for the short-term treatment of duodenal ulcer, prophylaxis against recurrence of duodenal ulcer, short-term treatment of benign gastric ulcer, gastroesophageal reflux disease, and long-term treatment of the Zollinger-Ellison syndrome. Other uses not yet FDA approved are under study and include prophylaxis against stress-related mucosal damage, ulceration and bleeding, and gastroesophageal reflux disease.

Famotidine is indicated for the short-term treatment of duodenal ulcer in a dose of either 20 mg twice a day or 40 mg at bedtime. Although more potent on a milligram-per-milligram basis than either cimetidine or ranitidine, famotidine is no more efficacious. Simon and associates showed that, after 4 weeks of therapy with famotidine, 20 mg twice a day, 35 of 42 patients (83%) were healed according to endoscopic criteria. Pain relief was prompt, with 70 percent of patients pain-free after 2 weeks of therapy. These figures are comparable to healing and pain relief rates seen with cimetidine and ranitidine. In Simon's study, one patient in the famotidine group was withdrawn from therapy because of skin rash. In another study of famotidine, Lyon found that the most common side effect from oral famotidine therapy was headache, reported in 2 percent of patients.

Of patients treated with famotidine, Reynolds found four risk factors associated with nonhealing of duodenal ulcer. Alcohol use before documented duodenal ulcer, a history of upper gastrointestinal bleeding, and a duodenal ulcer greater than 10 mm in diameter were independently associated with nonhealing after 4 weeks of therapy. Because Collen and associates have shown that bleeding duodenal ulcers are associated with idiopathic gastric acid hypersecretion, one could justify gastric analysis and increased drug dosages (i.e., 40 mg twice a day) in this subset of duodenal ulcer patients at risk for nonhealing. Extension of Collen's recommendations to other patients at risk for nonhealing awaits further research, but is logical from the results of currently available studies.

Famotidine is currently indicated for the treatment of benign gastric ulcer. As with the other H_2-receptor antagonists, treatment success is more a function of duration of drug therapy than of drug selection or dosage. Eight to 12 weeks are often required for complete healing of benign gastric ulcer: The healing rate of benign gastric ulcer is 2 to 3 mm/week regardless of ulcer size or drug therapy. Cessation of smoking and the use of nonsteroidal anti-inflammatory agents are necessary for optimal ulcer healing.

Although omeprazole is the drug of choice for the treatment of Zollinger-Ellison syndrome, famotidine may be useful as a second-line agent. In areas of the country where omeprazole is unavailable or if the patient is reluctant to travel to national referral centers such as the National Institutes of Health (phone 301-496-4201), famotidine is the agent of choice for Zollinger-Ellison syndrome. In previous studies by Collen and Jensen's groups, 25 percent of patients required more than 7 gm cimetidine or more than 3 gm ranitidine to control gastric acid secretion. Howard found that famotidine (mean daily dose 240 mg, range 80–480 mg) was effective in controlling symptoms and gastric acid output. It was free of significant side effects, had a duration of action approximately 30 percent longer than either cimetidine or ranitidine, and was more potent (32 times more potent than cimetidine, 9 times more potent than ranitidine). Despite this increased potency, Corleto and associates have demonstrated a loss of efficacy of famotidine in the control of gastric acid secretion in patients with Zollinger-Ellison syndrome. Control of basal acid output to levels less than 10 mEq/hour was lost in six of nine Zollinger-Ellison syndrome patients within 7 to 15 months after initiation of therapy. The authors do not offer an explanation for this loss of control, but comment that no significant increase in parietal cell mass occurred to cause the loss of efficacy of famotidine. In this study, omeprazole (a hydrogen ion–potassium adenosine triphosphatase inhibitor) did suppress acid completely in these six patients.

There is no known increase in serum HDL cholesterol during famotidine therapy, as there is during cimetidine treatment.

The use of famotidine to prevent stress-related mucosal damage, ulceration, and bleeding is the subject of an abstract by Welage and associates. In a study of 42 critically ill patients in the intensive care unit, better control of gastric pH (pH > 4) was achieved with famotidine, 20 mg intravenously every 12 hours, compared to cimetidine, 300 mg intravenously every 6 hours. Gastric pH readings were greater than 4 in 81 percent of measurements among the famotidine-treated patients, compared to only 31 percent among the cimetidine-treated patients. Gross gastrointestinal bleeding, length of stay in the intensive care unit, transfusion requirements, and cost of hospitalization were not commented on in this study.

ADMINISTRATION

The dosages for famotidine are listed in Table 2-6. The use of one-time-a-day dosing for acute duodenal ulcer disease and benign gastric ulcer improves patient compliance. The drug is best given at dinnertime instead of at bedtime in order to suppress more completely the evening and nighttime surge of gastric acid secretion.

We prefer to give famotidine as a continuous infusion for the prevention of stress-related mucosal damage and as an adjunct to the treatment of upper gastrointestinal hemorrhage from peptic ulcer disease. Famotidine, 50 mg in 250 ml of 5% dextrose in water delivered at a rate of 10 ml/hour gives 2 mg famotidine per hour. This dosage is sufficient to suppress gastric acid secretion to a pH of greater than 4 in over 85 percent of patients. It is necessary to check the gastric pH at least twice in the first 24 hours of therapy to confirm this level of acid suppression. If gastric pH is less than 4, an increase in infusion rate to 15 ml/hour (3 mg famotidine/hour) is justified. The addition of antacids should be reversed for those rare patients in whom parenteral infusion of potent H_2-receptor antagonists fails to achieve adequate control of gastric acid secretion.

PEARLS AND PITFALLS

1. Famotidine is approximately 25 times more potent than cimetidine and 10 times more potent than ranitidine.
2. To date, no study has demonstrated greater efficacy of famotidine than cimetidine or ranitidine in the treatment of duodenal ulcer disease or benign gastric ulcer disease.
3. Famotidine does not bind to any appreciable degree to the cytochrome P-450 system and does not alter significantly the serum concentration of drugs known to be metabolized via this system (diazepam, Dilantin, phenytoin, theophylline).
4. Famotidine has no antiandrogenic side effects.
5. The incidence of famotidine-induced headache can be as high as 5 percent of patients.
6. Famotidine does not alter ethanol absorption in nonalcoholic, well-nourished men.

Nizatidine

Nizatidine is the newest competitor in the histamine H_2-receptor antagonist category. Introduced in the spring of 1988, it is approved for treatment of active duodenal ulcer; healed duodenal ulcer (maintenance therapy); endoscopically diagnosed reflux, erosive, or ulcerative esophagitis; and heartburn. In controlled studies, it has been shown to be as effective as cimetidine, ranitidine, and famotidine in the rate of healing and relief of symptoms in duodenal ulcer disease and gastroesophageal reflux disease. Its application to other acid-related conditions awaits further study.

MECHANISM OF ACTION, PHARMACODYNAMICS, AND PHARMACOKINETICS

Nizatidine, a structural analogue of histamine, contains a thiazole ring (see Fig. 2-1) and is a competitive antagonist of histamine for parietal cell H_2-receptors. Ninety percent of the drug is available for tissue absorption, with peak plasma concentration occurring 0.5 to 3.0 hours after ingestion (700–1800 μg/liter for a 150-mg dose; 1400–3600 μg/liter for a 300-mg dose). The drug is chiefly excreted in the urine via active tubular secretion (90%). About 7 percent of the drug is metabolized to N_2-monodesmethylnizatidine. Sixty percent of an oral dose of the drug is found unchanged in the urine. People with normal kidney function accumulate minimal amounts of the drug. Because of its rapid clearance, the drug's half-life is only 1 to 2 hours (see Table 2-2). The half-life in people with renal impairment is prolonged up to 3.5 to 11.0 hours.

While a 300-mg dose of nizatidine suppresses 90 percent of nocturnal gastric acid secretion for up to 10 hours, a 150-mg dose inhibits 98 percent of meal-stimulated gastric acid output for 4 hours. Normal doses do not have any effect on serum gastrin levels or gastric pepsin concentration. The rate of nizatidine absorption is decreased by 10 percent with concurrent use of simethicone-containing antacids, but is unaffected by ingestion of propantheline.

INDICATIONS

For acute duodenal ulcer disease and for maintenance therapy of healed duodenal ulcer (see Table 2-6), the recommended dosage is 150 mg twice a day or 300 mg at bedtime. Maintenance dosage is 150 mg at bedtime. Patients with abnormal creatinine clearance (< 50 ml/min but > 20 ml/min) should receive a reduced dosage of nizatidine, 150 mg orally every 24 hours, for treatment of acute duodenal ulcer disease, and patients with a creatinine clearance of less than 20 ml/day should be dosed every other day.

A double-blind, prospective, endoscopically guided study of 43 patients with duodenal ulcer receiving either nizatidine, 150 mg orally twice a day for 8 weeks, or placebo showed healing rates of 82 percent in the nizatidine group versus 50 percent in the placebo group. The only statistically significant laboratory event was an increase in serum creatinine from 1.05 to 1.1 mg/dl in the active therapy group. Healing correlated with symptomatic relief of ulcer pain.

Bovera and associates reported similar healing rates of duodenal ulcers and ulcer pain relief when comparing nizatidine, 300 mg at bedtime, and ranitidine, 300 mg at bedtime, for acute duodenal ulcer disease. The nizatidine group had ulcer healing rates of 78 percent and 91 percent, respectively, at 4 and 8 weeks, while the ranitidine group showed 78 percent and 95 percent healing.

Simon and associates' European study concluded that nizatidine and ranitidine were equally effective in duodenal ulcer healing, with 92 percent and 93 percent of ulcers healed, respectively, after 8 weeks of therapy. No serious complications were reported.

A 1-year maintenance study by Cerulli and associates showed recurrent ulcer rates of 34 percent in the nizatidine group, as opposed to 64 percent for the placebo group, figures similar to previously published figures for cimetidine, ranitidine, and famotidine. Although treatment of gastric ulcer is not currently an approved indication in the United States, Naccarato and colleagues treated 275

Table 2-8. H_2-antagonists: Pregnancy and breast-feeding

Agent	FDA pregnancy category	Risk vs benefit (by trimester)			Breast-feeding category
		1st	2nd	3rd	
Cimetidine	B2	?	B > R	B > R	IV
Famotidine	B1	?	?	?	IV
Nizatidine	B1	?	?	?	IV
Ranitidine	B1	?	?	?	IV

Food and Drug Administration (FDA) pregnancy categories:
A = Well-controlled studies fail to demonstrate risk to the fetus.
B1 = Animal studies fail to demonstrate risk to the fetus but no human studies are available.
B2 = Animal studies show some risk to the fetus but this is not confirmed in human studies.
C1 = Animal studies show risk to the fetus but no human studies are available.
C2 = Animal and human studies are unavailable.
D = Drug is associated with birth defects but has potential benefits that may outweigh known risks.
X = Drug is associated with birth defects and with potential risk that clearly outweighs potential benefit.
Risk vs benefit: R >> B = Proven or potential risk outweighs potential benefits.
B > R = Potential benefits outweigh potential risks.
R >> B? = Risks may be outweighed by benefits in some circumstances.
? = Risk-to-benefit ratio is unknown.
Breast-feeding categories:
I = Drug does not enter breast milk.
II = Drug enters breast milk but is not known to be harmful in therapeutic doses.
IIIA = Drug may or may not enter breast milk but no adverse effects are expected.
IIIB = Drug may or may not enter breast milk but drug is systemically absorbed.
IV = Drug enters breast milk and poses a potential risk to the neonate.

gastric ulcer patients in Italy with either nizatidine, 150 mg twice a day; nizatidine, 300 mg at bedtime; or ranitidine, 150 mg twice a day. Patients underwent routine endoscopic evaluation every 4 weeks. Healing rates after 8 weeks of therapy were: nizatidine, 150 mg twice a day, 90 percent; nizatidine, 300 mg at bedtime, 86.5 percent; and ranitidine, 150 mg twice a day, 86.7 percent.

SIDE EFFECTS AND UNTOWARD ACTIONS

The most frequently reported side effects include sweating (1%), urticaria (0.5%), and somnolence (0.3%). These figures are higher than those reported in placebo-treated groups.

ANTIANDROGENIC SIDE EFFECTS

Gynecomastia and impotence were reported at the same rate as in placebo-treated groups.

Drug-related elevations in liver-associated enzymes have been reported. One case of an elevation of the serum glutamic pyruvic transaminase (SGPT) to greater than 2000 IU/liter has been seen. With discontinuation of the drug, the liver enzyme returned to normal. With market introduction, rare cases of cholestatic and mixed hepatocellular/cholestatic jaundice have been reported.

PEARLS AND PITFALLS

1. The dose of nizatidine should be reduced to 150 mg/day orally for treatment of acute duodenal ulcer disease in patients with chronic renal failure.
2. Drug-induced hepatitis is rare but possible with oral nizatidine therapy.
3. Patients with severe renal disease (creatinine clearance < 20 ml/min) should receive 150 mg nizatidine orally every other day for treatment of acute duodenal ulcer disease, and 150 mg nizatidine orally every third day for maintenance therapy.
4. Nizatidine does not facilitate ethanol absorption.

Suggested Reading

CIMETIDINE

Caballerai J, et al. Effects of cimetidine of gastric alcohol dehydrogenase activity and blood ethanol levels. Gastroenterology 1989; 96:388–392.

Cimetidine may enhance alcohol absorption from the stomach.

Campbell NRC, et al. Ferrous sulfate reduces cimetidine absorption. Dig Dis Sci 1993; 38:950–954.

Cimetidine appears to bind iron and is thus less absorbable. A dose of 150 mg iron sulfate decreases cimetidine absorption by 63 percent.

Capurso L, et al. Comparison of cimetidine, 800 mgs once daily and 400 mgs twice daily, in acute duodenal ulceration. Br Med J 1984; 289:1418–1420.

A seven-center trial of 187 patients with acute duodenal ulcer entered prospectively in a double-blind fashion to receive either 800 mg cimetidine at night or 400 mg cimetidine twice a day. After 4 weeks of therapy, 76 of 91 (84%) patients receiving 800 mg cimetidine at night and 65 of 96 (68%) patients receiving 400 mg cimetidine twice a day were healed.

Choonara JA, et al. Stereoselective interaction between the R enantiomer of warfarin and cimetidine. Br J Clin Pharmacol 1986; 21:271–277.

Although it is recognized that serum warfarin levels are increased with concurrent cimetidine therapy, drug interaction occurs only with the R(+) enantiomer. Because the R(−) enantiomer is a more potent anticoagulant, accumulation of the less potent R(+) enantiomer may explain the observed increase (20–40%) in warfarin blood levels without a corresponding increase in prothrombin time.

Cohen A, Fabre L. Tolerance to repeated intravenous doses of ranitidine HCl and cimetidine HCl in normal volunteers. Curr Ther Res 1983; 34:475–482.

A prospective evaluation of 100 normal volunteers receiving intravenous bolus injections and infusions of ranitidine and cimetidine for 7 to 10 days. Drug-induced hepatitis with transaminase values less than 100 units/liter were noted typically after 5 to 7 days of therapy in 24 percent of the ranitidine-treated and 19 percent of the cimetidine-treated subjects.

Craven DE, Driks MR. Nosocomial pneumonia in the intubated patient. Semin Resp Infect 1987; 2:20–33.

The etiology of nosocomial pneumonia in intubated patients is postulated to result from gastric colonization, transgression of the lower esophageal sphincter, erosion of esophageal and oropharyngeal mucosal surfaces enhancing gram-negative bacillary adherence, and aspiration of stagnant oropharyngeal secretions. Preliminary data from 95 patients show a 26.4 percent rate of pneumonia in 53 patients receiving antacids or H_2-receptor antagonists, compared to an 11.9 percent rate in 42 patients receiving sucralfate alone.

Dobbs JH, Muir JG, Smith RN. H2-antagonists and hepatitis. Ann Intern Med 1986; 103:803.

Hepatitis can be regarded as a rare (0.06–0.08%) and idiosyncratic complication of cimetidine and ranitidine therapy.

Driks MR, et al. Nosocomial pneumonia in intubated patients given sucralfate compared with antacids or histamine type-2 blockers: The role of gastric colonization. N Engl J Med 1987; 317: 1376–1382.

A study of 130 intubated patients receiving sucralfate, antacids, H_2-receptor antagonists, or both antacids and H_2-receptor antagonists for stress-related mucosal defense, which showed that pneumonia developed in 7 of the 61 patients (11.5%) treated with sucralfate, in 9 of the 39 patients (23%) treated with antacids, in 1 of the 17 patients (5.9%) treated with H_2-receptor antagonists, and in 6 of the 13 patients (46%) treated with a combination of antacids and H_2-receptor antagonists.

Evreux M, et al. Endoscopic and clinical evaluation of cisapride and cimetidine in reflux esophagitis. Gastroenterology 1988; 94:A120.

Cisapride, 10 mg 4 times a day, and cimetidine, 400 mg 4 times a day, were equivalent in the treatment of patients with gastroesophageal reflux disease (GERD) in terms of symptoms and ulceration healing.

Feely J, Wilkinson GR, Wood AJ. Reduction of liver blood flow and propranolol metabolism by cimetidine. N Engl J Med 1981; 304: 692–695.

Feldman M, Burton ME. Histamine-2-receptor antagonists. N Engl J Med 1990; 323:1672–1680 and 1749–1755.

Comprehensive review of this class of agents.

Frank WO, et al. Continuous cimetidine infusion regimens—effects on intragastric pH in ulcer patients (abstr). Gastroenterology 1988; 94:A134.
Primed, continuous infusion regimens of cimetidine, 37.5 mg/hour (900 mg/24 hr), maintained gastric pH greater than 4 for more time than a 300-mg cimetidine IV bolus every 6 hours.

Gollapudi P, Sontag S, Miller T. Surgery for complications of peptic ulcer before and after availability of cimetidine. Gastroenterology 1988; 94:A150.

Halloran LG, et al. Prevention of acute gastrointestinal complications after severe head injury: A controlled trial of cimetidine prophylaxis. Am J Surg 1980; 139:44–48.
A prospective, randomized study of 50 patients with severe head injury from 1977 to 1979 who received corticosteroids, a prophylactic anticonvulsant, and either cimetidine, 300 mg every 4 hours, or placebo for stress ulcer prophylaxis. Only 2 of the 26 cimetidine-treated group required blood transfusion for acute upper gastrointestinal hemorrhage, whereas 8 of 24 placebo-treated patients required 2 or more units of packed red blood cells to maintain a stable hematocrit.

Hasan M, Sircus W. The factors determining success or failure of cimetidine treatment of peptic ulcer. J Clin Gastroenterol 1981; 3:225–229.
A retrospective study of 80 cimetidine-treatment failures showing that early age of onset, smoking, continued nonsteroidal anti-inflammatory agent use, and heavy alcohol intake (> 5 pt of beer a day) correlated with treatment failure.

Hentschel E, et al. Effect of cimetidine treatment in the prevention of gastric ulcer relapse: A 1-year double-blind, multicenter study. Gut 1983; 24:853–856.
Of 130 patients with benign gastric ulcer, 112 (86%) were healed after 8 weeks of cimetidine therapy, 200 mg 3 times a day with 400 mg qhs. Of the 112, 84 were followed for 1 year, half on cimetidine, 400 mg qhs, and half on placebo. On maintenance therapy, 86 percent of the cimetidine group remained in remission by endoscopic criteria, compared to 45 percent on placebo.

Jensen RT, et al. Cimetidine-induced impotence and breast changes in patients with gastric hypersecretory states. N Engl J Med 1983; 308:883–887.
A total of 11 of 22 men (50%) with Zollinger-Ellison syndrome or idiopathic hypersecretion taking a mean daily cimetidine dose of 5.3 gm/day had reversible impotence, breast changes (gynecomastia or breast tenderness), or both. Gynecomastia may take longer than 3 months to resolve after cessation of drug.

Kingsley AN. Prophylaxis for acute stress ulcers: Antacids or cimetidine. Am Surg 1985; 51:545–547.
With a regimen of 50 mg/hour cimetidine, the author found the lowest frequency of bleeding (1 of 59, or 1.7%).

Krag E. Cimetidine treatment of protein-losing gastropathy (Ménétrier's disease). Scand J Gastroenterol 1978; 13:635–639.
The use of cimetidine in this case of Ménétrier's disease was associated with an increase in serum albumin, a decrease in gastric protein loss, and a decrease in gastric hyperrugosity.

Lieberman DA. Medical therapy for chronic reflux esophagitis. Long-term follow-up. Arch Intern Med 1987; 147:1717–1720.
A series of 20 patients with a 13-year mean duration of symptoms,

followed prospectively for a mean of 26 months after remission induced by 1.2 gm cimetidine and 40 mg metoclopramide daily, showed that both drugs were able to be gradually tapered and then discontinued after an average of 8 weeks of full-dose therapy. Early relapse was associated with a lower esophageal sphincter (LES) pressure. Intensive short-term therapy may be adequate treatment for patients without decreased LES pressures.

Mitchell MC, et al. Cimetidine protects against acetaminophen hepatotoxicity in rats. Gastroenterology 1981; 81:1052–1060.

Rats given cimetidine 4 and 10 hours after intraperitoneal installation of toxic doses of acetaminophen were compared to controls given placebo. Cimetidine resulted in significant improvement in survival (75% versus 40%) and decreased transaminase elevation (mean SGOT 3800 units/liter versus 7200 units/liter in placebo-treated rats). The postulated mechanism is cimetidine binding of the cytochrome P-450 system with inhibition of production of toxic acetaminophen metabolites.

Ostensen H, et al. Smoking, alcohol, coffee, and familial factors: Any associations with peptic ulcer disease? Scand J Gastroenterol 1985; 20:1227–1235.

An epidemiologic study showing that cigarette smoking and a positive family history correlated in a positive manner with the development of both gastric and duodenal ulcers. Coffee drinking and moderate intake of alcohol were of no importance in this regard.

Ostro MJ, et al. Control of gastric pH with cimetidine: Boluses versus primed infusions. Gastroenterology 1985; 89:532–537.

A study of 23 acutely ill patients receiving cimetidine for stress mucosal ulceration prophylaxis. The gastric pH was maintained continuously above 4 in only 5 patients given 300 mg IV every 6 hours, whereas 14 of the 23 maintained a gastric pH greater than 4 on 37.5 mg cimetidine per hour. An additional 6 patients achieved pH values greater than 4 when the infusion was increased to 50 mg/hour. Thus, 20 of 23 patients (87%) achieved continuous gastric pH values greater than 4 with cimetidine infusions of 50 mg/hour or less. No patient bled during the study period.

Peura DA, Johnson LF. Cimetidine for prevention and treatment of gastroduodenal mucosal lesions in patients in an intensive care unit. Ann Intern Med 1985; 103:173–177.

Bleeding persisted or developed in only 1 of 21 patients in the cimetidine group, compared to 7 of 18 patients in the placebo group.

Porter JB, et al. Long-term follow-up study of cimetidine. Pharmacotherapy 1984; 4:381–384.

A retrospective analysis of 8553 recipients of cimetidine found one possible case of cimetidine-induced hepatitis, which reversed over 6 months when cimetidine was discontinued.

Rudnick MR, et al. Cimetidine-induced renal failure. Ann Intern Med 1982; 96:180–182.

Two cases of acute, partially reversible interstitial nephritis developed after cimetidine use. In case A, rechallenge with cimetidine caused fever, chills, azotemia, pyuria, and eosinophilia. Cessation of cimetidine was associated with a prompt reversal of azotemia. In case B, renal biopsy showed interstitial plasma cells, macrophages, lymphocytes, and polymorphonuclear leukocytes with focal fibrosis.

Saeed ZA, et al. Management of gastric hypersecretion with intravenous antisecretory medication in patients with Zollinger-Ellison

Syndrome (ZES) (abstr). Gastroenterology 1988; 94:A393.
A study of 47 ZES patients demonstrating a clear correlation (r = 0.94) between the total daily oral dose and the continuous IV dose of cimetidine required to decrease basal acid output to less than 10 mEq/hour. This degree of acid suppression was necessary to allow an uncomplicated perioperative clinical course.

Siepler J, Trudeau W. Treatment of UGIH by constant versus intermittent infusion of cimetidine in the intensive care unit (abstr). Gastroenterology 1984; 86:1251.
A prospective study of 46 indigent patients admitted for upper gastrointestinal hemorrhage to an ICU. One-third received 50 mg/hour cimetidine intravenously, while two-thirds received 300 mg cimetidine every 6 hours intravenously. All patients received 30 ml antacids every 2 hours. Rebleeding (17 of 30 versus 3 of 15) and mortality (23.8% versus 6.6%) were significantly higher in the intermittent bolus group compared to the constant infusion group.

Simpson CJ, et al. Effect of cimetidine on prognosis after simple closure of perforated duodenal ulcer. Br J Surg 1987; 74:104–105.
A randomized, prospective study of the benefits of cimetidine on the postoperative course of 60 patients with perforated duodenal ulcer. Although cimetidine had no effect on the 12-month mortality, re-operation (second perforation or rebleeding) and symptoms were significantly more common in the control group.

Sontag S, et al. Cimetidine, cigarette smoking, and recurrence of duodenal ulcer. N Engl J Med 1984; 311:689–693.
Symptomatic ulcer recurrence occurred in 13 percent of the nonsmokers receiving placebo, 4 percent of the nonsmokers receiving cimetidine, 51 percent of the smokers receiving placebo, and 22 percent of the smokers receiving cimetidine. When all recurrences were grouped together (symptomatic and asymptomatic), nonsmokers receiving placebo had a lower recurrence rate than did smokers receiving cimetidine (21% versus 34%).

Tanner LA. Bradycardia and H_2 receptor antagonists (Hr). Ann Intern Med 1988; 109:434.
A review of 39 spontaneous domestic reports of bradycardia associated with H_2 receptor antagonists.

Terruzzi V, et al. The influence of cimetidine and ranitidine on the plasma lipid pattern. Br J Clin Pharmacol 1985; 19:846–848.
A potential benefit of the antiandrogenic activity of cimetidine is the observed increase (14%) in serum HDL cholesterol after 5 weeks of cimetidine, 800 mg/day, an effect not observed with ranitidine.

Thorens J, et al. Higher incidence of bacterial overgrowth during treatment with omeprazole as compared to cimetidine. Gastroenterology 1994; 106:A197.
Greater acid suppression was associated with higher rates of bacterial overgrowth.

Tytgat GNJ, Nicolai JJ, et al. Efficacy of different doses of cimetidine in the treatment of reflux esophagitis. Gastroenterology 1990; 99:629–634.
Cimetidine, 800 mg at dinner, is the authors' preferred initial regimen in reflux esophagitis.

Villeneuve JP, Warner HA. Cimetidine hepatitis. Gastroenterology 1979; 77:143–144.
A case report of a hypersensitivity type of allergic reaction to cimetidine in an 83-year-old white woman.

RANITIDINE

Abdulian JD, Chen YK, Collen MJ. Gastroesophageal reflux in the elderly. Gastroenterology 1994; 106:A35.

Effective therapy of GERD in the elderly often requires marked increases in ranitidine dose—as high as 3000 mg a day!

Bardham KD, Walker RR, Miller JP. A comparison of enprostil versus ranitidine in the treatment of gastric ulcer (abstr). Gastroenterology 1988; 94:A22.

A study of 156 patients with gastric ulcer treated for 8 weeks with either enprostil, a prostaglandin E_2 analogue, 35 μg twice a day, or ranitidine, 150 mg twice a day. Healing rates at 8 weeks were 72 and 80 percent, respectively. Diarrhea occurred in 10 and 6 percent, respectively.

Bredfeldt JE, et al. Ranitidine, acetaminophen, and hepatotoxicity. Ann Intern Med 1984; 101:719.

A letter to the editor presenting a case of cholestatic liver disease associated with concurrent ranitidine and acetaminophen usage. One possible explanation is that both drugs compete for hepatic glutathione.

Cohen A, Fabre L. Tolerance to repeated intravenous doses of ranitidine HCl and cimetidine HCl in normal volunteers. Curr Ther Res 1983; 34:475–482.

A prospective evaluation of 100 normal volunteers receiving intravenous bolus infusions of ranitidine and cimetidine 4 times a day for 7 to 10 days. Drug-induced hepatitis with transaminase values less than 100 IU/liter were noted, typically after 5 to 7 days of therapy, in 24 percent of the ranitidine- and 19 percent of the cimetidine-treated subjects.

Cole AT, et al. Ranitidine, aspirin, food, and the stomach. Br Med J 1992; 304:544–545.

Ranitidine protects the empty stomach from aspirin-induced erosions.

Colin-Jones DG, et al. Reducing overnight secretion of acid to heal duodenal ulcers. Am J Med 1984; 77 (suppl 5B): 116–122.

A prospective double-blind, double-placebo trial of 102 patients treated with either 150 mg ranitidine twice a day or 300 mg ranitidine at bedtime. Healing rates were 48 of 57 (84%) and 43 of 45 (96%), respectively.

Collen MJ, et al. Gastric acid hypersecretion is refractory gastroesophageal reflux disease. Gastroenterology 1990; 98:654–661.

Patients with refractory GERD are more likely to have Barrett's esophagus, are more likely to be acid hypersecretors, and are more likely to require higher doses of ranitidine.

Danilewitz M, Tim LO, Hirschowitz B. Ranitidine suppression of gastric hypersecretion resistant to cimetidine. N Engl J Med 1982; 306:20–22.

Three cases of idiopathic gastric acid hypersecretion unresponsive to intravenous cimetidine (1200–2400 mg/day) are presented. All three patients (aged 59, 76, and 83 years) were given intravenous ranitidine, 300 mg/day, which provided adequate control of acid output. Two patients developed pneumonia, one of whom died with Pseudomonas *pneumonia and septicemia.*

Dawson J, Cockel R. Ranitidine in acute upper gastrointestinal hemorrhage. Br Med J 1982; 285:476–477.

A double-blind study of 158 consecutive patients with acute upper gastrointestinal hemorrhage comparing ranitidine, 150 mg orally

3 times a day, to placebo in ability to decrease the incidence of recurrent hemorrhage. Although the overall results were comparable for the two treatment groups, 14 of 76 ranitidine-treated and 21 of 75 placebo-treated patients rebled. Among patients with duodenal ulcer, the rate of rebleeding with ranitidine treatment, 3 of 27, was significantly lower than the rate of rebleeding with placebo, 11 of 26.

di Stefano R, et al. A positive pulmonary aspiration test predicts a favorable response to ranitidine in patients with non-allergic asthma or chronic cough (abstr). Gastroenterology 1988; 94:A101.
In patients with nonallergic asthma or cough, a positive pulmonary aspiration test (egg labeled with 4.5 μCi of 99m Tc–DTPA) was a better predictor of a favorable clinical response to ranitidine, 150 mg/day orally, than 24-hour esophageal pH probe testing.

Dobbs JH, Muir JG, Smith RN. H2-antagonists and hepatitis. Ann Intern Med 1986; 103:803.
Hepatitis can be regarded as a rare (0.06–0.08%) and idiosyncratic complication of cimetidine and ranitidine therapy.

El-Omar E, et al. Marked rebound acid hypersecretion in healthy volunteers following ranitidine. Gastroenterology 1994; 106:A74.
Rebound hypersecretion of acid occurs in the 48 hours after cessation of ranitidine and is independent of gastritis.

Fiorucci S, et al. Effect of omeprazole and high doses of ranitidine on gastric acidity and gastroesophageal reflux in patients with moderate-severe esophagitis. Am J Gastroenterol 1990; 85:1 458–1464.
High doses of ranitidine, 300 mg orally twice a day, can achieve acid suppression similar to that seen with omeprazole.

Hentschel E, et al. Effect of ranitidine and amoxicillin plus metronidazole on the eradication of *H. pylori* and the recurrence of duodenal ulcer. N Engl J Med 1993; 328:308–312.
Eradication of ulcer-associated H. pylori *decreases ulcer recurrences significantly.*

Karachalios GN. Ranitidine and hepatitis. Ann Intern Med 1985; 103: 634–635.
A case report of a 65-year-old man admitted for an upper GI bleed secondary to a duodenal ulcer. Admission SGOT and SGPT were normal. Ranitidine, 300 mg/day, was begun. Renal function was normal. Three weeks later SGPT was 920 units/liter, and the bilirubin level was 11.9 mg/dl. Liver biopsy showed cholestasis. All abnormalities resolved with discontinuation of ranitidine.

Lanza F, et al. A multicenter double-blind comparison of ranitidine versus placebo in the prophylaxis of nonsteroidal anti-inflammatory drug–induced lesion in gastric and duodenal mucosa (abstr). Gastroenterology 1988; 94:A250.
A prospective, endoscopically controlled study of patients receiving nonsteroidal anti-inflammatory agents (NSAIADs) for rheumatologic conditions showing that ranitidine, 150 mg orally twice a day, was effective in the prevention of duodenal ulcer compared to placebo (0 of 62 patients receiving ranitidine versus 4 of 57 patients on placebo had evidence of duodenal ulceration, $p < 0.01$).

Offit K, Sojka DA. Possible ranitidine-induced granulomatous hepatitis. N Engl J Med 1984; 310:1603–1604.
A case report of a 66-year-old man receiving ranitidine, 150 mg/qhs for 4 weeks, who presented with fever and malaise. Liver test values were SGOT 128 units per liter, SGPT 145 units per liter,

alkaline phosphatase 466 units per liter, and gamma-glutamyl transpeptidase 535 units per liter. Biopsy showed granulomatous inflammation with eosinophilia. Fever and liver test abnormalities abated 1 week after discontinuation of the drug.

Penston JG, Wormsley KG. Long-term treatment of duodenal ulcers. Gastroenterology 1988; 94:A349.
Long-term treatment of patients with previously documented duodenal ulcers (DU) with either ranitidine or cimetidine was associated with symptomatic recurrences in only 16 percent at 3 years (12% for ranitidine, 27% for cimetidine). Although 82 of the 432 patients (19%) presented with an upper gastrointestinal hemorrhage, only 5 of the 432 patients (1.1%) receiving maintenance therapy had a recurrent DU with hemorrhage.

Rauws EAJ, Tytgat GNJ. Cure of duodenal ulcer associated with eradication of *H. pylori.* Lancet 1990; 335:1233–1235.
Ranitidine with amoxicillin, metronidazole, and bismuth led to ulcer healing and marked decrease in ulcer recurrence.

Reid SR, Baycliff CD. The comparative efficacy of cimetidine and ranitidine in controlling gastric pH in critically ill patients. Can Anaesth Soc J 1986; 33:287–293.
A randomized, prospective study of 71 patients admitted to an ICU, designed to evaluate the effectiveness of a primed infusion of cimetidine, 300-mg bolus with a 50-mg/hour infusion, compared to a primed infusion of ranitidine, 50-mg bolus with a 12.5-mg/hour infusion. Thirteen of the 38 patients in the cimetidine group (34.2%) and three of the 33 patients in the ranitidine group (9.1%) were "poorly" controlled (pH < 5 on more than 25% of the readings). One cimetidine and two ranitidine patients had clinical evidence of bleeding. No significant adverse effects attributable to the drugs occurred. Both agents effectively prevent stress-induced UGI hemorrhage.

Rigaud D, et al. Intragastric pH profile during acute respiratory failure in patients with chronic obstructive pulmonary disease. Chest 1986; 90:58–62.
A prospective evaluation of the ability of ranitidine, 35-mg loading dose and 17.5-mg/hour continuous infusion, to elevate gastric pH in 12 chronic obstructive pulmonary disease (COPD) patients with respiratory failure. Gastric pH was maintained above 4 for 65 percent of the time.

Ruiz-Santana S, et al. Stress-induced gastroduodenal lesions and total parenteral nutrition in critically ill patients. Crit Care Med 1991; 19:887–891.
Stress-related gastritis and hemorrhage are prevented equally well by total parenteral nutrition, sucralfate, and ranitidine.

Siepler J, et al. Prophylaxis of stress ulceration in the ICU: A comparison of cimetidine and ranitidine constant infusion (abstr). Gastroenterology 1987; 93:1639.
A nonrandomized, prospective study of 227 patients receiving continuous infusion cimetidine (N = 77), 300-mg bolus with 50 mg/hour, or ranitidine (N = 150), 50-mg bolus with 8 mg/hour. The amount of time with pH greater than 5 (66–71%), the amount of time with pH greater than 6 (32–34%), the number and percentage of upper GI bleeds (2/2.5% and 1/1.6%), and transfusion requirements (3 and 2) were equivalent.

Wyeth JW, et al. GR122311X (ranitidine bismuth citrate) with antibiotics for the eradication of *H. pylori.* Gastroenterology 1994: 106:A212.

GR, in combination with either amoxicillin or clarithromycin, eradicated H. pylori *in 83 percent of patients.*

Zimmerman TW, et al. Ranitidine treatment of gastroesophageal reflux disease in the elderly. Gastroenterology 1985; 88:1644.

A retrospective analysis of the response of 64 patients 60 years old or older to ranitidine or placebo treatment of gastroesophageal reflux disease. Improvement of symptoms and endoscopic healing of esophageal abnormalities were significantly more likely to occur in the ranitidine (150 mg po bid) group than in the placebo group. No significant untoward effects were seen.

FAMOTIDINE

Aono M, et al. Effect of famotidine and cimetidine on high density lipoprotein cholesterol levels in peptic ulcer patients (abstr). Dig Dis Sci 1986; 31:493S.

There is no known associated increase in serum HDL cholesterol with famotidine.

Chiverton SG, Hunt RH. Pharmacokinetics and pharmacodynamics of treatment for peptic ulcer disease in the elderly. Am J Gastroenterol 1988; 83:211–215.

A review of the drug therapy of peptic ulcer disease in the elderly. The authors emphasize:

If a patient is taking warfarin, phenytoin, or theophylline, and is stable, the addition of cimetidine requires dose reduction of warfarin, phenytoin, and theophylline and measurement of prothrombin time and serum drug levels.

Decreased renal tubular excretion of procainamide by concurrent cimetidine administration has an especially noteworthy propensity for toxicity.

Decreased acid secretion may inhibit iron and ketoconazole absorption.

Famotidine does not influence drugs eliminated by the P-450 mixed-function oxidase system.

Long-term treatment of elderly patients with impaired renal function with the basic aluminum salt sucralfate raises the specter of aluminum and dialysis dementia, even though long-term treatment of patients with normal renal function was not *associated with elevation of plasma aluminum levels.*

Colloidal bismuth compliance may be limited by its ammoniacal taste, blackening of the stool, and darkening of the tongue. Theoretical concern about increased plasma bismuth levels (toxic > 100 μm/liter) in renal failure patients has not been observed.

Corleto V, et al. Loss of efficacy of famotidine in the control of gastric acid secretion in patients with Zollinger-Ellison syndrome, reversed by omeprazole (abstr). Gastroenterology 1988; 94:A79.

The authors studied nine patients with Zollinger-Ellison syndrome (ZES) and found that BAO increased to greater than 10 mEq/hour, despite initial control with 80 to 400 mg/day famotidine, in six of the nine within 7 to 15 months of starting the drug. Complete acid suppression was achieved with omeprazole, 20 to 60 mg/day.

Howard JM, Chernios AN, Collen MJ. Famotidine, a new, potent, long-acting histamine H_2-receptor antagonist: comparison with cimetidine and ranitidine—the treatment of Zollinger-Ellison syndrome. Gastroenterology 1985; 88:1026.

A mean daily dose of famotidine of 240 mg, range 80–480 mg, controlled abdominal pain and pyrosis.

Klotz U, Arvela P, Rosenkranz B. Famotidine, a new H2-receptor antagonist, does not affect hepatic elimination of diazepam or tubular secretion of procainamide. Eur J Clin Pharmacol 1985; 28:671–675.

In contrast to cimetidine, an agent known to delay hepatic clearance of diazepam and renal tubular secretion of procainamide, famotidine did not alter significantly the half-life of diazepam (t1/2 = 45.6 hours pre- and 39.0 hours postfamotidine) or procainamide (t1/2 = 2.9 hours pre- and 3.0 hours postfamotidine) in eight healthy male volunteers.

Locniskar A, et al. Interaction of diazepam with famotidine and cimetidine, two H2-receptor antagonists. J Clin Pharmacol 1986; 26:299–303.

Eleven volunteers received diazepam concurrently with either famotidine, 40 mg 2 times a day, or cimetidine, 300 mg 4 times a day. Cimetidine increased significantly the elimination half-life of diazepam (55 to 72 hr). Famotidine did not alter diazepam pharmacokinetics. In this article, no comments were made about clinically significant changes in subject performance.

Lyon DT. Efficacy and safety of famotidine in the management of benign gastric ulcers. Am J Med 1986; (suppl 4B):33–41.

The most common side effect of famotidine is headache, reported in 2 percent of these patients treated for gastric ulcer.

McCallum RW, et al. MK-208, a novel histamine H2-receptor inhibitor with prolonged antisecretory effect. Dig Dis Sci 1985; 30: 1139–1144.

MK-208 (famotidine, Pepcid) is a guanidinothiazole derivative that is a potent H_2-blocker devoid of antiandrogenic activity with a longer duration of action than cimetidine (up to 7 hr). MK-208, 5 mg, was equipotent to 300 mg cimetidine in suppressing pentagastrin-stimulated acid output.

Raufman J-P, Francesco V, et al. Histamine-2 receptor antagonists do not alter serum ethanol levels in fed, non-alcoholic men. Ann Intern Med 1993; 118:488–493.

Famotidine, 20 mg orally twice a day for 7 days, did not alter ethanol absorption ingested in conjunction with a meal.

Reynolds JC. Four independent variables predict duodenal ulcer healing by famotidine in a relatively unselected patient population: A multivariate analysis of a prospective, multicenter study (abstr). Gastroenterology 1988; 94:A374.

A prospective evaluation of 135 patients that identified four risk factors associated with nonhealing of duodenal ulcer at 4 weeks: (1) alcohol use (3.9-fold increased risk over normal of not being healed); (2) prior DU (2.7-fold increased risk over normal of not being healed); (3) history of bleeding (1.9-fold increased risk over normal of not being healed); and (4) ulcer size greater than 10 mm (6.2-fold increased risk over normal of not being healed). Use of NSAIDs or aminosalicylic acid (ASA) before entry increased the odds of healing.

Simon B, et al. Famotidine versus ranitidine for the short-term treatment of duodenal ulcer. Digestion 1985; 32 (suppl 1):32–37.

A prospective, randomized trial of three famotidine regimens compared to ranitidine. Famotidine was given at dosages of 40 mg at bedtime, 20 mg twice a day, and 40 mg twice a day. Ranitidine was given at 150 mg twice a day. At 4 weeks, the healing rates for the four treatment regimens were 91, 83, 90, and 93 percent. At 8 weeks, these healing rates were 98, 95, 100, and 93 percent.

Smith JL, et al. Famotidine, a new H2-receptor antagonist. Dig Dis Sci 1985; 30:308–312.
Famotidine decreases dramatically acid output from parietal cells with parallel decrements in pepsin production. Nonparietal cell secretion (bicarbonate) is not decreased significantly. Pentagastrin-stimulated acid secretion remained decreased (50% of control) 12 hours after a 20-mg oral dose of famotidine.

Taha AS, Hudson N, et al. Prevention of NSAID-related gastric and duodenal ulcers by famotidine. Gastroenterology 1994; 106:A190.
Famotidine, 40 mg orally twice a day, reduced the incidence of ulceration in 285 rheumatoid arthritis patients from 26 percent (placebo) to 9 percent ($p<0.002$).

Welage LS, et al. An evaluation of intravenous famotidine versus cimetidine therapy in the critically ill (abstr). Gastroenterology 1988; 94:A491.
In this study of 42 critically ill ICU patients, famotidine-induced acid suppression (20 mg IV q12h) was greater than cimetidine-induced acid suppression (300 mg IV q6h). Among the famotidine-treated patients, 81 percent of the gastric pH readings were greater than 4, whereas among the cimetidine-treated cohort, only 31 percent of the gastric pH measurements were greater than 4.

NIZATIDINE

Bonfils S. Nizatidine versus ranitidine: Evolution of drug antisecretory efficacy over a 28-day period. Curr Ther Res 1992; 52:859–862.
Although tolerance to ranitidine with decreased acid suppression was observed during a 28-day period, no tolerance to nizatidine was seen and acid suppression was maintained.

Bovera E, et al. Nizatidine in the short-term treatment of duodenal ulcer—an Italian multicenter study. Hepatogastroenterology 1987; 34:269–271.
A double-blind study comparing nizatidine, 300 mg at bedtime, to ranitidine, 300 mg at bedtime, for treatment of active duodenal ulcer disease showed them to be similar in healing response.

Cerulli MA, et al. Nizatidine as maintenance therapy of duodenal ulcer disease in remission. Scand J Gastroenterol 1987; 136 (suppl):79–83.
Nizatidine, 150 mg, versus placebo was superior in prevention of duodenal ulcer disease in a 1-year study.

Cloud ML, Offen WW, Robinson M. Nizatidine versus placebo in gastroesophageal reflux disease: A 12-week multicenter, randomized, double-blind study. Am J Gastroenterol 1991; 86:1735–1742.
Nizatidine, 150 mg orally twice a day, is superior to placebo and nizatidine, 300 mg orally qhs, in healing erosive and ulcerative esophagitis and in relieving heartburn.

Dyck WP, et al. Treatment of duodenal ulceration in the United States. Scand J Gastroenterol 1987; 136(suppl):37–55.
A dose-response study showing equivalent healing rates of nizatidine, 300 mg at bedtime and 150 mg twice a day, significantly better than nizatidine, 25 mg twice a day, and placebo.

Hentschel E, et al. Nizatidine versus ranitidine in the prevention of duodenal ulcer relapse. Six-month interim results of a European multicenter study. Scand J Gastroenterol 1987; 136(suppl):84–88.

Statistically similar recurrence rates of duodenal ulcer were seen when comparing nizatidine, 150 mg at bedtime, and ranitidine, 150 mg at bedtime.

Levendoglu H, Mehl B, Wait C. Nizatidine, a new histamine blocker in the treatment of active duodenal ulcers. Am J Gastroenterol 1986; 12:1167–1170.

Nizatidine, 150 mg twice a day, compared with placebo was more effective in healing duodenal ulcer (82% versus 50%, respectively) after 8 weeks of treatment.

Naccarato R, et al. Nizatidine versus ranitidine in gastric ulcer disease: A European multicenter trial. Scand J Gastroenterol 1987; 136(suppl):71–78.

Benign gastric ulcer healing rates were similar when comparing nizatidine, 150 mg/day; nizatidine, 300 mg at bedtime; and ranitidine, 150 mg twice a day (90% and 86.5%, respectively) at 8 weeks.

Simon B, et al. 300 milligrams nizatidine at night versus 300 milligrams ranitidine at night in patients with duodenal ulcer: A multicenter trial in Europe. Scand J Gastroenterol 1987; 136 (suppl):61–70.

A large (859 patients), six-center trial of patients with duodenal ulcer showing equivalent rates of healing (92–93%) and nocturnal pain relief (>90% in both) in patients treated with either nizatidine or ranitidine (both 300 mg at bedtime).

Cytoprotective Agents

J. Thomas Dorsey III

Sucralfate

Sucralfate (Carafate) was introduced in Japan by the Chugai Pharmaceutical Company in 1968 for therapy of peptic ulcer disease. The drug was approved for use in the United States in 1981.

Sulfated saccharides such as heparin and chondroitin sulfate have been known since early in this century to inhibit peptic activity, and in 1932 the concept was advanced that chondroitin sulfate in the gastric mucus was the major factor protecting the stomach from autodigestion. In 1954, Levy demonstrated that chondroitin sulfate inhibited pepsin activity and protected against experimental gastric ulceration in an animal model. Other agents such as amylopectin sulfate were developed. This drug also showed evidence of activity in animal studies but was limited by side effects common to this group of compounds, including anticoagulation and the induction of colonic ulceration. Subsequent efforts to produce a compound with the same activity but without the side effects led to the development of sucralfate.

PHARMACOLOGY

The base compound of sucralfate is sucrose, which has its eight alcohol groups sulfated forming sucrose octasulfate. This substance is then complexed with polyaluminum hydroxide $[Al(OH)]^+$ to form sucralfate. The compound is a white amorphous powder insoluble in water and alcohol. It is poorly absorbed from the gut because of its high polarity, low solubility, and propensity for binding protein and bile acids. Ninety-five to 97 percent is excreted in the stool. Three to 5 percent of a dose is dissociated into sucrose octasulfate and aluminum base, which are absorbed. Sucrose octasulfate cannot be metabolized by the human and is excreted unchanged in the urine, as is the aluminum salt.

MECHANISM OF ACTION

Sucralfate's mechanism of action is multifactorial and differs from that of the antisecretory and acid-neutralizing drugs. Upon entering the acid environment of the stomach ($pH < 3–4$), some of the aluminum ions are dissociated and the compound becomes negatively charged. Polymerization occurs via intra- and intermolecular bridging, forming a viscous adhesive gel that retains its form even if the pH is subsequently raised (i.e., on entering the duodenum).

Sucralfate binds to normal mucosa, erosions, and ulcers. Binding to damaged areas of epithelium is more avid by a factor of 6 to 7 times than binding to normal mucosa. In addition, binding is better to duodenal than to gastric ulcers.

Sucralfate binds strongly to albumin, fibrinogen, and other proteins found in the ulcer base. Most of these proteins are positively charged at an acidic pH. Pepsin is negatively charged at this pH, as is sucralfate; thus, the binding of sucralfate proteins in the ulcer base prevents the binding of pepsin and subsequent digestion. In addition, it forms a physical barrier preventing diffusion of hydrogen ions from the gastric lumen to the gastric mucosa and acts as an antacid in the local microenvironment by slowly dissociating aluminum ions. The barrier also prevents bile acids from contacting the ulcer base.

Macroscopically, sucralfate binds for at least 6 hours. Although food removes sucralfate from normal mucosa, it does not affect sucralfate binding to damaged tissue other than by attaching to the luminal surface of the sucralfate patch. All traces of sucralfate are gone from the mucosa by 24 hours after a single dose.

Newer studies have shown that sucralfate binding is less acid dependent than previously thought. Aside from the barrier effect, sucralfate has a variety of luminal effects. It absorbs pepsin; 1 gm sucralfate decreases pepsin activity by 32 to 55 percent. Bile acids are also absorbed and sucralfate is as effective as cholestyramine in this regard. Aluminum ions also form an insoluble complex with bile acids.

Despite these luminal effects, there is no significant alteration in the volume or pH of gastric secretions and no change in the pepsin concentration. Thus, the barrier of gastric acid is maintained, preventing infection or colonization, as can occur with therapy using antacids or H_2-antagonists. In addition, there is evidence that sucralfate may have a direct antibacterial effect against *Escherichia coli* and *Pseudomonas*. Sucralfate interfered with the binding of *Helicobacter pylori* to the gastric mucosa, but not to a clinically significant degree.

The final mechanism of actions falls under the concept of cytoprotection, which refers to enhancement of mucosal defense mechanisms (mucus, bicarbonate secretion, epithelial cell renewal, and microcirculatory effects) by prostaglandin-dependent or -independent mechanisms without alterations of gastric secretion. An example of the prostaglandin-dependent mechanisms includes increases in both gastric and duodenal mucosal bicarbonate production. Two nonprostaglandin-mediated effects are an increased secretion of soluble mucus and binding of epidermal growth factor and fibroblast growth factor at the ulcer base, keeping them in contact with the underlying mucosa for a prolonged period of time.

INDICATIONS

1. Peptic ulcer disease. In duodenal ulcer, sucralfate has been demonstrated to be equivalent to H_2-receptor antagonists in healing at 6 to 8 weeks. Dosages of 1 gm orally 4 times a day or 2 gm twice a day are both effective. There may be less immediate pain relief with sucralfate. Maintenance of healed ulcer is effective at a dosage of 1 gm orally twice a day, but not 2 gm orally. Sucralfate has no effect on the natural history of duodenal ulcer. In gastric ulcer, healing rates are equivalent to those of H_2-receptor antagonists, but these may be slightly more effective in maintenance therapy. Natural history is not affected. There may be increased efficacy of sucralfate in smokers.
2. Stress-related mucosal damage. Sucralfate, at a dosage of 1 gm orally every 6 hours, is superior to placebo and equivalent to antacids and H_2-receptor antagonists in prevention of significant bleeding from stress ulceration. It has been suggested that by preservation of the gastric acid barrier and perhaps by direct antibacterial action, sucralfate decreases gastric colonization and subsequent nosocomial pneumonia. This was shown in a st[illegible]

by Driks and associates and more recently by Prod'hom and colleagues.

3. Nonsteroidal anti-inflammatory agent (NSAID)–induced ulcers. Sucralfate will heal NSAID-related duodenal or gastric ulcers and healing rates are improved by stopping the NSAID. Sucralfate is not effective as prophylaxis of NSAID-induced ulcers or their complications.
4. Nonulcer dyspepsia. In this heterogeneous population, several studies have shown sucralfate to be superior to placebo in relief of symptoms. The means for identifying the subset that would respond is not available at present.
5. Bile reflux gastritis. The bile-absorbing action and barrier effects of sucralfate make it an attractive option in the therapy of bile reflux gastritis. One study has shown significant improvement in histology without significant endoscopic or symptomatic improvement. More studies are needed.
6. Gastroesophageal reflux disease (GERD). Twelve studies have shown sucralfate to be effective in symptomatic relief and endoscopic healing of esophagitis. This requires 4-times-a-day dosing, and sucralfate's use with H_2-receptor antagonists has not shown additive benefit. Sucralfate is ineffective in maintenance therapy of GERD. Its use in sclerotherapy-induced ulcerations and radiation esophagitis needs to be studied further.
7. Miscellaneous uses. Sucralfate after meals has been used with success in a small number of patients with chemotherapy-induced oral stomatitis. Several articles, including one by Pera and associates, have investigated the use of technetium 99m–labeled sucralfate in the localization of peptic ulcers; however, it seems unlikely that this method would supplant currently existing diagnostic modalities. Several authors have shown that sucralfate is effective in lowering the serum phosphate level in patients with renal failure. However, like other phosphate binders, sucralfate causes an elevation in the serum aluminum levels. Finally, in a preliminary study by Carling and colleagues, sucralfate was shown to adhere to colitic mucosa and, when labeled with technetium 99m, may be useful in the determination of the extent of disease. A small number of patients were treated with a 10% sucralfate enema, 100 ml per rectum twice a day for 6 weeks. A large percentage of these patients had symptomatic improvement. These findings are preliminary and must be further investigated before sucralfate can be recommended in this setting.

SIDE EFFECTS

Side effects are uncommon, occurring in fewer than 5 percent of patients in most series; they are usually transient and seldom require discontinuation of the drug. The most common side effect is constipation, which occurs in 2 to 4 percent of patients. Other side effects, which occur in fewer than 1 to 2 percent of patients, are not significantly different from those reported while on placebo and include dry mouth, nausea, dyspepsia, headache, rash, dizziness, drowsiness, diarrhea, back pain, and vertigo. One case of bezoar formation has been reported. In animals, no evidence of mutagenicity or carcinogenicity has been found, and lethal overdosage (LD-50) could not be induced.

LABORATORY ABNORMALITIES

No changes have been noted in coagulation parameters or hematologic, renal, or liver biochemical values. There are no electrocardiographic changes or changes in fecal occult blood positivity. As noted, in patients with renal failure, aluminum levels may increase and phosphate levels may normalize. There are rare reports of hypophosphatemia in otherwise normal patients.

DRUG INTERACTIONS

Sucralfate decreases the bioavailability of tetracycline, ketoconazole, quinolone antibiotics, H_2-antagonists, digoxin, quinidine, theophylline, warfarin (Coumadin), phenytoin (Dilantin), levothyroxine, and penicillamine by binding these agents in the gut and decreasing their absorption. Sucralfate should not be given within 2 hours of administration of other drugs.

PREGNANCY

Sucralfate did not decrease fertility in animal studies. Chronic high doses of sucralfate did not cause birth defects in the mouse, rat, or rabbit models. There are no human studies, but sucralfate is probably safe for use in pregnancy. No studies in nursing women are available, but significant levels are unlikely in breast milk. There are no data on the use of sucralfate in children.

DOSAGE AND ADMINISTRATION

Sucralfate is available as a 1-gm tablet and as a suspension with a concentration of 1 gm/10 mg.

There are no known contraindications to the use of sucralfate. In the adult, recommended dosage is 1 gm orally 4 times a day given 1 hour before meals and at bedtime, or 2 hours after meals and at bedtime. Two grams twice a day has been shown to be effective in short-term healing of duodenal ulcer. Antacid should not be given within 30 minutes of sucralfate.

PEARLS AND PITFALLS

1. Sucralfate is a nonsystemic drug with few side effects aside from constipation, which is seen in 2 to 4 percent of patients.
2. It is as effective as cimetidine in the healing of duodenal ulcer and gastric ulcer and maintenance of duodenal ulcer healing. Some practitioners use sucralfate for maintenance therapy of gastric ulcers.
3. Particular groups of individuals for whom sucralfate may offer advantages over the H_2-blockers include patients with chronic renal failure, smokers, and pregnant patients.
4. Sucralfate has shown efficacy in gastroesophageal reflux disease, drug-induced gastritis, stress-related mucosal damage, and nonulcer dyspepsia.
5. The usual dose is 1 gm orally 4 times a day 1 hour before meals and at bedtime. Two grams twice a day has been shown to be as effective as the traditional dose in healing duodenal ulcer. Antacids should not be given within 30 minutes of a dose. Sucralfate can also interfere with the absorption of other drugs; administration of sucralfate and another agent should be separated by 2 hours.

Table 3-1. Cytoprotective agents: Pregnancy and breast-feeding

Agent	FDA pregnancy category	Risk vs benefit (by trimester)			Breast-feeding category
		1st	2nd	3rd	
Misoprostol	C1	R >> B	R >> B	R >> B	IV
Sucralfate	B1	B > R	B > R	B > R	IIIA

Food and Drug Administration (FDA) pregnancy categories:
A = Well-controlled studies fail to demonstrate risk to the fetus.
B1 = Animal studies fail to demonstrate risk to the fetus but no human studies are available.
B2 = Animal studies show some risk to the fetus but this is not confirmed in human bodies.
C1 = Animal studies show risk to the fetus but no human studies are available.
C2 = Animal and human studies are unavailable.
D = Drug is associated with birth defects but has potential benefits that may outweigh known risks.
X = Drug is associated with birth defects and with potential risk that clearly outweighs potential benefit.
Risk vs benefit: R >> B = Proven or potential risk outweighs potential benefits.
B > R = Potential benefits outweigh potential risks.
R >> B? = Risks may be outweighed by benefits in some circumstances.
? = Risk-to-benefit ratio is unknown.

Breast-feeding categories:
I = Drug does not enter breast milk.
II = Drug enters breast milk but is not known to be harmful in therapeutic doses.
IIIA = Drug may or may not enter breast milk but no adverse effects are expected.
IIIB = Drug may or may not enter breast milk but drug is systemically absorbed.
IV = Drug enters breast milk and poses a potential risk to the neonate.

Misoprostol

Prostaglandins are naturally occurring 20-carbon oxygenated fatty acids found in a wide variety of mammalian tissues. These compounds have widely varying biologic activities; for example, prostaglandins of the E and F_2 types stimulate contraction of uterine smooth muscle; prostaglandins of the A, E, and I type are potent vasodilators; and prostaglandins of the E type are bronchodilators. Naturally occurring E_2 and prostacyclin I_2 are found in gastric mucosa and regulate gastric mucosal blood flow and acid secretion; they exhibit cytoprotective properties (as defined by Roberts), including stimulation of mucous and bicarbonate secretion.

Synthesized prostaglandin E_1, misoprostol, has these cytoprotective properties as well as gastric acid antisecretory effects. It has been shown to protect the mucosa of the stomach from inflammatory and noxious stimuli.

MECHANISM OF ACTION

Misoprostol is a synthetic prostaglandin E_1 methyl ester analogue with gastric cytoprotective activity at low doses, gastric antisecretory activity at higher doses, and few systemic actions.

PHARMACODYNAMICS AND PHARMACOKINETICS

When given orally, misoprostol blocks histamine-, pentagastrin-, and meal-stimulated gastric acid output. It does not interfere with gastrin release or alter serum gastrin levels. The primary acid-inhibiting effect is to lower the concentration of acid, with little effect on the volume of gastric output. Misoprostol binds to the E-type prostaglandin receptors, which number approximately 8000 per parietal cell.

In rat ulcer models, the dose of misoprostol that prevented gastric ulceration (10–150 μg/kg) was well below the dose (1000 μg/kg) required to inhibit gastric acid secretion. Aspirin- and ethanol-induced ulcerations in dog and rat models were reduced by low-dose misoprostol administration.

Oral misoprostol has no significant effects on blood pressure, heart rate, or electrocardiogram measurements. Transient hypotension can accompany intravenous bolus administration.

Misoprostol does not inhibit platelet aggregation in a muscarinic receptor-binding assay. It has no antiestrogenic, progestational, or androgenic activity.

Peak concentrations of misoprostol are reached one-half hour after dosing, with an elimination half-life of 1½ hours. The tissue-plasma ratio for misoprostol for the stomach is about 70.

Savarino and associates have shown that misoprostol, 400 μg twice a day, was inferior to ranitidine, 150 mg twice a day, in decreasing gastric acid output. Utilizing 24-hour pH probes, the area under the curve was no different for misoprostol and placebo, whereas the area under the curve for the ranitidine-treated group was significantly less than was seen in either the misoprostol or placebo group.

INDICATIONS

1. NSAID-induced injury. Misoprostol is the only drug approved for prophylaxis of NSAID-induced lesions of the stomach and duodenum. It has been shown to be effective in decreasing the incidence of both duodenal and gastric ulcers in patients receiv-

NSAIDs. The incidence of gastric ulcer with placebo; misoprostol, 100 μg 4 times a day; and misoprostol, 200 μg 4 times a day, was 21.7, 5.6, and 1.4 percent, respectively, in one study by Graham and associates, versus 7.7 and 1.9 percent in a second study. The corresponding numbers for duodenal ulcer were 6.5/1.1 percent and 4.6/0.6 percent.

Appropriate populations to receive prophylaxis include the elderly (over 65 years of age), women with prior peptic ulcer disease or complications, and those with frequent rapid recurrences, slow healing ulcer, or comorbid conditions. Limiting side effects include diarrhea, 39 percent at 200 μg versus 25 percent at 100 μg and abdominal cramping. Effects on NSAID-induced injury of the small bowel and colon are not well studied, although a recent report has shown improvement of anemia in patients with NSAID enteropathy treated with misoprostol.

2. Stress-related mucosal damage. Zenner and associates have shown that misoprostol, 200 μg every 4 hours, is as effective as antacids in prevention of bleeding in patients with stress ulcer. There is a high incidence (25%) of diarrhea.
3. Peptic ulcer disease. In both duodenal and gastric ulcers, cytoprotective doses of misoprostol do not accelerate healing. Acid-suppressing doses are needed and are equivalent to those of H_2-receptor antagonists (H_2-RA). Pain relief is inferior and the side effect profile of cramps and diarrhea is increased. Misoprostol has no effect on relapse and no benefit in subgroups (smokers).

   Gonvers and associates have shown that misoprostol, 800 μg/day, was comparable to ranitidine, 300 mg/day, in the treatment of benign gastric ulcer. In this endoscopically guided, randomized, double-blind study, 21 of 37 ranitidine-treated patients (56%) and 16 of 42 misoprostol-treated patients (38%) were healed after 4 weeks of therapy. After 8 weeks of therapy, 86 percent of the ranitidine group and 74 percent of the misoprostol group were healed. Interestingly, in smokers, ranitidine was superior to misoprostol, with a higher healing rate at 4 weeks (73% versus 20%). This fact counters the argument that misoprostol is cytoprotective at these antisecretory doses and can overcome the negative effects of cigarette smoking on ulcer healing.

   Misoprostol at a cytoprotective dose of 50 μg orally every 6 hours healed only 42 percent of ulcers in a study by Brand and associates. Given what is known about the pathogenesis of duodenal ulcers, that is, relative gastric acid hypersecretion, it is not surprising that an antisecretory dose of the drug, 200 μg 4 times a day, is required for healing of duodenal ulcer.

   In patients with refractory duodenal ulcer disease—defined by persistence of a duodenal ulcer crater after 4 weeks of conventional doses of cimetidine or ranitidine—misoprostol, 200 μg 4 times a day, was associated with healing in about 40 percent of cases, compared to a placebo healing rate of about 20 percent ($p = 0.02$). Comparison of misoprostol to continued or adjusted doses of H_2-receptor antagonists or to omeprazole was not performed.
4. Acute upper gastrointestinal bleeding. In a review of the humanitarian use of misoprostol for severe, life-threatening, upper gastrointestinal hemorrhage refractory to cimetidine, ranitidine, antacids, and sucralfate, Corboy and associates have shown a "favorable" clinical outcome in 52 of 83 treatment courses (63%). Analyzing the outcome by diagnosis, they found favorable out-

comes in 20 of 28 duodenal ulcer patients (71%), 24 of 41 gastric ulcer patients (58%), 14 of 23 reflux esophagitis patients (61%), and 39 of 63 hemorrhagic gastritis patients (62%).

5. Dosage and administration. Misoprostol is available as 100-μg and 200-μg tablets, given after meals to minimize side effects.
6. Gastroesophageal reflux disease. There is no role for misoprostol in the treatment of GERD.

SIDE EFFECTS

1. The most common side effects include diarrhea (13%) and abdominal pain (7%). These are usually self-limited and can be minimized by administration after meals or by dose reduction; however, discontinuation is required in 2 percent.
2. Misoprostol is an abortifacient. Precautions when using the drug in women with childbearing potential are warranted. The patient should be using contraception and have a negative serum pregnancy test within 2 weeks of initiation of therapy. The drug should be started on the second or third day of the next normal menstrual period. The patient should receive both oral and written documentation of the above effects. The use of informed consent should be considered.
3. Misoprostol does not interfere with the absorption or action of aspirin or NSAIDs.
4. No dose adjustment is required in patients with renal failure or in the elderly.

PEARLS AND PITFALLS

1. In low doses, misoprostol has only cytoprotective action (increased mucous and bicarbonate secretion), while at high doses the drug has gastric acid and pepsin antisecretory effects.
2. In patients with refractory duodenal ulcer disease, misoprostol has been shown to heal 40 percent of ulcers.
3. In a short-term study of the effect of aspirin on the gastric mucosa, misoprostol has been shown to be more efficacious than sucralfate in the prevention of gastric erosions.
4. Extragastric side effects of misoprostol are uncommon except for diarrhea (10% incidence). Cardiovascular, hematologic, and hormonal side effects are very rare.

Suggested Reading

SUCRALFATE

Aarimaa M, et al. Mucosal defense in ulcer disease. Scand J Gastroenterol 1987; 23:1.

A current review of actions of sucralfate and its use in peptic ulcer disease (symposium).

Brooks WS. Sucralfate: Non-ulcer uses. Am J Gastroenterol 1985; 80:206.

Reviews use of sucralfate in esophagitis, drug-induced gastritis, and bile reflux gastritis, as well as miscellaneous other uses.

Cannon LA, et al. Prophylaxis of upper gastrointestinal tract bleeding in mechanically ventilated patients. Arch Intern Med 1987; 147:2101.

Sucralfate is as efficacious as antacids or cimetidine.

Carling L, Kageri I, Borvall E. Sucralfate enema: Effective in inflammatory bowel disease. Endoscopy 1986; 18:115.
A preliminary report of a potential new use for sucralfate.

Driks MR, Craven DE, Bartolome MD. Nosocomial pneumonia in intubated patients given sucralfate as compared with antacid or histamine type-2 blockers. N Engl J Med 1987; 317:1376.
The sucralfate group suffered less nosocomial pneumonia in intubated patients.

Hameeteman W, et al. Sucralfate versus cimetidine in reflux esophagitis. J Clin Gastroenterol 1987; 9:390.
Sucralfate is equivalent to cimetidine in therapy of reflux esophagitis.

Lam SK, et al. Sucralfate overcomes adverse effects of cigarette smoking on duodenal ulcer healing and prolongs subsequent remission. Gastroenterology 1987; 92:1193.
Sucralfate is superior to cimetidine in duodenal ulcer in smokers.

Leung ACT, et al. Aluminum hydroxide versus sucralfate as a phosphate binder in uraemia. Br Med J 1983; 286:1379.
Sucralfate is as effective as Al(OH) in decreasing serum phosphate, but both cause elevated serum aluminum levels.

Marks IN, et al. Second International Sucralfate Symposium. Scand J Gastroenterol 1983; 18:1.
Symposium on sucralfate mechanism of action and use in ulcer healing and maintenance therapy.

Marks IN, Samloff IM. Third International Sucralfate Symposium. Am J Med 1985; 79:1.
Symposium on use of sucralfate in peptic ulcer disease, reflux gastritis, and stress bleeding.

Pera A, et al. Gastric ulceration localization by direct in vivo labelling of sucralfate. Radiology 1985; 156:783.
Early work on using sucralfate to image ulcers.

Prod'hom G, et al. Nosocomial pneumonia in mechanically ventilated patients receiving antacid, ranitidine or sucralfate as prophylaxis for stress ulcer. Ann Intern Med 1994; 120:653–662.

Sabesin SM, Lam SK. International Sucralfate Research Conference. Am J Med 1987; 83:1.
Symposium stressing cytoprotection activities of sucralfate and its use in reflux esophagitis, nonulcer dyspepsia, and drug-induced mucosal damage.

Samloff IM. Gastritis, duodenitis, and peptic ulcer disease. J Clin Gastroenterol 1983; 3:103.
Development, pharmacology, mechanism, and safety of sucralfate in peptic ulcer disease.

MISOPROSTOL

Agrawal NM, et al. Healing of benign gastric ulcer: A placebo-controlled comparison of two dosage regimens of misoprostol, a synthetic analog of prostaglandin E1. Dig Dis Sci 1985; 30:164S.
A multicenter, randomized, double-blind, parallel-group comparison of two doses of misoprostol and placebo showed 8-week healing rates in the intent-to-treat cohort of misoprostol, 100 μg 4 times a day (62%); misoprostol, 25 μg 4 times a day (50%); and placebo (45%). Diarrhea was experienced by 10 percent of patients.

Brand DL, et al. Misoprostol, a synthetic PGE1 analog, in the treatment of duodenal ulcers: A multicenter double-blind study. Dig Dis Sci 1985; 30:147S.

After 4 weeks of therapy, 77 percent of patients taking misoprostol, 200 μg 4 times a day; 43 percent of patients taking misoprostol, 50 μg 4 times a day; and 51 percent of patients taking placebo were healed.

Bright-Asare P, et al. Efficacy of misoprostol (twice-daily dosage) in acute healing of duodenal ulcer. A multicenter, double-blind controlled trial. Dig Dis Sci 1986; 31:63S.
Three hundred thirty patients with duodenal ulcer received either placebo; misoprostol, 200 μg; or misoprostol, 400 μg 2 times a day for 4 weeks. Healing rates at 4 weeks for a total of 280 evaluable patients were: misoprostol, 400 μg 2 times a day, 65 percent; misoprostol, 200 μg 2 times a day, 53 percent; and placebo, 42 percent. Interestingly, the percentage of nonsmokers who healed at 4 weeks was higher than that of smokers in both misoprostol treatment groups.

Corboy ED, et al. Humanitarian use of misoprostol in severe refractory upper gastrointestinal disease. Am J Med 1987; 83:49.
In humanitarian clinical trials, misoprostol was frequently associated with symptomatic relief and improvement in upper gastrointestinal hemorrhage from a variety of causes, including peptic ulcer disease, esophagitis, and hemorrhagic gastritis.

Dajani EZ. Overview of the mucosal protective effects of misoprostol in man. Prostaglandins 1987; 33:117.
Beneficial effects of misoprostol include reducing aspirin-induced gastric bleeding, aspirin-induced fecal occult blood loss, and ethanol-induced gastric damage. In the ethanol study, the mucosal protective effect was greater than that given by cimetidine.

Fich A, et al. Effect of misoprostol and cimetidine on gastric cell labelling index. Gastroenterology 1985; 89:57.
The number of antral and fundic labeled cells was significantly lower after misoprostol as compared to pretreatment, whereas the number of antral and fundic labeled cells was significantly higher after cimetidine than before therapy. The authors conclude that the decreased gastric cell turnover induced by misoprostol indicates that the trophic effect of prostanoids on gastric mucosa is not due to an increase in cellular kinetics.

Fich A, et al. Effect of misoprostol and cimetidine on gastric cell turnover. Dig Dis Sci 1985; 30:133S.
Misoprostol significantly decreased the number of labeled cells in antral and fundic gastric pits. Cimetidine significantly increased the number of labeled cells. The authors conclude that the decreased cell turnover induced by misoprostol does not appear to be a mechanism responsible for its mucosal protective and healing activity.

Gonvers JJ, et al. Gastric ulcer: A double-blind comparison of 800 micrograms misoprostol versus 300 milligrams ranitidine. Hepatogastroenterology 1987; 34:233.
In 79 gastric ulcer patients who received either ranitidine or misoprostol, the 8-week healing rates were 86 percent for ranitidine and 74 percent for misoprostol. In smokers, ranitidine was superior to misoprostol, leading to a higher 4-week healing rate (73% versus 20%). There is no evidence that misoprostol overcomes the negative effect of smoking on gastric ulcer healing.

Graham DY, et al. Prevention of NSAID induced gastric ulcers with misoprostol. Lancet 1988; 2:1277–1280.

Graham DY, et al. Duodenal and gastric ulcer prevention with miso prostol in arthritis patients taking NSAID's. Ann Intern Med 1993; 119:257–262.

Herting RL, Clay GA. Overview of clinical safety of misoprostol. Dig Dis Sci 1986; 31:47S.
Misoprostol has a dose-related antisecretory effect that lasts 3 to 5 hours. Use of the drug does not result in rebound ulcer recurrence in the first 12 months after therapy. There is a tropic effect on the pregnant uterus. No significant effects on blood pressure, pulse, platelets, the immune system, pulmonary vasculature, or endocrine system were found.

Lam SK, et al. Prostaglandin E1 (misoprostol) overcomes the adverse effect of chronic cigarette smoking on duodenal ulcer healing. Dig Dis Sci 1986; 31:68S.
A double-blind, randomized trial of 229 patients with duodenal ulcer receiving either placebo; misoprostol, 200 μg 4 times a day; or misoprostol, 300 μg 4 times a day, showing 4-week ulcer healing rates for the misoprostol groups of 61 and 71 percent, respectively. The time-healing curves for smokers and nonsmokers overlapped, implying that smoking is not a factor in the rate of healing of duodenal ulcers of patients treated with misoprostol.

Lanza F, et al. A blinded, endoscopic comparative study of misoprostol versus sucralfate and placebo in the prevention of aspirin-induced gastric and duodenal ulceration. Am J Gastroenterol 1988; 83:143.
Thirty healthy volunteers were randomized into three equal groups receiving either misoprostol, 200 μg; sucralfate, 1 gm; or placebo, co-administered with 650 mg aspirin, 4 times a day for 7 days. A clinically significant degree of protection of the gastric mucosa was achieved with misoprostol (10/10, 100%) compared to sucralfate (2/10, 20%) or placebo (0/10, 0%). In the duodenum, 9 of 10 subjects taking misoprostol showed no damage, compared to only 5 of 10 taking sucralfate and 3 of 10 taking placebo.

Londong W. Anti-ulcer drugs in antisecretory doses for "cytoprotection" in arthritic patients? Klin Wochenschr 1986; 64:32.
No study reviewed by the author of cytoprotective use of misoprostol, pirenzepine, or H_2-receptor antagonists corresponds to Roberts' definition of cytoprotection because all are being given in antisecretory doses in clinical trials.

Mazure PA. Comparative efficacy of misoprostol and cimetidine in the treatment of acute duodenal ulcer: Results of major studies. Am J Med 1987; 83:22.
Misoprostol has potent antisecretory activity in addition to a mucosal protective action at low doses. In one study reviewed by the author the rate of disappearance of mucosal erosions was significantly greater for misoprostol than for cimetidine.

McGuigan JE, Chang Y, Dajani EZ. Effect of misoprostol, an antiulcer prostaglandin, on serum gastrin in patients with duodenal ulcer. Dig Dis Sci 1986; 31:120S.
No significant difference in fasting serum gastrin or in integrated gastrin responses was found in duodenal ulcer patients after treatment with placebo or misoprostol, 50, 100, or 200 μg 4 times a day for 4 weeks.

Monk JP, Clissold SP. Misoprostol: A preliminary review of its pharmacodynamic and pharmacokinetic properties, and therapeutic efficacy in the treatment of peptic ulcer disease. Drugs 1987; 33:1.
In this large review, the author notes that duodenal ulcer pain

relief from misoprostol therapy is less than pain relief resulting from cimetidine therapy. There are no studies to date on the use of misoprostol for maintenance therapy after documented ulcer healing.

Morris AJ, et al. The effect of misoprostol on the anemia of NSAID enteropathy. Aliment Pharmacol Ther 1994; 8:343–346.

Newman RD, et al. Misoprostol in the treatment of duodenal ulcer refractory to H2-blocker therapy: A placebo-controlled multicenter, double-blind, randomized trial. Am J Med 1987; 83:27.

A study of 225 patients with duodenal ulcer persisting after at least 4 weeks of adequate, conventional therapy with cimetidine or ranitidine. Misoprostol, 200 μg 4 times a day, was significantly superior to placebo in healing duodenal ulcers (37% versus 20%, respectively).

Ogawa M, et al. Inhibitory effects of prostaglandin E1 on T-cell mediated cytotoxicity against isolated mouse liver cells. Gastroenterology 1988; 94:1024.

The cytotoxicity of mouse T cells for mouse hepatocytes in a model for chronic autoimmune liver disease was significantly decreased in vitro by the addition of prostaglandin E_1 at concentrations greater than 10 μM. This study suggests a possible new and exciting role for prostaglandin E_1 in the treatment and modulation of "lupoid" hepatitis.

Quimby QF, et al. Active smoking depresses prostaglandin synthesis in human gastric mucosa. Ann Intern Med 1986; 104:616.

The accumulation in culture medium of prostaglandin E_2 and F_{1a} from fundic, antral, and duodenal mucosa was significantly depressed by active smoking. This depression may help explain slower ulcer healing and predisposition to ulcer recurrence in smokers.

Rachmilewitz D, Chapman JW, Nicholson PA. A multicenter, international, controlled comparison of two dosage regimens of misoprostol with cimetidine in treatment of gastric ulcer in outpatients. Dig Dis Sci 1986; 31:75S.

On an intent-to-treat basis, ulcer healing rates for misoprostol, 50 and 200 μg 4 times a day, and cimetidine, 300 mg 4 times a day, were 39, 51, and 58 percent, respectively. Cimetidine, 300 mg 4 times a day, relieved global pain significantly better than did misoprostol, 200 μg, at 2 weeks but not at 4 weeks.

Roberts A. Cytoprotection by prostaglandins. Gastroenterology 1979; 77:761.

Hypothetical mechanisms by which cytoprotection occurs are (1) mucous secretion, (2) restoration of the sodium pump, (3) activation of the enzyme adenyl cyclase, (4) alteration of gastric blood flow, and (5) protection of the gastric mucosal barrier by decreased transmucosal fluxes of sodium, potassium, and hydrogen ion.

Savarino V, et al. Evaluation of antisecretory activity of misoprostol in duodenal ulcer patients using long-term intragastric pH monitoring. Dig Dis Sci 1988; 33:293.

Ranitidine, 150 mg twice a day, was significantly more effective in decreasing gastric acidity than was misoprostol, 400 μg twice a day.

Wildeman RA. Focus on misoprostol: Review of worldwide safety data. Clin Invest Med 1987; 10:243.

Misoprostol has been released for use in 12 countries and reports from over 100,000 patients reveal only mild adverse side effects.

including a 7 percent incidence of diarrhea and a 13 percent incidence of abdominal pain, only rarely (<1%) so severe as to warrant discontinuation of the drug.

Zenner MJ, et al. Misoprostol versus antacid titration for preventing stress ulcers in postoperative surgical ICU patients. Ann Surg 1989 210:590–595.

Bismuth

Margaret Andrea Wise and Michael M. Van Ness

For years bismuth preparations have been recognized to have antidiarrheal and antipeptic properties, but more recently selective antibacterial actions have been recognized. Although the literature contains few clinical trials and much is unknown about potential mechanisms of action, renewed interest in the potential benefits of bismuth compounds has sparked further research in its application to the problem of refractory and recurrent peptic ulcer disease and inflammatory bowel disease.

MECHANISM OF ACTION AND PHARMACOKINETICS

Bismuth salts have numerous and varied actions in the gastrointestinal tract.

All salts of bismuth are fluid-absorptive.

Bismuth oxide, precipitated from bismuth salts by acid present in the digestive system, forms a tenacious layer on the digestive mucosa. Bismuth oxide has particular affinity for granulation tissue (i.e., ulcer base).

Bismuth salts fix chloride ion with the formation of insoluble bismuth oxychloride.

Bismuth compounds inhibit the growth of enterococci, staphylococci, and *Pseudomonas* species.

Bismuth decreases gastric and intestinal motility, reduces intestinal spasticity, and prolongs intestinal transit time.

Bismuth ion increases directly the secretion of mucus in both the stomach and the intestine.

Bismuth ion attenuates the role of pepsin by chelation of the protein and protein precursor.

Although bismuth is not well absorbed systemically after an oral dose, the amount of salicylate absorbed when one 8-ounce bottle is taken over 3.5 hours (the recommended dose) is equivalent to taking eight 325-mg aspirin tablets.

The mean inhibitory concentration of colloidal bismuth subcitrate for *Helicobacter pylori* is less than 25 mg/liter.

INDICATIONS

Bismuth subsalicylate (Pepto-Bismol) is approved by the Food and Drug Administration for the symptomatic treatment of indigestion, nausea, and diarrhea.

Hamilton and associates treated 80 duodenal ulcer patients with either tripotassium dicitrato bismuthate (TDB), one tablet 4 times a day, or cimetidine, 200 mg 3 times a day with 400 mg at bedtime. After 6 weeks of therapy, ulcers were healed in 75 percent of both treatment groups. However, duodenal ulcers recurred in 43 percent of patients in the 12 months after treatment with TDB and in 78 percent of patients after cimetidine treatment.

Martin and associates have shown similar ulcer relapse rates to those reported by Hamilton's group. In a study of 55 patients treated with either TDB or cimetidine and followed for a year after documented healing of duodenal ulcers, 23 of 27 cimetidine-treated patients relapsed, compared to 11 of 28 placebo-treated patients. The mechanism of this difference is unknown, although it is known that ultrastructural abnormalities of the duodenal epithelial cell found in ulcer patients return to normal more often with TDB than with cimetidine.

Boyes and associates treated 20 gastric ulcer patients with either TDB, 5 ml 4 times a day, or placebo for 4 weeks. Endoscopic healing of the ulcer was documented in 9 of 10 patients receiving bismuth, compared to only 3 of 10 who received placebo.

Goldenberg and associates have shown that tripotassium dicitrato bismuthate (De-Nol) prevents stress-, alcohol-, and aspirin-induced mucosal damage.

The use of bismuth-containing compounds for the treatment of gastritis (nonimmune, type B) with or without concurrent or sequential antibiotic therapy is controversial. Although Bizzozero (1893), Salomon (1896), and Doenges (1939) described spiral bacteria in the stomachs of animals and humans in the late-nineteenth and early-twentieth centuries, it was not until the reports of Marshall and Warren in 1983 and 1984 that renewed interest developed in this area. An etiologic relationship between spiral-shaped organisms *(H. pylori)* and gastritis was suggested by their results. Likewise, Buck and associates found a strong correlation between the presence of gastritis (27 of 39, or 67%) and curved or spiral gram-negative bacilli. One proposed mechanism of injury caused by *H. pylori* is the rapid hydrolysis of urea at intercellular junctions with back-diffusion of hydrogen ion.

A 1994 National Institutes of Health (NIH) Consensus Conference concluded that *H. pylori* was an important etiologic factor in the development of peptic ulcer disease and should be sought and eradicated when found.

The treatment of ulcerative colitis with bismuth has been studied in the United Kingdom. Pullan and associates treated 63 patients who had distal ulcerative colitis with either 5-aminosalicyclic acid (5-ASA) or bismuth citrate. Clinical remission rates, sigmoidoscopic appearance of colonic mucosa, and histology were equally improved in the two treatment groups.

ADMINISTRATION

Each tablespoon (15 ml) of Pepto-Bismol liquid contains 262 mg bismuth subsalicylate. Each tablet of Pepto-Bismol contains 300 mg bismuth subsalicylate. The tablets have none of the ammoniacal taste or smell characteristic of the liquid.

For symptomatic treatment of indigestion, nausea, and diarrhea, the usual dosage is 2 tablespoons or two tablets every one-half to one hour, not to exceed eight doses per day. Children are dosed according to age: 3 to 6 years, 1 teaspoon or one-half tablet; 6 to 10 years, 2 teaspoons or one tablet; 10 to 14 years, 4 teaspoons or one-and-a-half tablets. Tablets may be chewed or allowed to dissolve in the mouth.

For prevention of traveler's diarrhea, bismuth subsalicylate (Pepto-Bismol), 60 ml (2 oz) 4 times a day, is indicated.

For treatment of duodenal ulcer disease, De-Nol (colloidal bismuth, tripotassium dicitrato bismuthate, TDB) in doses ranging from 15 to 60 ml/day (5–10 ml orally 3–6 times a day) can be justified based on the results of studies done by Shreeve, Salmon, and Hamilton.

For treatment of gastric ulcer disease, use of TDB, 5 ml diluted in 15 ml water, is justifiable based on the results of work by Boyes, Sutton, and Tanner.

The use of combination antibiotic and bismuth therapy is justifiable for the treatment of *H. pylori* gastritis. The highest published rates of clearance of *H. pylori* in patients with gastritis were put forward by Borsch and colleagues. They used bismuth subsalicylate, 600 mg 3 times a day; amoxicillin suspension, 500 mg 3 times a day; and metronidazole, 500-mg tablets 3 times a day, for 2 weeks and achieved 100 percent (23 of 23) clearance after 2 weeks of therapy, with 90 percent remaining clear after an additional 2 weeks of observation.

Compliance with this type of prolonged therapy has led others to develop alternative regimens. Labenz and associates advocate use of omeprazole, 20 mg twice a day, with amoxicillin suspension, 500 mg 4 times a day, both for 2 weeks. This regimen will eradicate *H. pylori* in 80 percent of patients. Tucci and colleagues treat for one day with omeprazole, 40 mg; amoxicillin suspension, 2 gm 4 times; metronidazole, 500 mg 4 times; and Pepto-Bismol tablets, two tablets 4 times. *Helicobacter pylori* eradicate rates of 70 to 75 percent are reported.

SIDE EFFECTS

Side effects of bismuth subsalicylate include blackening of the stool; salicylate-induced tinnitus from rapid ingestion, prolonged use, or concurrent aspirin use; and bleeding due to salicylate-induced platelet inhibition.

There are no known drug interactions or inhibition of drug absorption from bismuth compounds. As a practical matter, it is prudent to avoid concurrent drug and bismuth administration.

There are acute or chronic toxic effects of high-dose bismuth salts. Although there is no established LD-50 for bismuth subsalicylate, a retrospective analysis of toxicity of oral bismuth salts showed a syndrome of reversible bismuth encephalopathy, characterized by confusion, dysarthria, myoclonus, and coma.

Long-term use of the bismuth congeners, bismuth subnitrate, and bismuth subgallate is associated with neurotoxicity.

PEARLS AND PITFALLS

1. Bismuth is considered to act at a pH of 1 to 6, with optimum pH of 4 or less, requiring dosing at least an hour before or after meals.
2. Given the systemic absorption of aspirin with bismuth subsalicylate (Pepto-Bismol), the use of Pepto-Bismol in children 12 years of age or younger for viral syndromes such as influenza and varicella may risk the development of Reye's syndrome.

Suggested Reading

Borsch G, Mai U, Opferkuch W. Oral triple therapy may effectively eradicate *Campylobacter pylori* in man: A pilot study (abstr). Gastroenterology 1988; 94:A44.

An aggressive and intensive antibiotic regimen cleared C. pylori *from 100 percent of patients as judged by CLOtest and culture.*

Boyes BE, et al. Treatment of gastric ulceration with a bismuth preparation. Postgrad Med J 1975; 51(S5):29–33.

Twenty patients with gastric ulcer were selected to receive either placebo or a bismuth preparation (TDB). The mean percentage reduction in the cross-sectional area of the ulcer by radiographic criteria was 91 percent in the TDB treatment group and 36 percent in the control group. Ninety percent of the ulcers were healed at endoscopy, compared to only 30 percent healing in the control group.

Buck GE, et al. Relation of *Campylobacter pylori* to gastritis and peptic ulcer. J Infect Dis 1986; 153:664–669.

Of 39 biopsies of the gastric mucosa of patients with gastritis, 27 showed spiral gram-negative bacilli compatible with C. pylori.

Dooley CP, Cohen H. The clinical significance of *Campylobacter pylori.* Ann Intern Med 1988; 108:70–79.

Although eradication of the organism is associated with healing of gastritis and a lower relapse rate in duodenal ulcer disease, the authors conclude that a role for the organism in other upper gastrointestinal diseases is unproven.

Goldenberg MM, et al. Protective effect of Pepto-Bismol liquid on the gastric mucosa of rats. Gastroenterology 1975; 69:636.

Bismuth subsalicylate may prove useful, like sucralfate and H_2-receptor antagonists, in the prevention of stress-, alcohol-, and aspirin-induced gastric mucosal damage.

Hamilton I, et al. Healing and recurrence of duodenal ulcer after treatment with tripotassium dicitrato bismuthate (TDB) tablets or cimetidine. Gut 1986; 27:106–110.

Eighty patients with duodenal ulcer were randomized to receive either TDB or cimetidine. Healing occurred in 78 and 74 percent of the two treatment groups. The percentage of recurrences in the 12 months after treatment in the patient groups was 78 percent in the cimetidine group but only 43 percent in the bismuth group.

Hornick RB. Peptic ulcer disease: A bacterial infection? N Engl J Med 1987; 316:1598–1599.

The prospects in this area of research are exciting, intriguing, and promising, but unproven.

Labenz J, et al. Amoxicillin plus omeprazole versus triple therapy for eradication of *Helicobacter pylori* in duodenal ulcer disease. Gut 1993; 34: 1167–1170.

Group 1 (amoxicillin, 2 gm/day plus omeprazole, 40 mg/day) patients had better pain relief, ulcer healing, and medication tolerance than group 2 (bismuth subsalicylate, 1800 mg/day, plus metronidazole, 1200 mg/day, plus tetracycline, 1500 mg/day, plus ranitidine, 300 mg at bedtime) patients.

Marshall BJ, Warren JR. Unidentified curved bacilli in the stomach of patients with gastritis and peptic ulceration. *Lancet* 1984; 2: 1311–1314.

An association between the presence of spiral-shaped bacilli and chronic gastritis, duodenal ulcer, or gastric ulcer is postulated by the author.

Martin DF, et al. Difference in relapse rates of duodenal ulcer after healing with cimetidine or tripotassium dicitrato bismuthate. *Lancet* 1981; 1:7–10.

Although no difference was noted in ulcer healing rates after 1 and 2 months of therapy between cimetidine and TDB, the relapse rate was higher in the cimetidine-treated group (23 of 27 patients) compared to the bismuth group (11 of 28).

Pullan RD, et al. Comparison of bismuth citrate and 5-aminosalicylic acid enemas in distal ulcerative colitis: A controlled trial. Gut 1993; 34:676–679.

Bismuth citrate enemas give as good a response in patients with distal ulcerative colitis as 5-ASA.

Salmon PR, et al. Evaluation of colloidal bismuth (De-Nol) in the treatment of duodenal ulcer employing endoscopic selection and follow-up. Gut 1974; 15:189–193.

A greater number of patients (9 of 10) treated with colloidal bismuth showed endoscopic and symptomatic improvement than those receiving placebo (6 of 10).

Shreeve DR. A double-blind study of tripotassium dicitrato bismuthate in duodenal ulcer. Postgrad Med J 1975; 51(S5), 33–36.

A double-blind study of duodenal ulcer patients treated with either TDB or placebo. The healing rate after 4 weeks of therapy by endoscopy was 14 of 19 in the TDB group and 4 of 19 ($p < 0.005$) in the placebo group.

Shreeve DR, Klass HJ, Jones PE. Comparison of cimetidine and tripotassium dicitrato bismuthate in healing and relapse of duodenal ulcers. Digestion 1983; 28:96–101.

In a comparison of healing and relapse rates of cimetidine-treated and bismuth-treated patients with duodenal ulcers, the rate of healing at 4 weeks was 75 percent in the bismuth-treated patients and 54 percent in the cimetidine-treated group. The relapse rate at 1 year was 47 percent for the bismuth-treated patients and 60 percent for the cimetidine group.

Simko V, Michael S. Retrospective analysis of toxicity of oral bismuth (BIS) medications. Gastroenterology 1994; 106:A 181.

A serum bismuth concentration of 50 to 100 μg/liter can cause bismuth toxicity.

Sutton DR. Gastric ulcer healing with tripotassium dicitrato bismuthate and subsequent relapse. Gut 1982; 23:621–624.

Gastric ulcer healing occurred in 18 of the 25 (72%) patients given TDB and in 9 (36%) of the patients given placebo. During a follow-up period of 44 months, relapse occurred in 13 of 29 (45%) reevaluated patients.

Tanner AR, et al. Efficacy of cimetidine and tripotassium dicitrato bismuthate (De-Nol) in chronic gastric ulceration: A comparative study. Med J Austr 1979; 1:1–2.

Of 57 patients with gastric ulcer evaluated endoscopically after 6 weeks of therapy, 20 of 30 bismuth-treated patients (67%) were healed, compared to 17 of 27 patients (63%) treated with cimetidine.

Tucci A, et al. One-day therapy for treatment of *Helicobacter pylori* infection. Dig Dis Sci 1993; 38:1670–1673.

One-day, high-dose combination therapy (amoxicillin, 2 gm orally 4 times a day; metronidazole, 500 mg orally 4 times a day; bismuth subcitrate, 240 mg orally 4 times a day, in combination with omeprazole, 40 mg orally) eradicated H. pylori *in 23 of 32 patients (72%).*

Wilson TR. The pharmacology of tripotassium dicitrato bismuthate (TDB). Postgrad Med J 1975; 51:18–21.

TDB is a colloidal bismuth preparation that is free from toxicity and capable of facilitating the healing of gastric ulcers in both humans and experimental animals.

Metoclopramide and Erythromycin

J. Thomas Dorsey III

Metoclopramide

Since its initial approval by the Food and Drug Administration (FDA) in 1981 for diabetic gastroparesis, the prokinetic agent metoclopramide has been applied to a variety of clinical situations, leading to broader usage. This drug is a prototype of a class of medications, including cisapride and dazopride, that is likely to extend dramatically the ability of the clinician to treat patients with altered gastrointestinal motility.

MECHANISM OF ACTION

Developed in the early 1960s, metoclopramide (2-methoxy-5-chloroprocainamide) is a procainamide derivative with clinically insignificant anesthetic and antidysrhythmic effects. Although the exact mechanism of action is not understood, extensive research over the last 20 years suggests that it is a potent dopamine-receptor antagonist with cholinomimetic properties.

Stimulation of dopamine receptors in the gastrointestinal tract results in gastric relaxation and decreased forward passage of a tracer-labeled food bolus from the stomach into the proximal small bowel. This effect is vagally mediated and is abolished by vagotomy. Pharmacologic inhibition of this effect occurs with metoclopramide and can be counterantagonized by administration of levodopa. The prokinetic effect of metoclopramide is also explained by an apparent cholinomimetic effect on the gastrointestinal tract thought to be secondary to enhanced acetylcholine release, resulting in increased smooth-muscle contraction. Unlike other cholinomimetic agents such as bethanecol, metoclopramide has not been shown to increase acid secretion or gastrin release.

Metoclopramide coordinates forward propulsion of esophagogastric contents in an effective manner. Use of this drug in normal human volunteers results in increased lower esophageal sphincter pressure, increased amplitude and duration of esophageal peristalsis, increased antral peristaltic contractions, relaxation of the pyloric sphincter, and decreased proximal small bowel transit time. Although little physiologic response in the distal small bowel or colon was documented in the early research, subsequent investigators have reported an increase in the amplitude of colonic contractions and a decrease in the transit time of the colon in both normal volunteers and patients with severe diabetic enteropathy.

Metoclopramide is rapidly absorbed into the gastrointestinal tract, with peak serum levels appearing in 1 hour. The normal half-life ranges from 3 to 6 hours and is increased to as long as 24 hours in patients with renal impairment due to almost complete renal excretion. Because of weak protein binding, drug removal can be effectively achieved by dialysis.

INDICATIONS

Current indications for metoclopramide include treatment of diabetic gastroparesis and gastroesophageal reflux, reduction of cancer chemotherapy–associated emesis, and the facilitation of small-bowel intubation and radiographic examination of the stomach and small bowel. In addition, a number of as yet unapproved uses have been identified. The use of metoclopramide to reduce the risk of aspiration of gastric contents in the patient facing emergent surgery and to treat patients with the gastrointestinal complications of scleroderma, dystrophica myotonica, and adynamic or chemotherapy-induced ileus is justified by reports in the medical literature.

Diabetic Gastroparesis

Diabetic gastroparesis is a condition characterized by decreased gastric emptying and generalized gastric atony. The diagnosis is suspected on clinical grounds in patients with long-standing diabetes who have early satiety, nausea, vomiting, and weight loss, but it is confirmed by radiographic or scintigraphic examination. Ricci and associates described significantly increased gastric emptying in these patients and a marked reduction of symptoms following oral administration of metoclopramide. A subsequent case report suggests responsiveness to a rectal suppository form in a patient intolerant of oral dosages. The long-term efficacy and symptomatic benefit of metoclopramide in this setting have not been documented completely.

Gastroesophageal Reflux

Gastroesophageal reflux results from decreased lower esophageal sphincter pressure, regurgitation of acid from the stomach to the esophagus, and inadequate clearance of regurgitated material. In a number of clinical trials, the prokinetic effects of metoclopramide have resulted in diminution of symptoms compared with placebo, but have not correlated with a decreased incidence of esophagitis on endoscopic follow-up examination.

Chemotherapy-Induced Emesis

The etiology of emesis in the setting of cancer treatment is multifactorial. Stimulation of the chemoreceptor trigger zone, apomorphine (a dopamine agonist) release, and delayed gastric emptying have all been observed following the administration of chemotherapeutic agents. Cisplatin, one of the most emetogenic agents, has been shown to disrupt normal smooth muscle pacemaker potentials in the stomachs of dogs and to result in gastrointestinal retroperistalsis. Metoclopramide, in this model, corrects such dysmotility by peripherally enhancing forward motility and centrally inhibiting the dopamine agonist effect at the chemoreceptor trigger zone activity.

Small Bowel Radiographic Examination

Metoclopramide has long been recognized to decrease the transit time of barium- or tracer-labeled meals through the small bowel. When studied in a double-blinded fashion with other prokinetic agents such as domperidone, metoclopramide shortened the radiographic examination to a greater extent, caused no difference in technical quality of the study compared with controls, and resulted [illegible]ess radiation exposure to the patient.

Nonapproved Indications

The rationale for application of metoclopramide to other clinical problems or diseases is based on the ability to enhance esophagogastric motility. A beneficial effect in patients with esophageal dysmotility and delayed gastric emptying due to both progressive systemic sclerosis or dystrophica myotonica has been reported and appears to address a primary pathophysiologic defect. In addition, metoclopramide has reported efficacy in reducing the risk of aspiration in patients in whom reflux of gastric contents may be more common, such as the chronically debilitated nursing home occupant or the patient in need of emergent surgery. The future role for this and similar prokinetic agents requires further study to determine long-term benefit, the limitations of side effects, and the extent of drug-drug interactions.

CONTRAINDICATIONS

Metoclopramide should not be used in patients with suspected or known mechanical intestinal obstruction, gastrointestinal perforation, or known sensitivity or intolerance, or in known epileptic patients or those likely to be treated with drugs that cause extrapyramidal side effects. The presence of pheochromocytoma is believed to be an absolute contraindication since metoclopramide can result in increased catecholamine release from the tumor. If this situation should occur, the appropriate treatment of the resultant hypertension is an alpha-receptor blocking agent such as phentolamine. Because of inadequate controlled studies, the use of metoclopramide is relatively contraindicated in the pregnant patient (see Table 5-1).

ADMINISTRATION

Metoclopramide is dispensed in 10-mg tablets. It is also available in syrup (5 mg/ml) and injectable forms (5 mg/ml). Treatment for gastroesophageal reflux is 10 to 15 mg 4 times a day 30 minutes before meals, and at bedtime as needed, for control of symptoms. Diabetic gastroparesis is usually treated with 10 mg before meals but may require parenteral administration depending on the severity of symptoms. Once gastric emptying improves, conversion to an oral regimen is usually possible. Chronic self-administered subcutaneous injection for gastroparesis has been described at a dosage of 5 to 10 mg SQ every 4 to 6 hours.

Significant relief of symptoms may be experienced early in the course of therapy and continue to improve for up to 3 weeks. The dosage for small bowel intubation and radiographic examination is 10 mg intravenously. To prevent chemotherapy-induced emesis, a loading dose of 1 to 2 mg/kg body weight is used, with 0.5 to 1.0 mg/kg given every 3 to 4 hours subsequently while the patient is receiving chemotherapy.

PEARLS AND PITFALLS

1. Because metoclopramide decreases gastric emptying time as well as gastrointestinal transit time, insulin-dependent diabetic patients may need to increase the amount of regular insulin and decrease the amount of NPH; or other long-acting insulin preparations used. When metoclopramide is begun, close attention must be given to blood glucose levels.
2. Drowsiness and central nervous system depression seen with metoclopramide are substantially increased in patients who con(

Table 5-1. Metoclopramide and erythromycin: Pregnancy and breast-feeding

Agent	FDA Pregnancy Category	Risk vs Benefit (by trimester)			Breast-feeding Category
		1st	2nd	3rd	
Erythromycin	C	B > R	B > R	B > R	IV
Metoclopramide	B1	?	?	?	IV

Food and Drug Administration (FDA) pregnancy categories:
A = Well-controlled studies fail to demonstrate risk to the fetus.
B1 = Animal studies fail to demonstrate risk to the fetus but no human studies are available.
B2 = Animal studies show some risk to the fetus but this is not confirmed in human studies.
C1 = Animal studies show risk to the fetus but no human studies are available.
C2 = Animal and human studies are unavailable.
D = Drugs associated with birth defects but with potential benefits that may outweigh known risks.
X = Drugs associated with birth defects and with potential risk that clearly outweighs potential benefit.
Risk vs benefit: R >> B = Proven or potential risk outweighs potential benefits.
B > R = Potential benefits outweigh potential risks.
R >> B? = Risks may be outweighed by benefits in some circumstances.
? = Risk-to-benefit ratio is unknown.

Breast-feeding categories:
I = Drug does not enter breast milk.
II = Drug enters breast milk but is not known to be harmful in therapeutic doses.
IIIA = Drug may or may not enter breast milk but no adverse effects are expected.
IIIB = Drug may or may not enter breast milk but drug is systemically absorbed.
IV = Drug enters breast milk and poses a potential risk to the neonate.

tantly receive dopamine antagonists such as phenothiazines.
3. Dystonic reactions associated with metoclopramide should be treated immediately with 50 mg diphenhydramine intravenously.

The efficacy of metoclopramide versus placebo antacid regimens was studied in a double-blind fashion. Metoclopramide was significantly more effective than placebo and antacid in improving symptoms and increasing gastric emptying, which was delayed in reflux patients, but did not result in an increased rate of healing in patients with esophagitis on endoscopy.

Erythromycin

Erythromycin, a product of *Streptomyces erythreus,* was introduced in 1952 by McGuire and has found a role as a broad-spectrum antimicrobial agent. Although scattered reports of its effects on gut motility appeared as early as 1960, intensive investigation did not occur until 1984. The first human study demonstrating clinical benefit was performed in 1989.

Erythromycin is a macrolide antibiotic. The chemical structure consists of a 14-member lactone ring to which are attached two deoxysugars. Specifically, the ring is composed of 13 carbon atoms and 1 oxygen atom. At C3 is attached clandinose and, at C5, decosamine with a dimethylamino group. Ring size seems to be an important determinant of prokinetic activity, as 16-membered rings have no activity whereas other 14-member ring compounds without antibiotic effect do.

PHARMACOLOGY

Erythromycin base is inactivated by gastric acid and is therefore administered as an ester or enterically coated. Food decreases absorption except with the estolate ester. Two to 5 percent of an oral dose is excreted unchanged in the urine. The drug is 70 percent protein bound. Cleared by the liver, a fraction undergoes demethylation and the remainder is excreted in bile in an active form. Plasma half-life is 1.4 hours. The drug is not removed by peritoneal fluid or hemodialysis. It readily diffuses into the extracellular fluid, with the exception of cerebrospinal fluid. It traverses the placenta, and fetal plasma concentrations are 5 to 20 percent those of maternal plasma.

MECHANISM OF ACTION

Erythromycin was thought initially to act by increasing concentrations of motilin, a 22–amino acid peptide discovered in 1967 and found in enterochromaffin cells of the duodenal mucosa. Motilin receptors are found in the antrum and proximal small bowel. Subsequently, erythromycin was found to bind directly to motilin receptors with agonist effect. However, another mechanism of action, not dictated by motilin receptors, has been proposed to explain additional effects.

INDICATIONS

Gastroparesis

In a double-blind, placco-controlled cross-over trial, Janssens and associates demonstrated that erythromycin normalized both solid and liquid emptying in patients with diabetic gastroparesis. Richards and colleagues confirmed the efficacy of parenteral and oral erythromycin in both diabetic and idiopathic gastroparesis. However, in this trial, 29 percent of patients discontinued the drug.

Postoperative Uses

Yeo and associates demonstrated that parenteral erythromycin decreased the incidence of postoperative delayed gastric emptying in a controlled trial of patients undergoing Whipple procedures. Bonacini and colleagues, in a controlled trial, failed to show benefit.

Uncontrolled studies have proposed efficacy in gastroparesis associated with vagotomy, scleroderma, and chemotherapy, as well as benefit in Roux en Y syndrome, gastroesophageal reflux disease (GERD), anorexia nervosa, and chronic idiopathic intestinal pseudo-obstruction. It also has been shown to increase gallbladder contraction and emptying.

SIDE EFFECTS

Erythromycin is well known for its gastrointestinal side effects, including nausea, vomiting, abdominal pain, and diarrhea. Parenteral administration can lead to phlebitis.

There have been reports linking erythromycin to hypertrophic pyloric stenosis, raising questions about its use in children. Its use in pregnant and breast-feeding patients is listed in Table 5-1.

With more widespread use, the possibility exists that resistant bacterial strains may be induced.

DOSAGE AND ADMINISTRATION

Oral dosages of 250 mg orally 3 times a day to 500 mg orally 4 times a day have been used. Intramuscular injection is not given because of severe pain at the injection site. Intravenous erythromycin lactobionate at a dose of 200 mg every 6 hours was used in the trial by Yeo and associates. There is also a report of administration via peritoneal dialysis catheter of 100 mg erythromycin/2 liters dialysate. Pediatric dosages range from 30 to 50 mg/kg/day given 4 times a day.

PEARLS AND PITFALLS

1. Erythromycin has shown prokinetic effects especially in the setting of diabetic gastroparesis. Use in other settings shows promise, but is unproven.
2. Parenteral dosage seems more effective than oral use. The long-term efficacy has not been well documented. Side effects can limit its use.
3. Currently, it is best utilized when other prokinetics are not tolerated or are ineffective.

Suggested Reading

METOCLOPRAMIDE

Akwari OE. The gastrointestinal tract in chemotherapy induced emesis: A final common pathway. Drugs 1983; 25:18–34. *Metoclopramide is effective in preventing emesis by direct gastrointestinal as well as central effects.*

Alphin RS, et al. Antagonism of cisplatin induced emesis by metoclopramide and dazopride through enhancement of gastric motility. Dig Dis Sci 1986; 31:524–529.

The authors further investigate the antiemetic effects of metoclopramide and dazopride by studying the central and peripheral sites of action in nonhuman subjects treated with cisplatin. They conclude that metoclopramide acts predominantly by enhancing gastrointestinal motility and inhibiting apomorphine-induced emesis, but has little antagonistic effect at central dopamine receptors (e.g., at the chemoreceptor trigger zone) in clinically used doses.

Battle WM, et al. Colonic dysfunction in diabetes mellitus. Gastroenterology 1980; 79:1217–1221.

The authors investigate the myoelectrical and motility abnormalities seen in the colons of diabetic patients with constipation. They conclude that these patients have evidence of an autonomic enteropathy with absent postprandial gastrocolonic response that responds to the use of neostigmine and metoclopramide.

Beam L, Bianchi C, Crema C. Effects of metoclopramide on isolated colon: 1. Peripheral sensitization to acetylcholine. Eur J Pharmacol 1970; 12:320–331.

The authors report the augmentation of acetylcholine release from postganglionic nerve terminals and sensitization of muscarinic receptors in gastrointestinal smooth muscle in isolated human smooth muscle and guinea pig colon. This study expands the understanding of metoclopramide as an unconventional cholinergic drug that relies on intrinsic stores of acetylcholine.

Gipson SL, et al. Pharmacologic reduction of the risk of aspiration. South Med J 1986; 79:1356–1358.

Forty women undergoing gynecologic surgery received metoclopramide, cimetidine, a combination of the two, or no treatment at all. A resultant decrease in gastric volume and increase in gastric pH are documented and support the use of this drug in reducing the risk of gastric content aspiration in the preoperative patient.

Horowitz M, et al. Gastric and esophageal emptying in dystrophica myotonica: Effect of metoclopramide. Gastroenterology 1987; 92: 570–577.

Dystrophica myotonica is associated for this reason with abnormal esophageal and gastric emptying. This paper documents the prokinetic effects of metoclopramide in these patients and supports its use in treating gastroparesis.

Johnson DA, et al. Metoclopramide response in patients with progressive systemic sclerosis: Effects on esophageal and gastric motility abnormalities. Arch Intern Med 1987; 147:1597–1601.

Metoclopramide improved lower esophageal pressure and gastric emptying in 12 patients with progressive systemic sclerosis.

McCallum RW. Review of the current status of prokinetic agents in gastroenterology. Am J Gastroenterol 1985; 80:1008–1016.

This review article details the evolution of prokinetic agents in gastroenterology, including metoclopramide and its congeners dazopride and cisapride.

Morewood DJW, Whitehouse GH. A comparison of three methods for performing barium follow through studies of the small intestine. Br J Radiol 1986; 59:971–993.

Gastric emptying time is decreased in patients pretreated with either domperidone or metoclopramide before barium examination of the stomach or small bowel.

Ricci DA, et al. Effect of metoclopramide in diabetic gastroparesis. J Clin Gastroenterol 1985; 7:25–32.
Gastric emptying time by scintigraphic study showed a significant improvement in diabetic patients receiving metoclopramide compared with those receiving placebo.

Trapnell BC, et al. Metoclopramide suppositories in the treatment of diabetic gastroparesis. Arch Intern Med 1986; 146:2278–2279.
Diabetic patients with symptoms of severe gastroparesis who are intolerant of oral dosages of metoclopramide may respond to a rectal route of administration.

Winnan J, et al. Double blind trials of metoclopramide versus placebo antacid in symptomatic gastroesophageal reflux. Gastroenterology 1980; 78:1292.
The efficacy of metoclopramide versus placebo-antacid regimens was studied in a double-blind fashion. Metoclopramide was significantly more effective than placebo and antacid in improving symptoms and increasing gastric emptying, which was delayed in patients with reflux, but did not result in an increased rate of healing in patients with esophagitis on endoscopy.

ERYTHROMYCIN

Bonacini M, et al. Effect of intravenous erythromycin on postoperative ileus. Am J Gastroenterol 1993; 88:208.
No benefit seen.

Gwee KA, Read NW. Rolling review: Disorders of gastrointestinal motility; therapeutic potentials and limitations. Aliment Pharmacol Ther 1994; 8:105–118.
An up-to-date review.

Janssens J, et al. Improvement of gastric emptying in diabetic gastroparesis by erythromycin. N Engl J Med 1990; 332:1028–1031.
Erythromycin normalized both solid and liquid gastric emptying.

Peeters TL. Erythromycin and other macrolides as prokinetic agents. Gastroenterology 1993; 105:1886–1889.
Best reserved as second-time agents.

Richards RD, et al. The treatment of idiopathic and diabetic gastroparesis with acute intravenous and chronic oral erythromycin. Am J Gastroenterol 1993; 88:203.
Compliance less than ideal.

Weber FH, Richards RD, McCallum Rw. Erythromycin: A motilin agonist and gastrointestinal prokinetic agent. Am J Gastroenterol 1993; 88:485–490.
Mechanism of action explored.

Yeo CJ, et al. Erythromycin accelerates gastric emptying after pancreaticoduodenectomy. Ann Surg 1993; 218:229–238.
Postoperative gastric emptying improved.

Omeprazole

Michael Carboni and Michael M. Van Ness

Omeprazole is the first member of a new class of potent gastric acid inhibitors for the treatment of peptic ulcer disease, Zollinger-Ellison syndrome, and erosive reflux esophagitis. Early results indicate that omeprazole is more potent, more convenient, more expensive, and as safe as traditional H_2-receptor antagonists.

MECHANISM OF ACTION, PHARMACODYNAMICS, AND PHARMACOKINETICS

Omeprazole is a substituted benzimidazole. It inhibits gastric acid secretion by noncompetitive inhibition of the H+/K+ adenosine triphosphatase (ATPase) proton pump. This proton pump is the final step in gastric acid secretion and lies within the secretory membrane of parietal cells. Omeprazole is not only a powerful inhibitor of basal acid output but, unlike the H_2-receptor antagonists, also inhibits stimulated gastric acid output.

Omeprazole is a lipid-soluble weak base. It is acid labile, necessitating formulation as enteric-coated granules in order to reach the small intestine. As omeprazole is absorbed and gastric acid secretion is inhibited, intragastric pH rises, increasing its absorption and bioavailability.

The plasma half-life of omeprazole is about 50 minutes. Because omeprazole accumulates in parietal cells, its effective half-life is considerably longer (18–24 hours). Omeprazole's inhibition of acid secretion is dose-dependent and increases over time because of increasing absorption. A single dose reaches peak inhibitory effect in 2 to 4 hours, while repeated daily doses require 3 to 5 days for maximum acid inhibition. With repeated daily doses, inhibition of acid output remains for days even with cessation of drug therapy. Eventually complete recovery of acid output occurs.

Twenty-four–hour intragastric acidity studies demonstrate that oral omeprazole in doses of 20 to 80 mg inhibits gastric acid secretion by 50 to 100 percent within hours of drug ingestion. Repeated dosing with 20 mg gradually increases the level of inhibition to nearly 100 percent. With a single morning dose, nocturnal secretion is decreased by 50 percent, as is meal-stimulated and pentagastrin-stimulated acid secretion. Intravenous dosing is under investigation and is equally effective in its inhibition of gastric output.

Other physiologic effects include elevation of serum gastrin. Hypergastrinemia from endogenous production, as seen in Zollinger-Ellison syndrome, is not aggravated by omeprazole therapy. Although Freston has chosen a two- to fourfold increase in plasma gastrin levels in patients treated for one year, it is impractical and unnecessary to screen all patients for this change, which is of little, if any, clinical significance. Omeprazole does not affect gastric emptying or secretion of intrinsic factor. It does appear to increase intragastric concentrations of bile acid, the significance of which is unknown.

INDICATIONS

Zollinger-Ellison Syndrome

A key indication for omeprazole therapy is Zollinger-Ellison syndrome (ZES). Patients with Zollinger-Ellison syndrome may be resistant to treatment with high doses of H_2-receptor antagonists. Because of its beneficial clinical effects and pronounced, long-lasting reduction in gastric acid secretion, omeprazole is the drug of choice for treatment of ZES patients.

Since omeprazole is such a potent gastric acid inhibitor, anticholinergic therapy is not needed, as it may be with H_2-receptor antagonists. No irreversible adverse effects in humans have been noted, even with long-term therapy of Zollinger-Ellison patients.

Recommended doses for the treatment of ZES are not fixed but are titrated to keep basal acid output less than 10 mEq/hr. Dosages range from 20 to 80 mg/day.

Erosive Reflux Esophagitis

Omeprazole has been shown to be better than H_2-receptor antagonists in a study of eight patients with erosive esophagitis. Seven of these patients were healed with 30 mg/day omeprazole for 4 weeks. The remaining patient had a 95 percent reduction in the area of erosion.

In a study by Bell and Hunt, omeprazole healed 67 to 92 percent of patients, even those with grade IV esophagitis.

Gastric Ulcer Disease

Omeprazole (20 mg/day) has been found to be equal in potency and efficacy to daily ranitidine therapy (150 mg twice a day). Healing rates are not affected by smoking.

Duodenal Ulcer Disease

With once-daily dosing, it is possible to almost completely inhibit 24-hour intragastric acidity in most patients with duodenal ulcer. Direct comparative studies indicate that omeprazole is superior to H_2-receptor antagonists in short-term treatment of duodenal ulcers. The majority of patients heal within 2 to 4 weeks with faster and more pronounced pain relief on omeprazole. Optimum recommended therapy is 20 to 30 mg for 4 weeks. Omeprazole (40 mg) in combination with amoxicillin suspension (2 gm 4 times a day), metronidazole (500 mg 4 times a day), and bismuth subcitrate (240 mg 4 times a day) for one day is well tolerated and associated with *Helicobacter pylori* eradication in 75 percent of patients. Ulcers diagnosed concurrently would require standard therapy and follow-up.

Intravenous therapy is also available if immediate reductions in acidity are needed. A single bolus injection of 10 mg omeprazole is comparable to the inhibition provided by 20 mg of a single oral dose. Intravenous injections reach peak inhibitory effects within 2 hours. Brunner and Chang have shown that intravenous omeprazole seems to be associated with decreased continued bleeding in patients with peptic ulcers—even those in whom ranitidine therapy has failed.

Healing rates of duodenal ulcers treated with omeprazole are impaired by smoking. Sixty percent of the smokers studied endoscopically healed in 6 to 8 weeks.

The recurrence rate of duodenal ulcers treated with omeprazole is approximately 50 percent within 1 year, comparable to that seen with H_2-receptor antagonists.

Table 6-1. Omeprazole: Pregnancy and breast-feeding

Agent	FDA Pregnancy Category	Risk vs Benefit (by trimester)			Breast-feeding Category
		1st	2nd	3rd	
Omeprazole	B1	?	?	?	IV

Food and Drug Administration (FDA) pregnancy categories:
A = Well-controlled studies fail to demonstrate risk to the fetus.
B1 = Animal studies fail to demonstrate risk to the fetus but no human studies are available.
B2 = Animal studies show some risk to the fetus but this is not confirmed in human studies.
C1 = Animal studies show risk to the fetus but no human studies are available.
C2 = Animal and human studies are unavailable.
D = Drugs associated with birth defects but with potential benefits that may outweigh known risks.
X = Drugs associated with birth defects and with potential risk that clearly outweighs potential benefits.
Risk vs benefit: R >> B = Proven or potential risk outweighs potential benefits.
B > R = Potential benefits outweigh potential risks.
R >> B? = Risks may be outweighed by benefits in some circumstances.
? = Risk-to-benefit ratio is unknown.

Breast-feeding categories:
I = Drug does not enter breast milk.
II = Drug enters breast milk but is not known to be harmful in therapeutic doses.
IIIA = Drug may or may not enter breast milk but no adverse effects are expected.
IIIB = Drug may or may not enter breast milk but drug is systemically absorbed.
IV = Drug enters breast milk and poses a potential risk to the neonate.

SIDE EFFECTS

Because it is specific for the H+/K+ ATPase of parietal cells, omeprazole lacks any systemic effects beyond that of gastric acid inhibition. In addition, it has been well tolerated and has few adverse clinical effects. One case of fulminant hepatic failure has been reported, as well as impaired vitamin B_{12} absorption, esophageal candidiasis, and one case of hemolytic anemia. Mild liver enzyme elevation is common at higher omeprazole dosages (greater than 40 mg/day).

Studies in rats and rabbits have shown no fetal toxicity, teratogenicity, or mutagenicity with omeprazole. Pregnancy does not appear to be an absolute contraindication. Omeprazole's use in pregnant and breast-feeding patients is addressed in Table 6-1. No hepatic or renal toxicity has been demonstrated. Studies done in patients with chronic renal failure indicate that omeprazole is safe, effective, and nondialyzable.

Omeprazole does have an association with gastric carcinoids, established by 2-year oncogenicity studies in rats. Doses 10 times those used therapeutically in humans have produced low-malignant carcinoid tumors from the ECL cells of rat gastric mucosa. These tumors may have arisen from direct effects of omeprazole, but they more likely arose from ECL-cell hyperplasia induced by secondary hypergastrinemia. Humans do not respond in this manner and ECL hyperplasia has been seen only in association with omeprazole use in an MEN-1 patient with ZES.

Suggested Reading

Archambult AP, et al. Omeprazole (20 mg daily) versus cimetidine (1200 mg daily) in duodenal ulcer healing and pain relief. Gastroenterology 1988; 94:1130–1134.
A study of 169 patients with acute duodenal ulcers comparing omeprazole with cimetidine.

Bell NJ, Hunt RH. Role of gastric acid secretion in the treatment of gastroesophageal reflux disease. Gut 1992; 33:118–124.
The authors note that improved healing rates in gastroesophageal reflux disease are achieved best with a high degree of prolonged acid suppression.

Berlin RG. Omeprazole. Gastrin and gastric endocrine cell data from clinical studies. Dig Dis Sci 1991; 36:129–136.
The author concludes in this review that the rat model is a false indicator of risk in humans of enterochromaffinlike cell hyperplasia, as omeprazole is not *associated with changes in gastric oxyntic cell population.*

Brook CW, et al. Relapse of duodenal ulceration after healing with omeprazole. Med J Aust 1987; 147:595–597.
During a 12-month period, the recurrence rate of duodenal ulcers was documented in 55 patients previously healed with omeprazole.

Brunner G, Chang J. Intravenous therapy with high doses of ranitidine and omeprazole in critically ill patients with bleeding peptic ulcerations of the upper intestinal tract. Digestion 1990; 45: 217–225.
Of 19 patients allocated to the omeprazole treatment group, 16 (84%) stopped bleeding. Of the 17 patients in the ranitidine group

who continued to bleed, 13 were controlled when treated with omeprazole (80 mg intravenously for 5 days).

Freston FW. Clinical significance of hypergastrinemia: Relevance to gastric monitoring during omeprazole therapy. Digestion 1992; 51S1:102–114.

Plasma gastrin levels usually rise two- to fourfold during omeprazole therapy. About 3.3 percent of patients treated with omeprazole for one year have plasma gastrin levels above 400 pg/ml.

Havu N. Enterochromaffinlike cell carcinoids of gastric mucosa in rats after life-long inhibition of gastric secretion. Digestion 1986; 35:42–55

Oncogenicity studies in rats showing an association with long-term inhibition of gastric acid secretion and compensatory rise in serum gastrin with hyperplasia of ECL cells and subsequent formation of gastric carcinoids.

Jansen JB, et al. Effect of single and repeated intravenous doses of omeprazole on pentagastrin-stimulated gastric acid secretion and pharmacokinetics in man. Gut 1988; 29:75–80.

Healthy male volunteers studied for the effect of single and repeated intravenous doses of omeprazole on gastric acid secretion.

Jochem V, et al. Fulminant hepatic failure related to omeprazole. Am J Gastroenterol 1992; 87:523–525.

Although heretofore the authors found that minimal elevations of hepatocellular enzymes were the only liver-associated omeprazole side effect, they believe omeprazole caused fulminant hepatic failure in this 62-year-old man. Centrizonal necrosis consistent with production of a toxic metabolite by an induced cytochrome P-450 system was seen.

Labenz J, et al. Amoxicillin plus omeprazole versus triple therapy for eradication of *Helicobacter pylori* in duodenal ulcer disease. Gut 1993; 34:1167–1170.

Group 1 (amoxicillin, 2 gm/day, plus omeprazole, 40 mg/day) patients had better pain relief, ulcer healing, and medication tolerance than group 2 (bismuth subsalicylate, 1800 mg/day, plus metronidazole, 1200 mg/day, plus tetracycline, 1500 mg/day, plus ranitidine, 300 mg at bedtime) patients.

Lamer AJ, Lendrum R. Esophageal candidiasis after omeprazole therapy. Gut 1992; 33:860–861.

Physiologic acid reflux may play a protective role in preventing Candida *infection.*

Lauritsen K, et al. Effect of omeprazole and cimetidine on duodenal ulcers: A double-blind comparative trial. N Engl J Med 1985; 312:958–961.

Treatment of 132 duodenal ulcer patients with omeprazole compared to cimetidine.

Marcuard SP, et al. Omeprazole therapy causes malabsorption of cyanocobalamin. Ann Intern Med 1994; 120:211–215.

Omeprazole therapy acutely decreased vitamin B_{12} absorption by about 75 percent in 10 healthy volunteers taking omeprazole, 20 mg/day.

Marks DR, et al. Hemolytic anemia associated with the use of omeprazole. Am J Gastroenterol 1991; 86:217–218.

A case report with spontaneous recovery after drug cessation.

Tucci A, et al. One-day therapy for treatment of *Helicobacter pylori* infection. Dig Dis Sci 1993; 38:1670–1673.

One-day, high-dose combination therapy (amoxicillin, 2 gm orally 4 times a day; metronidazole, 500 mg orally 4 times a day; bismuth subcitrate, 240 mg orally 4 times a day, in combination with omeprazole, 40 mg orally) eradicated H. pylori *in 23 of 32 patients (72%).*

Inflammatory Bowel Disease Drugs

Inflammatory bowel disease, with its unknown etiology and complicated pathogenesis, is a difficult and frustrating illness to treat. Whenever physicians and their patients are faced with the task of controlling an illness for which no cure is available, the therapeutic armamentarium is limited to agents that ameliorate signs and symptoms of the disease. Such is the case with ulcerative colitis and Crohn's disease, maladies that currently affect 2 million Americans, inflicting pain and causing altered life-style, extreme financial burden, and sometimes death.

A complete review of the pathophysiologic alterations and etiologic theories of inflammatory bowel disease is clearly beyond the scope of these chapters; however, several observations should be highlighted. Various effector cells of the inflammatory response have been found in increased number within the mucosa of patients with active ulcerative colitis and Crohn's disease. These include T and B lymphocytes, plasma cells, macrophages, epithelioid cells, neutrophils, mast cells, and eosinophils. Inflammatory mediators secreted by these cells, such as prostaglandins, kinins, leukotrienes, platelet-activating factors, immunoglobulins, and lymphokines, are found in high concentration in various tissues during active inflammation. Interleukin-2, known to stimulate secondary cytokine production, has been associated with exacerbation of quiescent Crohn's disease in two patients with renal cell carcinoma.

Within the gastrointestinal tract these agents cause proximate tissue injury leading to mucosal and transmural edema, vascular congestion, acute and chronic inflammatory cellular infiltration, cell death, and reactive fibrosis. While inflammatory bowel disease is not believed to be a classic autoimmune disorder, recent studies implicate an immunoregulatory defect as a major factor in its pathogenesis. As many as 50 percent of patients with early, mild Crohn's disease have been shown to have circulating T-lymphocyte populations possessing enhanced suppressor T-cell activity. In contrast, decreased suppressor T-cell activity has been demonstrated in late, severe disease. In light of evidence showing that some patients with Crohn's disease have increased B-and T-lymphocyte response to multiple mucosal and bacterial antigens, it is speculated that there is a tendency in these patients to initially mount an inappropriate immune response to one or more mucosal or microbial antigens.

Once inflammation becomes firmly entrenched, the suppressor T-cell response is incapable of turning off the immune activity. The exact role of corticosteroids in altering this process is unknown, but several of their anti-inflammatory actions have been elucidated. Corticosteroids diminish the levels of circulating leukocytes, inhibit the release of interleukin-I and -II, and reduce tissue levels of the inflammatory mediators and lymphokines. Both the proliferative response of T lymphocytes to antigenic and mitogenic stimuli and their cytotoxic activity are profoundly diminished. Besides affecting cellular mediators, corticosteroids inhibit prostaglandin and leukotriene production by their inhibition of phospholipase A_2. Prednisolone has been shown to reduce synthesis and to lower tissue levels of prostaglandin E_2 (PGE_2) in cultured rectal biopsies of patients with ulcerative colitis. The result is a reduction in vasodilation, capillary permeability, chemotaxis, and neutrophilic enzyme release within the gastrointestinal mucosa.

Ulcerative Colitis

Corticosteroids are currently recognized as the most effective agents in the treatment of ulcerative proctosigmoiditis, moderate ulcerative colitis, and severe colitis unresponsive to other agents.

Multiple clinical trials have proved their efficacy compared to placebo. A retrospective analysis in 1964 by Korelitz and Lindner of patients with ulcerative colitis before and after the advent of steroid use showed significant reductions in overall morbidity and mortality, a decrease in complications, and a shift from emergent to more elective surgery since these agents came into common use. Along with the clinical and gross endoscopic improvement, histologic examination of rectal biopsies of patients with active colitis shows resolution of neutrophilic infiltration of the lamina propria, an increase in mucous goblet cells, and a decrease in fragmented epithelial cells in response to steroid therapy.

Corticosteroids can be given intravenously, orally, or by rectal instillation as suppositories, rectal drip, retention enemas, and foam. They should be viewed as effective therapeutic agents for ulcerative colitis, restricted in their use to resolving new-onset attacks or recurrent exacerbations, and should not be utilized for long-term management.

Rectally instilled steroids have been demonstrated to spread retrograde as far as the splenic flexure by scintigraphy of technetium 99–labeled suspensions. Enemas have the most extensive spread, while foams may reach the midsigmoid colon. Spreading is more proximal in patients with active disease than in those with inactive colitis or in control subjects, and there seems to be a positive correlation between the extent of disease involvement and the degree of steroid spreading. Retention enemas should be used in patients with proximal sigmoid disease, while foams are as effective and are usually preferred for proctitis and distal sigmoiditis. They are especially helpful in relieving tenesmus and rectal urgency or incontinence. Most patients find foams easier to retain and more acceptable aesthetically than enemas. Steroid suppositories should be used for proctitis only. Oral agents should be used for refractory proctitis, colitis that extends to the proximal sigmoid colon, or colitis associated with systemic symptoms, significant diarrhea, or abdominal pain.

Severe colitis, necessitating hospitalization, requires parenteral corticosteroids or corticotropin (ACTH). Steroid therapy should be only one of several treatment modalities offered, and a protocol of medical management may include bed rest; correction of dehydration, electrolyte abnormalities, and anemia; nutritional supplementation; and appropriate use of sulfasalazine, antibiotics, or immunosuppressive agents.

Trials of intensive intravenous corticosteroid treatment for mild, moderate, and severe attacks of ulcerative colitis have demonstrated remission rates of 92, 87, and 56 percent, respectively.

The lowest remission rates occur in patients with chronic, continuous pancolitis. In the 1950s, Truelove, using a regimen of intravenous and rectal steroids, predetermined that the absence of any improvement after 5 days of treatment constituted an absolute indication for colectomy. Further studies have shown that patients with severe colitis who receive treatment for longer than 5 days have a mean time of remission of between 8 and 10 days. Prolonging treatment for longer than 10 days or changing drugs (e.g., from hydrocortisone to ACTH) does not improve remission rates. Thus, patients who fail to respond to 10 days of high-dose, intravenous steroids should have a total abdominal colectomy.

A small number of patients present with or progress to fulminant colitis or toxic megacolon. There have been no good, controlled trials of steroid therapy in these life-threatening cases. It is accepted practice to give at least a short trial of corticosteroids while stabilizing the patient preoperatively. There is no evidence that steroids adversely affect surgical outcome as long as they do not lead to a delay in performing an indicated colectomy. Systemic corticosteroid therapy that is successful in inducing remission of the bowel disease usually resolves flares of colitis-associated complications. Axial arthropathy and hepatic complications (pericholangitis, chronic active hepatitis, sclerosing cholangitis, and postnecrotic cirrhosis) follow an independent course, may antedate the onset of bowel disease, and do not respond well to medical therapy.

In the treatment of ulcerative colitis, sulfasalazine and the newer 4–aminosalicylic acid (ASA) and 5-ASA compounds are useful in inducing remission in mild flares of the disease and in the maintenance of remission.

More exotic therapy with fish oil and bismuth has been reported in the treatment of ulcerative colitis. Stenson used fish oil (eicosapentaenoic acid), 18 capsules a day, and found improved histology and decreased rectal dialysate leukotriene B_4 levels, but no change in steroid dosage or symptoms. Pullan and Ganesh found similar remission rates, sigmoidoscopic appearances, and histology in 63 patients treated with either 5–aminosalicylic acid enemas or bismuth citrate/polyacrylate (450 mg) enemas.

Crohn's Disease

Steroids were introduced as treatment for Crohn's disease in the early 1950s. Until 1979, only retrospective and uncontrolled trials evaluating efficacy were available. Most of these studies reported encouraging clinical improvement in patients treated with ACTH or corticosteroids, with greater than 50 percent of patients responding favorably. Much of the data from these early studies were conflicting, reporting progression of disease on therapy, increased complications and mortality in some treatment groups, and increased need for surgery after treatment. To answer the many questions regarding the natural history, optimal treatment, and complications of Crohn's disease, a multicenter drug study was initiated in 1971. A total of 1119 patients were entered into the study after fulfilling diagnostic criteria. The results of this National Cooperative Crohn's Disease Study (NCCDS) were published in 1979, detailing the effect of treatment with sulfasalazine, prednisone, and azathioprine compared to placebo. The conclusions drawn from this report have guided our use of steroids, anti-inflammatory agents, and immunosuppressives in Crohn's disease for the last 10 years.

The results of the NCCDS showed that in patients with active, symptomatic disease, prednisone was superior to placebo in inducing and maintaining improvement. Using the Crohn's disease activity index (CDAI) to evaluate improvement, 78 percent of patients achieved at least transient remission (CDAI < 150) during 17 weeks of prednisone treatment. Response was influenced by prior drug therapy. Patients taking sulfasalazine at the beginning of prednisone treatment responded no better to prednisone with sulfasalazine than to prednisone without sulfasalazine. Conversely, prior treatment with steroids precluded a significant improvement with the addition of sulfasalazine. Different responses were also noted depending on the location of active disease. Prednisone was superior to placebo only in patients with isolated ileal or ileocolonic disease. Patients with Crohn's colitis alone responded to prednisone no better than to placebo, although this group was quite small.

In a follow-up, controlled trial by Singleton in 1979, sulfasalazine was used in combination with prednisone for active and quiescent Crohn's disease to judge the former's adjunctive and steroid-sparing effect. The combination was less effective for active ileal disease than was prednisone alone and exhibited no prednisone-sparing effect. Thus, the addition of sulfasalazine to steroid therapy does not appear to improve substantially the response to treatment in active Crohn's disease.

In the NCCDS, steroid therapy was administered to 274 patients in remission to assess its prophylactic effect. Steroid therapy proved to be no better than placebo in preventing relapse of active disease. Another multicenter drug trial, the European Cooperative Crohn's Disease Study (ECCDS), confirmed the effectiveness of high-dose steroids for active disease, but also demonstrated beneficial results from maintenance methylprednisolone at a dosage of 12.5 mg/day. Unfortunately, no appropriate control group was used for the maintenance regimen.

Long-term corticosteroid therapy (> 6 months), high-dose corticosteroid therapy (> 15 mg prednisone daily), or significant corticosteroid side effects (diabetes, hypertension, cataracts, or osteoporosis) justify the use of steroid-sparing agents such as 6-mercaptopurine or azathioprine. Immunosuppressive agents require careful follow-up and intensive patient counseling.

Complications of Crohn's disease such as enterocutaneous fistulae often respond to antibacterial agents such as metronidazole, either alone or in combination with 6-mercaptopurine or 6-mercaptopurine and low-dose corticosteroids.

Refractory Crohn's disease may respond to either 6-mercaptopurine, methotrexate, or cyclosporine. These patients may benefit from decreased prednisone dosages but side effects are common, serious, and often unpredictable. Intravenous cyclosporine A (4 mg/kg/day for 6–10 days followed by oral dosing at 8 mg/kg/day) was associated with closure of fistulae in five patients with Crohn's disease that was unresponsive to previous medical and surgical therapy.

The use of 5-ASA in the treatment of Crohn's disease is gaining widespread favor. Initial studies suggest a benefit in maintenance of mild ileal or ileocolonic Crohn's disease. Oral 5-ASA appears to be safe in pregnancy.

Total parenteral nutrition remains a useful adjunct in the treatment of severe Crohn's disease, in the preparation of nutritionally depleted Crohn's patients for surgery, and as a life-sustaining therapy for patients with extensive Crohn's disease and nonfunctional gut.

W. Zack Taylor and Michael M. Van Ness

Suggested Reading

Brynskov, et al. A placebo-controlled double-blind, randomized trial of cyclosporine therapy in active chronic Crohn's disease. N Engl J Med 1989; 321:845–850.

Cyclosporine therapy resulted in improvement in 59 percent of patients with Crohn's disease compared to 32 percent of placebo-treated patients. Response was apparent within 2 weeks; side effects such as renal failure, hyperkalemia, and hyperfusion are common with long-term therapy.

Elson CO, et al. An evaluation of total parenteral nutrition in the management of inflammatory bowel disease. Dig Dis Sci 1980; 25:42–48.

Assessing the role of total parenteral nutrition (TPN) as an adjunct in the therapy of inflammatory bowel disease.

Haber CJ, et al. Nature and course of pancreatitis caused by 6-mercaptopurine in the treatment of inflammatory bowel disease. Gastroenterology 1986; 91:982–986.

The authors report the clinical course of 13 cases (3.25%) of pancreatitis attributable to 6-mercaptopurine (6-MP) in 400 patients with inflammatory bowel disease. The pancreatitis tends to occur early (within 30 days), is usually mild, and recurs with rechallenge.

Hanauer SB, Smith MB. Rapid closure of Crohn's disease fistulas with continuous intravenous cyclosporin A. Am J Gastroenterol 1993; 88:646–649.

Five patients with 12 fistulae unresponsive to all previous medical and surgical therapy were treated with intravenous cyclosporin A for 6 to 10 days, followed by oral therapy. Ten of 12 fistulae closed, with a mean time to closure of 8 days.

Korelitz BI, Lindner AE. The influence of corticotropin and adrenal steroids in the course of ulcerative colitis: A comparison with the presteroid era. Gastroenterology 1964; 46:671.

Impressive review of the positive impact of steroid therapy on the course of ulcerative colitis (UC).

Pullan RD, Ganesh S, Mani V, et al. Comparison of bismuth citrate and 5-aminosalicylic acid enemas in distal ulcerative colitis: a controlled trial. Gut 1993; 34(5):676–679.

Bismuth and 5-ASA per rectum work equally well.

Singleton JW. Steroids in chronic liver and inflammatory bowel diseases. Hosp Pract 1983; 12:97.

Good review of indications and regimens for steroid therapy in inflammatory bowel disease (IBD).

Sparano JA, et al. Symptomatic exacerbation of Crohn's disease after treatment with high-dose interleukin-2. Ann Intern Med 1993; 118:617–618.

An inflammatory sigmoid mass and jejunal obstruction with perforation were seen in two patients with quiescent Crohn's disease who had renal cell carcinoma treated with interleukin-2.

Stenson WF, Cort D, Beekan W, et al. A trial of fish oil supplemental diet in ulcerative colitis. Gastroenterology 1990; 98:A475.

A double-blind study suggesting both symptomatic and sigmoidoscopic benefit to dietary supplementation with eicosapentaenoic acid.

Sutherland LR, et al. 5–Aminosalicylic acid enema in the treatment of distal ulcerative colitis, proctosigmoiditis, and proctitis. Gastroenterology 1987; 92:1894–1898.

A randomized, double-blind, placebo-controlled study of 153 patients with left-sided ulcerative colitis. The patients who received 5-ASA had a clinical improvement rate of 63 percent from 4-gm nighttime enemas. The data are important in that dropouts were included in the final calculation of the intent-to-treat success rate.

Truelove SC. Treatment of ulcerative colitis with local hydrocortisone. Br Med J 1956; 2:1267.

Truelove's landmark article reporting the effectiveness of rectally instilled hydrocortisone in mild to moderately severe UC.

Truelove SC. Treatment of ulcerative colitis with local hydrocortisone hemisuccinate sodium. Br Med J 1958; 2:1072.

A controlled trial proving the efficacy of a water-soluble preparation of hydrocortisone for rectal instillation in UC.

Truelove SC. Systemic and local corticosteroid therapy in ulcerative colitis. Br Med J 1960; 1:464.

A combination of oral prednisolone, 5 mg 4 times a day, and hydrocortisone enemas for mild to moderately severe UC was more effective than either agent alone.

Truelove SC, Witts LJ. Cortisone in ulcerative colitis. Br Med J 1955; 2:1041.

Early landmark study showing favorable response of UC to oral cortisone.

Williams CN, Haber G, Aquino JA. Double-blind, placebo-controlled evaluation of 5-ASA suppositories in active distal proctitis and measurement of extent of spread using 99m Tc–labeled 5-ASA suppositories. Dig Dis Sci 1987; 32:71S–75S.

This study reiterates the utility of 5-ASA, 500-mg suppositories 3 times a day, in active proctitis. The suppositories deliver the 5-ASA to the rectum alone.

Corticosteroids

Michael M. Van Ness

Glucocorticoids are 21-carbon steroid molecules, structurally and functionally similar to cortisol, the principal circulating glucocorticoid in humans. Minor modifications in the structure of these compounds alter their potency, duration of action, and mineralocorticoid activity dramatically. Table 7-1 lists the most commonly used glucocorticoids by their relative potencies, dosage equivalents, and sodium-retaining potential. Two corticosteroids used to treat inflammatory bowel disease, cortisone and prednisone, lack functional activity until converted in vivo to cortisol and prednisolone, respectively. Other commercial preparations include cortisol (hydrocortisone), prednisolone, methylprednisolone, betamethasone, beclomethasone, dexamethasone, and tixocortol pivulate. In addition, corticotropin (ACTH), which is normally released from the anterior pituitary gland and regulates adrenal cortisol production, has been used with considerable success in the parenteral treatment of ulcerative colitis and Crohn's disease.

PHARMACOLOGY AND PHARMACOKINETICS

Corticosteroids are well absorbed after oral administration and clinically effective systemically when given by this route. Topical application to the skin and mucous membranes results in local activity and, in some instances, absorption and a systemic effect. Ninety percent of cortisol and its synthetic analogues is bound in plasma by two protein fractions, cortisol-binding globulin (CBG) and albumin. CBG has a high affinity for cortisol but low total binding capacity, while albumin provides for the majority of protein-bound steroid even though its affinity is less due to its considerably larger plasma pool.

The activity of glucocorticoids, as with all steroid hormones, depends on passive entry into the cell cytoplasm, binding to specific intracytosolic receptors, and ingress into the nucleus. Genomic expression is then modulated, with subsequent mRNA transcription, and translation to proteins that then govern metabolic and enzymatic pathways. Due to their intracellular location of action, the activity of glucocorticoids cannot be correlated to plasma levels. Likewise, circulating half-life and duration of action do not seem to be closely related. For example, the half-life of prednisone is 60 minutes and that of prednisolone is 115 to 252 minutes; however, their relative potency and equivalent dosage are identical. Glucocorticoids clearly exert many of their actions after disappearance from plasma and not all of these effects have an equal duration. It is clear that duration of action is a function of dose, and enhanced activity can be obtained by increasing the amount administered. The protein-free, unbound fraction of circulating steroid is believed to be the active moiety. Reduced levels of albumin and steroid-binding globulin increase the levels of this active, serum-free steroid. Even though the therapeutic effect of the drug may remain unaltered, the risk of side effects will increase.

Prednisone is the most commonly used glucocorticoid and owes its activity to its metabolite, prednisolone. The conversion of prednisone to prednisolone occurs in the liver and has led to recommend-

Table 7-1. Commonly used glucocorticoids

Duration of Action	Glucocorticoid Potency	Equivalent Glucocorticoid Dose (mg)	Mineralo-corticoid Activity
Short-acting			
Cortisol (hydro-cortisone)	1	20	yes
Cortisone	0.8	25	yes
Prednisone	4	5	no
Prednisolone	4	5	no
Methylpred-nisolone	5	4	no
Intermediate-acting			
Triamcinolone	5	4	no
Long-acting			
Betamethasone	25	0.60	no
Dexametha-sone	30	0.75	no

tions that only prednisolone be used in patients with hepatic dysfunction. Liver disease, however, prolongs prednisolone half-life and is usually accompanied by hypoalbuminemia, which increases the unbound fraction of circulating steroid. Thus, the reduced conversion and lower initial prednisolone concentration in such patients are compensated for by delayed clearance and higher levels of active steroid, preserving the effectiveness of prednisone regardless of hepatic function.

The overall steroid dose should be reduced in patients with significant liver disease who require long-term treatment, to reduce adverse side effects. Glucocorticoids are primarily metabolized in the liver and excreted in the urine as glucuronides, sulfates, and unconjugated compounds. Their elimination is not affected by alterations in renal function.

The absorption of prednisolone has been extensively studied in patients with inflammatory bowel disease. Wide absorptive variations in patients with Crohn's disease have been demonstrated, especially in patients with Crohn's disease of the ileum. Tanner found no significant difference in peak levels or total absorption of 20 mg prednisolone given orally, though the majority of his patients had predominantly colonic Crohn's disease. Some degree of corticosteroid malabsorption is possible in Crohn's disease, particularly when extensive small bowel inflammation is present. Mucosal integrity, surface area, and transit time of the small bowel are significant factors affecting the bioavailability of these agents. The total absorption of prednisolone does not differ between normal individuals and patients with ulcerative colitis after oral dosing. However, there is a lower peak level and a more gradual reduction of plasma levels in patients, possibly due to delayed absorption. The overall effect of drug does not seem to be altered.

The site of action of topically administered steroids is thought to be primarily local; however, systemic absorption occurs through the rectal mucosa with most agents. Fifty percent of administered hydrocortisone reaches the systemic circulation, and up to 90 percent absorption has been demonstrated, with retention times exceeding 8 hours. The rectally instilled steroids are classified according to this degree of absorption and concomitant adrenal suppression (Table 7-2). The largest group includes those that are highly absorbed with subsequent adrenal suppression, followed by the absorbable agents with no systemic effects, and the nonabsorbable compounds.

Several preparations have been developed that limit the systemic effects of rectal steroids. Beclomethasone dipropionate and budenoside are two compounds that are absorbed but undergo rapid first-pass hepatic metabolism. Prednisolone metasulfobenzoate is a large molecule that is poorly absorbed after rectal instillation. All of these compounds are equally or more effective than hydrocortisone and avoid adrenal suppression and steroid side effects. Tixocortol pivulate, a recently formulated, nonglucocorticoid, synthetic derivative of cortisol, is easily absorbed but has negligible systemic effects due to rapid first-pass metabolism, clearance, and elimination. It is also very effective in reducing colonic inflammation without reducing serum cortisol levels. These agents have been available for use in Europe for some time and may be approved in the United States.

MECHANISMS OF ACTION

Corticosteroids stabilize lysosomal membranes, reduce capillary permeability, function as inhibitors of chemotaxis and phagocytosis, and impair cell-mediated immunity in experimental models.

INDICATIONS AND ADMINISTRATION

Ulcerative Colitis

Oral

Several studies provide data on the most effective and least toxic dosage schedules. For attacks of mildly to moderately severe ulcerative colitis, a 40 to 60-mg dose is superior to a 20-mg/day dose for remission induction.

Powell-Tuck and Lennard-Jones showed that a single 40-mg dose of prednisolone given in the morning for active proctocolitis was as effective in inducing remission as 10 mg taken 4 times a day, with less adrenal suppression. There is a large body of anecdotal experience favoring twice-a-day over 4-times-a-day steroid dosing. For more severe cases that do not require intravenous therapy, it is prudent to split the dosage. No controlled trials have been performed to evaluate an alternate dose regimen of steroids for acute attacks, but most reports do not support its use.

Intravenous

Resistant cases of ulcerative colitis that do not respond to oral steroid therapy within 10 to 14 days and patients presenting with severe attacks (Table 7-3) should receive intravenous corticosteroids. The most frequently used agents include hydrocortisone, prednisolone, methylprednisolone, and ACTH. Because of its intense mineralocorticoid effect, necessitating intravenous potassium replacement of up to 200 mg/day, hydrocortisone has become less popular as an intravenous agent.

Table 7-2. Rectally administered topical steroids

Absorbable Steroids	Delivery Vehicle	Systemic Effects/Adrenal Suppression
Hydrocortisone hemisuccinate (Cortenema)	Enema: 100 mg in 60-ml aqueous solution	yes
Hydrocortisone acetate	Enema: 100 mg in 60-ml aqueous solution	yes
	Suppository: (Cort-Dome) 15 mg, 25 mg	yes
	Foam: (Cortifoam) 10% in 20-gm foam	yes
	Foam: (Proctofoam-HC) 1% in 10-gm foam	yes
Prednisolone 21-phosphate	Enema: 20 mg in 100-ml aqueous solution	yes
	Suppository: 5 mg	
Methylprednisolone acetate	Enema: 40 mg in water	yes
Prednisolone	Enema: 100 mg in oil	yes
Betamethasone 17-valerate	Enema: 5 mg in aqueous solution	yes
Tixocortol pivulate	Enema: 250 mg in 100-ml aqueous solution	no
	Suppository: 250 mg	no
Poorly absorbable steroids		
Prednisolone metasulfobenzoate	Enema and suppository	low
Beclomethasone dipropionate	Enema and suppository	low

Table 7-3. Criteria for severe colitis

1. *Diarrhea*: Six or more stools per day with macroscopic blood.
2. *Fever*: Mean evening temp. ≥ 37.5°C or a temp. of ≥ 37.8°C on at least 2 days out of 4.
3. *Erythrocyte sedimentation rate elevation* ≥ 30 mm/hr.
4. *Anemia*: Hemoglobin level ≤ 11.5 mg/liter
5. *Tachycardia*: Mean pulse rate ≥ 90/min.

From SC Truelove, DP Jewell, Criteria for severe colitis. Lancet 1974; 1:1067.

Early clinical studies suggested that ACTH was superior to corticosteroids, particularly for patients with a relapse of colitis. Kaplan and associates in 1975 and Meyers in 1982 found both agents equally effective; however, patients previously treated with steroids had a better response to hydrocortisone and those without prior treatment had significantly better improvement with ACTH. The lesser response of patients who had received prior steroid therapy to ACTH (25% improved with ACTH, compared to 53% with hydrocortisone) could not be explained by impaired adrenal responsiveness, since mean serum cortisol and dehydroepiandrosterone levels were similar in both groups. Given these data, one might treat severe, initial attacks of ulcerative colitis with ACTH and recurrent, previously treated episodes with corticosteroids. In reality, both agents are usually successful.

The recommended dosages are hydrocortisone, 300 to 400 mg/day; prednisolone, 60 to 80 mg/day; methylprednisolone, 60 to 80 mg/day; and ACTH, 120 U/day. They may be administered by intermittent bolus or continuous infusion; the latter method is preferred.

Once remission is obtained, an attempt should be made to advance to equivalent oral dosages with a subsequent taper of the drug. Generally, prednisone dosage is decreased at a rate of 5 mg/week down to a level of 20 mg/day. Flares are less common above 20 mg/day and side effects are infrequent below this dosage. Subsequent weaning should proceed at a slower pace (e.g., 2.5-mg reductions every 1–2 weeks). Further tapering in 2.5-mg weekly increments, perhaps using an alternate-day schedule, should be continued until the drug is stopped.

Alternate-day tapering once the daily dose reaches 10 to 15 mg may be attempted and is frequently successful. An example of this type of regimen would be converting a 15-mg daily dose to 30 mg every other day, then tapering in 5-mg increments every week to 10 days. Since adrenal suppression and systemic toxicity are negligible on alternate-day steroids, this may be a preferred regimen in patients with multiple side effects.

Topical

Proper use of rectally instilled steroids induces remission or improvement in more than 80 percent of patients with active ulcerative proctosigmoiditis. They should be administered in a single dose at bedtime. After instillation, patients should lie on the left side for at least 30 minutes, then turn to the supine and prone positions to ensure proper contact with the entire circumference of the distal colon. The solution should be retained as long as possible, preferably all night. The usual course of therapy lasts 14 to 21 days. An incomplete or partial response may dictate prolonging treatment for up to 8 weeks on a daily or alternate-day schedule, but systemic side effects and adrenal suppression should be anticipated, necessitating slow tapering.

If no response occurs after 2 weeks, twice-daily administration may be tried for up to 14 days. Lack of improvement after 1 month of treatment should prompt discontinuation of the agent and pursuance of systemic steroid or sulfasalazine treatment. If remission is achieved, treatment should be stopped or tapered off. Maintenance treatment with topical steroids is not recommended.

Crohn's Disease

Oral

A reasonable approach to the patient with Crohn's disease is to consider steroid therapy after implementing supportive care and administering sulfasalazine or 5–aminosalicylic acid (5-ASA) compounds without the desired therapeutic response. For patients with refractory disease and those with systemic symptoms such as fever, weight loss, and anorexia, steroids should be started at high doses (e.g., prednisone, 60–80 mg/day, or the equivalent, in four divided doses). A favorable response with resolution of fever, pain, and diarrhea, and improvement in appetite and sense of well-being usually occur within 10 days, at which point slow tapering of the dosage should begin. Optimally, one should make an attempt to wean the patient off steroids completely within 4 to 6 weeks.

Many patients experience an exacerbation of symptoms with attempts to lower or discontinue steroids. Any flare should prompt reinstituting a high dose, since small incremental dosage elevations may allow the inflammatory process to become less responsive and increasingly refractory. If patients are unable to taper down to a low dose (< 10 mg/day) of prednisone, alternate-day therapy, surgery, and use of a steroid-sparing agent should be considered. Alternate-day steroids are usually unsuccessful in Crohn's disease.

Intravenous

As with ulcerative colitis, high fever, severe diarrhea, bleeding, weight loss, anorexia, or bowel obstruction necessitates continuous intravenous therapy with either ACTH (120 U/day) or corticosteroids (methylprednisolone, 48–80 mg/day).

Topical

Topical application of steroids may be helpful in alleviating the symptoms of the colitis-related complications. Adjunctive therapy for oral ulceration includes topical application of triamcinolone acetonide dental paste (Kenalog in Orabase) 3 times a day after meals, or intralesional injections of triamcinolone acetonide, 10 mg/ml in a 0.1 to 0.5 dilutional mixture with 1 to 2% lidocaine hydrochloride (Xylocaine HCl).

Intraarticular injections of corticosteroids may give relief immediately, while waiting for the overall clinical picture to improve. The most frequently used drugs include short-acting, inexpensive agents such as hydrocortisone acetate (25 mg/ml) and the longer-acting betamethasone sodium phosphate (6 mg/ml), triamcinolone hexacetonide (20 mg/ml), or dexamethasone sodium phosphate (4 mg/ml). One may combine short- and long-acting agents or dilute them in 1–2% Xylocaine HCl. Ocular steroids such as dexamethasone, 0.1%, or prednisone, 1%, are sometimes necessary in cases of severe uveitis.

CONTRAINDICATIONS

There are very few absolute contraindications to steroid therapy. Colonic perforation, peritonitis, and abscess formation are frequently listed as absolute contraindications; however, in the context of steroid use in inflammatory bowel disease, most patients are already undergoing steroid treatment when these complications occur and an increase in dosage to cover surgical stress is required. Clearly, pyogenic, viral, and systemic fungal infection are relative contraindications to beginning steroids, but steroid therapy can be given concomitantly with the appropriate antibiotic, antiviral, or antifungal agent if the clinical situation dictates.

Corticosteroids may mask the signs and symptoms of intraabdominal or systemic sepsis, necessitating frequent, detailed evaluations of patient status. Wound healing may be delayed as a result of steroid use.

Early surgical reports indicated that preoperative steroid use increased the incidence of postoperative infection, wound dehiscence, anastomosis breakdown, and mortality. However, multiple reviews and controlled trials have proved otherwise.

All patients with latent tuberculosis or positive tuberculin reactivity should receive chemoprophylaxis during prolonged steroid therapy. Patients with previous peptic ulcer disease, diabetes mellitus, hypertension, diverticulitis, osteopenia, or myasthenia gravis may receive steroids, but close attention should be given to any flare or exacerbation of symptoms. Diuretics may be needed to offset fluid retention, and glucose homeostasis may be altered in diabetics, requiring an adjustment of diet, oral agents, or insulin. There is no need to place patients on antacids or H_2-antagonists for ulcer prophylaxis; however, patients with active or very recent peptic ulcers should probably receive continued acid suppression.

SIDE EFFECTS

The National Cooperative Crohn's Disease Study (NCCDS) provides the best data about steroid side effects in the treatment of inflammatory bowel disease. Prednisone, 0.25 to 0.75 mg/kg body weight, was used for up to 2 years. The most frequently occurring major side effects (peptic ulcer disease, hypertension, and psychiatric disturbances) occurred in 32 percent of patients. Only 1 patient in 85 suffered more than one major complication. The vast majority of complications resolved with reduction or withdrawal of treatment. The most common minor side effects were facial mooning, acne, and ecchymosis, which occurred after 100 days of treatment for active disease in 50, 35, and 16 percent, respectively. Evident side effects occurred in roughly one-third of patients receiving low-dose prednisone, 0.25 mg/kg/day, for prophylaxis. A total of 18 percent of steroid-treated patients had to be withdrawn from the study because of side effects.

Steroid-related osteonecrosis is a serious complication of treatment of inflammatory bowel disease. It appears that inflammatory bowel disease itself predisposes to osteonecrosis, as evidenced by the report of Freeman and Kwan in which two patients with Crohn's disease developed septic necrosis despite never having received corticosteroids. Arthralgia of steroid withdrawal and arthropathy of iflammatory bowel disease can be confused with the referred pain of early osteonecrosis. A mean cumulative lifetime dose of prednisone of 7 gm and mean daily doses of 26 mg/week for a mean of 42 weeks were seen in the series reported by Vakil and Sparberg. Bone scans or magnetic resonance imaging are most sensitive for early detection.

PEARLS AND PITFALLS

1. Most studies have shown neither Crohn's disease nor ulcerative colitis to be detrimental to the outcome of pregnancy. Some data indicate that active Crohn's disease increases the fetal risk. If inflammatory bowel disease flares during pregnancy, corticosteroids should be used to enhance a favorable outcome. No perinatal or fetal adverse effects have been associated with corticosteroid use. Appropriate routes of administration and dosage for the disease activity present should be utilized. Fetal and newborn hypopituitary adrenal axis (HPA) suppression does not occur.
2. If the recommended once-daily administration of prednisone for ulcerative colitis does not result in prompt improvement, splitting the dose into a twice-a-day or 4-times-a-day regimen should be tried. A 3- to 5-day trial should be sufficient to determine whether either will be effective.
3. Patients with underlying psychiatric disease are not at increased risk for development of steroid-related psychiatric side effects. If psychiatric-emotional symptoms develop they are more than likely to resemble the primary illness. The dosage of steroid used does not affect the time of onset, duration, or severity of psychiatric symptoms. If symptoms develop, reduction or discontinuation of steroid treatment should be attempted. Neuroleptics, lithium, and electroconvulsive therapy (ECT) may also be helpful.
4. Due to the increased nonprotein-bound, active steroid in plasma, corticosteroid dosage should be reduced in patients with hypoalbuminemia to lower the incidence of side effects and toxicity.
5. If disease activity flares during corticosteroid dosage tapering in ulcerative colitis or Crohn's disease, prednisone should be increased to previous high-dose levels (e.g., 60–80 mg/day), or intravenous treatment started. Small incremental increases in dosage usually fail to induce remission and reset the refractory-dosage level, entrenching disease activity at progressively higher doses of steroid.
6. Corticosteroids in high doses retard growth in children who have unfused epiphyses, and it is frequently recommended that steroid therapy be avoided in children under 15 years of age. It is important to remember that inflammatory bowel disease alone significantly delays linear growth, frequently before its diagnosis in children and adolescents. Corticosteroid treatment in doses necessary to arrest disease activity may very well be associated with accelerated growth as a result of controlling the inflammatory process. Low-dose and alternate-day schedules of treatment may suppress the disease without inhibiting growth and permit nutritional restitution and growth acceleration. Therefore, it is prudent to withhold corticosteroids in children and adolescents with further growth potential, if alternate forms of therapy are available and equally effective. One must recognize the growth-suppressing effect of active inflammatory bowel disease and give corticosteroids as a therapeutic trial to quiet the bowel inflammation if indicated. A paradoxical acceleration of growth may follow.

Long-term use of steroids should be avoided in children, as toxicity will eventually outstrip any beneficial effect produced.

7. For those patients who require low-dose (< 15 mg prednisone daily) steroid therapy for long periods of time, close attention should be given to the risk of developing cataracts and osteopenia. This is particularly important in older patients. Yearly ophthalmologic examination should be performed, and adequate calcium intake ensured. Low-dose vitamin D administration is advisable in most patients, to counter the inhibitory effect of steroids on calcium absorption and the increased bone resorption that occurs. Hip or knee pain should alert the physician to the possibility of aseptic necrosis of the femoral head.

Suggested Reading

Axelrod L. Glucocorticoid therapy. Medicine 1976; 55:39.
An extensive review of glucocorticoid pharmacology and a guide to steroid therapy.

Baiocco P, Korelitz BI. The influence of inflammatory bowel disease and its treatment on pregnancy and fetal outcome. J Clin Gastroenterol 1984; 6:211.
Steroids should be administered to pregnant patients with active inflammatory bowel disease (IBD) if indicated.

Farthing MJG, et al. Retrograde spread of hydrocortisone-containing foam given intrarectally in ulcerative colitis. Br Med J 1979; 2:822.
Technetium 99m–labeled hydrocortisone foam spread as far as the proximal sigmoid colon in active ulcerative colitis (UC).

Freeman HJ, Kwan WCP. Brief report: Non-corticosteroid–associated osteonecrosis of the femoral heads in two patients with inflammatory bowel disease. N Engl J Med 1993; 329:1314–1316.
The authors present two patients with ileocolonic Crohn's disease requiring hip replacement; neither patient had ever been treated with corticosteroids. The authors postulate that aseptic necrosis may be a rare extraintestinal skeletal manifestation of inflammatory bowel disease.

Friedman G. Clinical challenges in inflammatory bowel disease: Tixocortol pivulate. National Foundation for Ileitis and Colitis 1988: 8.
A brief review of the existing data regarding tixocortol pivulate.

Janowitz H. *Inflammatory Bowel Disease—A Personal View.* Chicago: Year Book, 1985. Pp 68, 73.
A practical review with many clinical "pearls" regarding steroid therapy for ulcerative colitis and Crohn's disease.

Jarnerot G, et al. Intensive intravenous treatment of ulcerative colitis. Gastroenterology 1985; 89:1005.
Results of the use of Truelove's intensive intravenous steroid regimen in mild, moderate, and severe UC.

Jeffries WM. Low-dosage corticosteroid therapy. Arch Intern Med 1967; 119:265.
Low-dose steroid treatment (60 mg or less hydrocortisone daily) is safe over a long period of time.

Kaplan HP, et al. A controlled evaluation of intravenous adrenocorticotropic hormone and hydrocortisone in the treatment of active colitis. Gastroenterology 1975; 69:91.

Adrenocorticotropic hormone and hydrocortisone are equally effective in acute UC.

Kirschner BS, et al. Growth retardation in inflammatory bowel disease. Gastroenterology 1978; 75:504.
Growth retardation, seen in 20 percent of children with Crohn's disease, may improve with appropriate treatment of the bowel disease.

Kozarek R. Extracolonic manifestations of inflammatory bowel disease. Am Fam Physician 1987; Feb, p 205.
An excellent review.

Lennard-Jones JE. Toward optimal use of corticosteroids in ulcerative colitis and Crohn's disease. Gut 1983; 24:177.
Excellent review of steroid therapy for IBD.

Meyers S, Janowitz H. The place of steroids in the therapy of toxic megacolon. Gastroenterology 1978; 75:729.
Steroid treatment does not worsen the prognosis of toxic megacolon.

Meyers S, Janowitz H. Systemic corticosteroid therapy of ulcerative colitis. Gastroenterology 1985; 89:1189.
An editorial review of parenteral corticosteroid use in severe UC.

Meyers S, et al. Predicting the outcome of corticoid therapy for acute ulcerative colitis. J Clin Gastroenterol 1987; 9:50.
An assessment of prognostic variables in 66 patients with UC treated with parenteral ACTH or hydrocortisone.

Mogadam M, et al. Pregnancy in inflammatory bowel disease: Effect of sulfasalazine and corticosteroids on fetal outcome. Gastroenterology 1981; 80:72.
Corticosteroid treatment of IBD in pregnancy does not adversely affect fetal morbidity or mortality.

Powell-Tuck J, Lennard-Jones JE. A comparison of oral prednisolone given as single or multiple daily doses for active proctocolitis. Scand J Gastroenterol 1978; 13:833.
A single, morning 40-mg dose of prednisolone for UC is as effective as 10 mg 4 times a day.

Powell-Tuck J, et al. A controlled trial of alternate-day prednisolone as a maintenance treatment for ulcerative colitis in remission. Digestion 1981; 22:263.
Prednisolone, 40 mg orally every other day, was superior to placebo in remission maintenance for UC.

Somerville KW, et al. Effect of treatment on symptoms and quality of life in patients with ulcerative colitis: Comparative trial of hydrocortisone acetate foam and prednisolone-21-phosphate enemas. Br Med J 1985; 2:866.
Quality of life is altered less by foams than by enemas in the treatment of distal UC.

Vakil N, Sparberg M. Steroid-related osteonecrosis in inflammatory bowel disease. Gastroenterology 1989; 96:62–67.
Osteonecrosis developed in 7 of 161 patients (4%) treated with corticosteroids over a 10-year period. Risk factors for development of osteonecrosis include a mean cumulative dose of prednisone of 7 gm, steroid use within 6 months of the development of either knee or hip pain, and the presence of inflammatory bowel disease. Patients with inflammatory bowel disease are younger and had received less prednisone for shorter durations of time than did patients for steroid-induced osteonecrosis in other disease states.

Sulfasalazine

John J. Vargo and D. Michael Jones

Sulfasalazine is the most widely used drug in the treatment of inflammatory bowel disease. It was discovered by a Swedish physician, Nana Svartz, who was looking for a drug for "rheumatic polyarthritis" in the late 1930s. She noted that her patients with ulcerative colitis experienced marked improvement in their symptoms. Multiple trials over the 5 decades since then have confirmed the efficacy of the drug in the treatment of inflammatory bowel disease.

ABSORPTION, METABOLISM, AND DISTRIBUTION

Sulfasalazine (SA) is a conjugate of 5–aminosalicylic acid (5-ASA), a salicylate analogue, and sulfapyridine (SP), a sulfonamide. These moieties are linked by a diazo bond. Approximately 20 to 30 percent of the ingested drug is absorbed from the upper gastrointestinal tract, with blood levels detectable within 1 to 2 hours of oral intake and steady-state serum levels achieved in 24 hours. Ninety percent of the absorbed drug is excreted unchanged in the bile; 10 percent is excreted unchanged in the urine. Sixty to 70 percent of the ingested drug passes directly into the colon without being absorbed.

Intestinal bacteria possessing an intracellular azoreductase that is inhibitable by oxygen reduce the diazo bond and release SP and 5-ASA. After azo bond reduction, most of the highly lipophilic SP is absorbed from the colon, partially metabolized, and excreted in the urine as the free sulfonamide or its acetyl or glucuronide metabolite. Sulfapyridine is subject to polymorphic acetylation. Slow acetylators tend to have higher serum levels of total SP and a higher incidence of side effects. The therapeutic moiety 5-ASA is poorly lipophilic and remains primarily in the colonic lumen. Only a small portion of this metabolite is absorbed and excreted in the urine as the acetylated derivative. The acetylation of 5-ASA in contrast to SP is not genetically polymorphic. Most 5-ASA is recovered unchanged in the feces, although small amounts are present in an acetylated form.

MECHANISM OF ACTION

Sulfasalazine and its breakdown products 5-ASA and SP have been shown to affect inflammatory cell function and the immune response at multiple levels. Despite a wealth of experimental information, it remains unclear which mechanism(s) are essential in the attenuation of inflammatory bowel disease activity.

Based on the hypothesis that increased production of prostaglandins may be involved in the pathogenesis of inflammatory bowel disease, SA and 5-ASA have been shown to inhibit the production of prostaglandins and other products of the cyclooxygenase pathway including prostacyclin and the thromboxanes. Interestingly, more potent prostaglandin inhibitors such as indomethacin not only show no benefit in the treatment of inflammatory bowel disease, but may cause an exacerbation of the disease. A decrease in the lipoxygenase product leukotriene B_4, a potent chemotactic mediator, has been attributed to SA and 5-ASA.

Sulfasalazine, 5-ASA, and SP can affect neutrophil, lymphocyte, monocyte, macrophage, and platelet function. At the level of th neutrophil, SA and SP can impair chemotaxis while the parent compound can attenuate phagocytosis. Lymphocyte production of immunoglobulins (Ig) G, M, and A is decreased by SA and 5-ASA while cell-mediated immunity is impaired by both SA and SP.

Mast cell degranulation and oxygen radical scavenging have been demonstrated with SA, 5-ASA, and, to a much lesser extent, SP.

INDICATIONS

Ulcerative Colitis

In controlled trials, SA is superior to placebo in the remission of mild to moderately active ulcerative colitis and in the maintenance of remission. Sulfasalazine is not recommended in the treatment of acute, severe ulcerative colitis. The optimal duration of maintenance therapy has never been determined.

Crohn's Disease

In controlled trials, SA is more effective than placebo in the treatment of mild to moderately active ileocolonic or colonic Crohn's disease. The efficacy of SA in ileocolonic disease appears to be less than with pure colonic involvement. It has not been shown to be effective in the treatment of small-bowel Crohn's disease or in the prevention of relapse. Therefore, maintenance therapy is not indicated. There appears to be no role for SA in severe, active Crohn's disease. Sulfasalazine is not effective as a steroid-sparing agent in patients with quiescent disease.

DOSAGE

The suggested dosage in acute inflammatory bowel disease is 1 gm/15 kg body weight per day in divided doses. The usual dosage is 3 to 4 gm/day. The risk of side effects or toxic reactions increases with dosages of 4 gm/day or more. To avoid side effects, the initial sulfasalazine dose should be low (1 gm/day), with gradual daily increases of 500 mg/day until the therapeutic range is reached. A therapeutic response is usually apparent by 1 month.

Once remission has been achieved in ulcerative colitis, the sulfasalazine may be gradually tapered to a maintenance dose of 2 gm/day. After remission has been induced in Crohn's disease, therapy should be continued for several months before the sulfasalazine is slowly tapered.

SIDE EFFECTS

Sulfasalazine-related side effects occur in approximately 15 percent of patients and are usually noted in the first 4 to 6 weeks of therapy. Side effects are usually related to the SP moiety either in a dose-related or an allergic/idiosyncratic fashion. Common symptoms of SA intolerance include dyspepsia, headache, anorexia, arthralgias, and myalgias, which are reversible following a reduction in the SA dose. Less common dose-related side effects include anosmia, alopecia, palpitations, and blue discoloration of the skin.

Allergic or idiosyncratic side effects, in contrast to their dose-related counterparts, are not related to serum SP levels or acetylator phenotype. These reactions are reversible with discontinuation of the medication and recur with a subsequent rechallenge.

A spectrum of dermatologic side effects can be seen, ranging from urticaria to the Stevens-Johnson syndrome. Hematologic side effects include neutropenia and agranulocytosis, megaloblastic anemia secondary to an effective folate deficiency, red cell aplasia, thrombocytopenia, hemolytic anemia, reticulocytosis, methemoglobinemia, and sulfhemoglobinemia. The occurrence of hemolysis appears to be directly related to sulfapyridine levels and to acetylator status. Some patients have experienced a generalized allergic reaction with fever, skin rash, arthralgias, and lymphadenopathy. Cyanosis unrelated to methemoglobinemia, sulfhemoglobinemia, and oxygen desaturation has been reported.

The SP moiety may lead to a reversible form of male infertility characterized by oligospermia and alterations in sperm morphology and motility. With SA discontinuation or the use of another 5-ASA analogue, an improvement in the semen analysis is seen within 3 months and fertility is restored. Extremely rare side effects include neurotoxicity, encephalopathy, pancreatitis, hair loss, hepatotoxicity, pulmonary fibrosis, a lupuslike syndrome, and hemorrhagic colitis.

USE DURING PREGNANCY AND LACTATION

The presence of SA and SP can be detected in breast milk, amniotic fluid, and umbilical cord serum. Extensive retrospective data indicate that the use of SA during pregnancy and the postpartum interval does not lead to increased fetal wastage, congenital abnormalities, growth retardation, or neonatal jaundice. Even though SA and SP displace bilirubin poorly, a low SA maintenance dose of 1.5 gm/day should be implemented early in the pregnancy (Table 8-1).

DESENSITIZATION

Over the past 5 years, the role of SA desensitization has decreased with the advent of other 5-ASA compounds. Approximately 80 to 90 percent of patients intolerant to SA are also intolerant to one of the other 5-ASA derivatives. Desensitization can be considered in patients who are intolerant of SA or who demonstrate minor allergic or idiosyncratic side effects. Desensitization should not be attempted in patients who have previously experienced agranulocytosis, frank hemolysis, hepatotoxicity, pulmonary toxicity, or toxic epidermal necrolysis.

Patients who have generalized side effects such as nausea, vomiting, headache, and malaise should have the medication stopped for 2 weeks. Sulfasalazine should then be restarted at 0.25 to 0.5 gm/day for a week, then gradually increased by 0.25 gm at weekly intervals until a dose of 2 gm/day is reached. Doses above 3 gm/day may not be tolerated in these patients.

Patients who have hypersensitivity or idiosyncratic reactions should be approached much more cautiously. The sulfasalazine should again be discontinued for at least 2 weeks. The patient should then be started on one-eighth tablet per day. The dose should be doubled every 7 days until a dose of 2 to 3 gm/day is reached. Minor recurrences of the sensitivity reaction (pruritus) may be treated with antihistamines with or without steroids. Close clinical follow-up is imperative during the desensitization period. Once desensitization has been achieved, the drug should be continued indefinitely to maintain the desensitized state. The drug should be discontinued if severe hypersensitivity reactions occur during the desensitization process.

Table 8-1. Sulfasalazine: Pregnancy and breast-feeding

Agent	FDA pregnancy category	Risk vs benefit (by trimester)			Breast-feeding category
		1st	2nd	3rd	
4-ASA, 5-ASA	B1	B > R	B > R	B > R	II
Sulfasalazine	B1	B > R	B > R	B > R	II

Food and Drug Administration (FDA) pregnancy categories:
A = Well-controlled studies fail to demonstrate risk to the fetus.
B1 = Animal studies fail to demonstrate risk to the fetus but no human studies are available.
B2 = Animal studies show some risk to the fetus but this is not confirmed in human studies.
C1 = Animal studies show risk to the fetus but no human studies are available.
C2 = Animal and human studies are unavailable.
D = Drugs associated with birth defects but with potential benefits that may outweigh known risks.
X = Drugs associated with birth defects and with potential risk that clearly outweighs potential benefit.
Risk vs benefit: R >> B = Proven or potential risk outweighs potential benefits.
B > R = Potential benefits outweigh potential risks.
R >> B? = Risks may be outweighed by benefits in some circumstances.
? = Risk-to-benefit ratio is unknown.

Breast-feeding categories:
I = Drug does not enter breast milk.
II = Drug enters breast milk but is not known to be harmful in therapeutic doses.
IIIA = Drug may or may not enter breast milk but no adverse effects are expected.
IIIB = Drug may or may not enter breast milk but drug is systemically absorbed.
IV = Drug enters breast milk and poses a potential risk to the neonate.

DRUG INTERACTIONS

Sulfasalazine, but not its metabolites, competitively inhibits the absorption of folic acid. Cholestyramine directly binds sulfasalazine in the gut lumen and markedly decreases the metabolism of the drug. A similar interaction has been reported between ferrous sulfate and sulfasalazine. Sulfasalazine decreases the bioavailability of digoxin. Sulfasalazine metabolism is diminished by the concurrent administration of broad-spectrum antibiotics.

NEW ANALOGUES

A discussion of the newer 5-ASA analogues is found in Chap. 11. However, a few points should be made with respect to the comparative efficacy of SA and these newer compounds. In ulcerative colitis, SA and the 5-ASA analogues in a dose of at least 2 gm/day appear to be equivalent in terms of remission rates of mild or moderately active disease and in maintenance of remission. Although some data indicate that patients with active Crohn's colitis or ileocolitis may benefit from 5-ASA compounds, issues of comparative efficacy to SA, maintenance of remission, and optimal dosage remain in question.

PEARLS AND PITFALLS

1. There is no place for sulfasalazine in the treatment of acute, severe flares of ulcerative colitis.
2. Sulfasalazine can be safely used in pregnant and nursing women.
3. Oligospermia and abnormal sperm motility can be seen while receiving SA therapy that can result in reversible male infertility. Sperm counts and morphology usually return to normal within 3 months of discontinuing SA. A 5-ASA analogue should be considered in male patients who are contemplating starting a family.
4. Desensitization should be attempted in patients who are intolerant of sulfasalazine or who have mild hypersensitivity or idiosyncratic reactions. Most patients can be successfully desensitized. 5-ASA analogues may be used in the patients who fail desensitization or exhibit severe allergic or idiosyncratic reactions.
5. 5-ASA analogues should be tried in patients with distal ulcerative colitis in whom oral sulfasalazine and steroid enemas have failed. These often obviate the need for oral steroids.
6. Sulfasalazine does not appear to be effective in Crohn's disease that is limited to the small bowel.
7. Megaloblastic anemia should alert the physician to the need to give supplemental folic acid (1 mg/day) to patients receiving SA. Other drugs capable of inducing megaloblastic anemia include ethanol, methotrexate, and phenytoin (Dilantin). Other conditions capable of causing megaloblastic anemia include tropical sprue, terminal ileitis, pernicious anemia, and cirrhosis.

Suggested Reading

Azad Khan AK. Optimum dose of sulphasalazine for maintenance treatment in ulcerative colitis. Gut 1980; 21:232–240.

A landmark clinical trial that established the optimum maintenance dose of sulfasalazine as 2 gm/day.

Collen MJ. Azulfidine-induced oligospermia. Am J Gastroenterol 1980; 74:441–442.

A case report and discussion.

Craven PA, Pfanstel J, Saito R. Actions of sulfasalazine and (5)–aminosalicylic acid as reactive oxygen scavengers in the suppression of bile acid–induced increases in colonic epithelial cell loss and proliferative activity. Gastroenterology 1987; 92:1998–2008.
The study examines the mechanism of protective action of sulfasalazine in a rat model in which colonic epithelial cell loss and subsequent increases in epithelial proliferative activity were induced by intracolonic instillation of sodium deoxycholate.

Das KM, Chowdhury R, Fara JW. Small bowel absorption of sulfasalazine and its hepatic metabolism in human beings, cats, and rats. Gastroenterology 1979; 77:280–284.
The absorption and hepatic metabolism of sulfasalazine are discussed at length.

Donaldson RM. Management of medical problems in pregnancy—inflammatory bowel disease. N Engl J Med 1985; 312:1616–1619.
An excellent discussion of pregnancy in relationship to clinical, diagnostic, and therapeutic aspects of inflammatory bowel disease.

Gaginella T, Walsh RE. Sulfasalazine, multiplicity of action. Dig Dis Sci 1992; 37:801–812.
An excellent review of the effects of sulfasalazine (Azulfidine) at the cellular level.

Haines JD. Hepatotoxicity after treatment with sulfasalazine. Postgrad Med 1986; 79:193–198.
A case report and discussion.

Hamadeh MA, Atkinson J, Smith LJ. Sulfasalazine-induced pulmonary disease. Chest 1992; 101:1003–1037.
A case report of two patients presenting with sulfasalazine-induced pulmonary toxicity and a review of the literature.

Jacobson IM, Kelsey PB, Blyden GT. Sulfasalazine-induced agranulocytosis. Am J Gastroenterol 1985; 80:118–121.
A case report and discussion.

Korelitz B, et al. Desensitization to sulfasalazine after hypersensitivity reactions in patients with inflammatory bowel disease. J Clin Gastroenterol 1984; 6:27–31.
A report of 40 of 47 patients with hypersensitivity reactions successfully desensitized.

Margolin ML, et al. Clinical trials in ulcerative colitis II. Historical review. Am J Gastroenterol 1988; 83:227–243.
An exhaustive review of clinical trials in ulcerative colitis, with insightful comments by the authors on their significance.

Miyachi Y, Yoshioka A, Imamura S. Effect of sulphasalazine and its metabolites on the generation of reactive oxygen species. Gut 1987; 28:190–195.
The in vitro anti-oxidant effects of sulfasalazine and its metabolites are studied.

Peppercorn MA. Sulfasalazine: Pharmacology, clinical use, toxicity, and related new drug development. Ann Intern Med 1984; 101: 377–386.
An excellent review article on all aspects of sulfasalazine.

Schoonjans R, Mast A, et al. Sulfasalazine-associated encephalopathy in a patient with Crohn's disease. Am J Gastroenterol 1993; 8:1416–1420.
The development of coma and upper extremity monoparesis is described in a patient who developed hepatitis and dermatitis while being treated with Azulfidine.

Schroder H, Campbell DE. Absorption, metabolism, and excretion of salicylazosulfapyridine in man. Clin Pharmacol Ther 1972; 13: 539–551.

A study of the pharmacology of sulfasalazine in nine healthy patients who received 4 gm/day for 10 days.

Shanahan F, Targan S. Sulfasalazine and salicylate-induced exacerbation of ulcerative colitis. N Engl J Med 1987; 317:455.

A letter attributing the rare acute hemorrhagic colitis side effect to the salicylate moiety.

Soldata PD, et al. A possible mechanism of action of sulfasalazine and 5-aminosalicylic acid in inflammatory bowel diseases: Interaction with oxygen-free radicals. Gastroenterology 1985; 89: 1215–1216.

The paper relates the in vivo anti-inflammatory action of sulfasalazine to its ability, through 5–aminosalicylic acid, to scavenge oxygen-free radicals.

Summers RW, et al. National Cooperative Crohn's Disease Study: Results of drug treatment. 1979; 77:847–869.

A double-blind, randomized trial that compared sulfasalazine (1 gm/15 mg body weight) to placebo over 4 months in patients with various degrees of involvement of Crohn's disease.

Sutherland LR, May GR, Shaffer EA. Sulfasalazine revisited: A meta-analysis of 5–aminosalicylic acid in the treatment of ulcerative colitis. Ann Intern Med 1993; 118:540–549.

Sulfasalazine and newer 5-ASA preparations are superior to placebo but are equivalent to each other in terms of treatment of active disease and maintenance of remission.

Taffet SL, Das KM. Desensitization in patients with inflammatory bowel disease to sulfasalazine. Am J Med 1982; 73:520–524.

A presentation of one method of desensitization.

Wu FC, Aitken RJ, Ferguson A. Inflammatory bowel disease and infertility: Effects of sulfasalazine and 5–aminosalicylic acid on sperm-fertilizing capacity and reactive oxygen species generation. Fertil Steril 1989; 52:842–845.

Sperm motility, density, and function are assayed. Poor sperm function in patients being treated with sulfasalazine was noted to improve when 5-ASA was utilized.

Antimetabolites

Michael M. Van Ness

The immunosuppressive drugs 6-mercaptopurine, azathioprine, and methotrexate may benefit a selected group of patients with inflammatory bowel disease. Their use requires careful consideration by the physician of their risks, benefits, and limitations. Detailed instruction to the patient cannot be overemphasized. Signing of a doctor-patient "contract" is a useful tool to ensure complete understanding of the risks and benefits of these agents.

Brooke and associates published the first anecdotal report of the benefit of azathioprine in six patients with Crohn's disease. Since then, seven controlled trials with azathioprine, one controlled trial with 6-mercaptopurine, and one open-labeled trial with methotrexate have been conducted and form the basis for use of these agents in inflammatory bowel disease.

PHARMACOLOGY

Both 6-mercaptopurine and azathioprine are antimetabolites that inhibit purine-ring biosynthesis, thereby decreasing deoxyribonucleic acid (DNA) synthesis and impeding cellular division. Azathioprine is produced by conjugation of a free SH group to 6-mercaptopurine. It was developed in the hope of decreasing the toxicity of 6-mercaptopurine without decreasing its effectiveness. By weight, 6-mercaptopurine accounts for 54 percent of a dose of azathioprine. Both 6-mercaptopurine and azathioprine are metabolized by enzymatic oxidation by xanthine oxidase. Allopurinol, a powerful inhibitor of xanthine oxidase, greatly potentiates the cytotoxic action and toxic side effects of 6-mercaptopurine and azathioprine. Concurrent administration of allopurinol necessitates a 75 percent dose reduction of 6-mercaptopurine so as to avoid untoward side effects.

Methotrexate is another antimetabolite. It is a folic acid analogue and acts to inhibit regeneration of tetrahydrofolate, which is necessary for methyl group transfer, and thereby inhibits de novo synthesis of purine nucleotides.

INDICATIONS

Based on the work of Present, Lennard-Jones, Korelitz, and Kozarek, indications for use of these drugs are strictly defined (Table 9-1). Patients who fail to achieve a remission on high-dose steroids (40–60 mg/day), patients who fail to maintain a remission on sulfasalazine or 5-ASA agents and require intermittent use of high-dose steroids, patients who respond to steroids but who experience multiple early relapses, and patients who have active fistulous disease that is unresponsive to corticosteroids and metronidazole (Flagyl) may be candidates for 6-mercaptopurine. Most authors favor use of 6-mercaptopurine instead of azathioprine, as 6-mercaptopurine is the active form of the pro-drug azathioprine and its effects are believed to be more predictable.

The largest clinical trial of 6-mercaptopurine in Crohn's disease was conducted by Present and his colleagues. They studied 83 patients with Crohn's disease that was active at the time of, or just

Table 9-1. Indications for use of 6-mercaptopurine in Crohn's disease

1. Active Crohn's disease unresponsive to maximal medical management, including sulfasalazine and corticosteroids.
2. Prolonged (> 6 mo) corticosteroid use or multiple, early relapses necessitating high-dose corticosteroid use.
3. Fistula unresponsive to maximal medical management, including metronidazole and corticosteroids.

before, entry into the study. These patients had had Crohn's disease for a mean of 4.3 years. Four groups were analyzed: patients with ileitis with fistulae, patients with ileitis without fistulae, patients with colitis or ileocolitis with fistulae, and patients with colitis or ileocolitis without fistulae. There was no arbitrary cessation of ongoing drug therapy at the time of entry into the study; in particular, corticosteroids were not arbitrarily stopped.

Overall, between 67 and 79 percent of patients taking 6-mercaptopurine improved, compared to only 13 percent of patients taking placebo. Fistulae healed in 31 percent of patients taking 6-mercaptopurine, versus only 6 percent of patients taking placebo. In patients receiving 6-mercaptopurine, steroids were able to be discontinued in 55 percent and reduced in another 20 percent (total 75%), compared to steroid cessation or reduction in only 36 percent of patients receiving placebo. Clinical improvement after steroid cessation or reduction was maintained in 64 percent of patients receiving long-term therapy (up to 2 years in this study, up to 5 years in another). The mean time to response was 3.1 months (range 2 weeks to 9 months). There was a somewhat higher frequency of response (77%) in patients with ileocolonic disease compared to ileitis or colitis alone. The response to 6-mercaptopurine did not appear to be dose-related, with a mean dose of 70 mg/day in responders, compared to 89 mg/day in nonresponders.

Subsequent studies have added to our understanding of therapy of Crohn's disease with 6-mercaptopurine. Patients who respond to the drug and subsequently stop the agent have a mean time to relapse of 12 months (0.5–42.0 months). Responders who stop the drug, relapse, and recommence therapy have a short mean time until a second response (1.5 months compared to 3.1 months initially). The risk of malignancy from use of 6-mercaptopurine does not appear to be increased. Unlike renal transplant patients, who also receive combination immunosuppressive therapy, these patients receive relatively modest amounts of drug.

Fistulae have been shown to improve with treatment with 6-mercaptopurine. In a series reported by Korelitz and Present, improvement with fistula closure was seen in 39 percent and improvement in fistulae without complete closure in another 26 percent. Fistulae were more likely to heal in patients with no prior surgical history. The site of intestinal involvement with Crohn's disease appeared unrelated to the likelihood of fistula healing. With continuous therapy, fistulae remained closed for up to 5 years.

Patients with disease that is refractory to high-dose corticosteroid therapy may be candidates for methotrexate. Kozarek and associates treated 14 Crohn's disease and 7 ulcerative colitis (UC) patients with 25 mg intramuscular methotrexate once a week for 12 weeks

Clinical and histologic improvement was seen in both diseases but was better in the Crohn's patients. None of the seven patients with UC achieved a complete remission.

CONTRAINDICATIONS

Antimetabolic agents are relatively contraindicated for use in the pregnant patient. Despite a dearth of knowledge about teratogenicity, therapeutic abortion was once recommended by some authors if a patient taking 6-mercaptopurine became pregnant. On the other hand, uncomplicated pregnancies resulting in normal children are reported in women with malignant disease treated with chemotherapeutic agents. Recently, Alstead and associates reported 16 uncomplicated pregnancies in 14 women taking azathioprine for inflammatory bowel disease. Therefore, the difficult question of termination of pregnancy remains unanswered in this population and must be individualized case by case.

6-Mercaptopurine is contraindicated for use in the patient with a previous episode of either azathioprine- or 6-mercaptopurine–induced pancreatitis. Pancreatitis is a rare complication of their use and is manifested by the development of abdominal pain, fever, nausea, and vomiting within the first month of therapy. In Haber and associates' report of thirteen 6-mercaptopurine–associated cases, the incidence was 3.25 percent, the onset was within 8 to 32 days, and the amylase elevation averaged 6 times normal. With cessation of the drug, all signs and symptoms resolved rapidly (range 1–11 days) without complication. Of the seven patients rechallenged with the drug, all developed recurrent pancreatitis. All efforts to desensitize the patients to the agent by initiating therapy with very small doses were unsuccessful and led to recurrent pancreatitis. The authors conclude that, once implicated as a cause of pancreatitis, neither azathioprine nor 6-mercaptopurine should be utilized again.

ADMINISTRATION

Before administration of antimetabolite therapy, a clear understanding of the indications, dosing, side effects, and duration of therapy must be reached between the physician and the patient. This "contract" is best signed, with copies retained by both parties. An example of such a document is given in Fig. 9-1.

6-Mercaptopurine is best administered as a single daily oral dose, 1.0 mg/kg body weight. There is little benefit to increasing the dose beyond this level, as there is no known dose-response curve. Azathioprine is best given as a single daily dose, 1.0 mg/kg, and increased within 2 weeks to a maximum of 2.5 mg/kg, once a day. Methotrexate, 25 mg intramuscularly once a week as an initial dose, can be continued for 12 weeks and then decreased slowly to a maintenance dose of 7.5 mg orally per week. The side effects of neutropenia and thrombocytopenia are seen with all three agents and are clearly dose-related. Before the first dose is given, a complete blood cell count, platelet count, and serum amylase determination, and serum levels of serum alanine aminotransferase, aspartate aminotransferase, and alkaline phosphatase are required. Thereafter, weekly complete blood and platelet counts should be monitored to guide dose adjustments so as to keep the white blood cell counts above 4500 cells per cubic millimeter and platelet counts above 100,000 per cubic millimeter. Once the patient's condition is stable, the frequency of blood studies can be decreased to a monthly basis. Abdominal pain,

DATE: ______________________

PATIENT'S NAME: ______________________

DIAGNOSIS: ______________________

MEDICATIONS: ______________________

I, ______________________
(patient's name)
have been informed by my doctor of the need to take the medication 6-mercaptopurine at a starting daily dose of

______________________ .
(number of the 50-milligram pills)

I understand that this drug can decrease the number of white blood cells in my blood.

I understand the need to have blood drawn weekly until my white blood cell count is stable.

I understand that this drug can cause pancreatitis and hepatitis.

I understand the need to inform my doctor as soon as possible of fever, abdominal pain, vomiting, or jaundice.

I understand that it may take as long as 3 to 6 months before I have any benefit from 6-mercaptopurine.

I understand that I may have no benefit whatsoever from this medication.

PATIENT'S SIGNATURE: ______________________

PHYSICIAN'S SIGNATURE: ______________________

Fig. 9-1. Patient contract for treatment with 6-mercaptopurine.

back pain, and elevated serum amylase, or fever alone, require abrupt cessation of 6-mercaptopurine therapy. If the diagnosis of pancreatitis is confirmed, 6-mercaptopurine should not be restarted. Rarely should 6-mercaptopurine be continued in the face of a known systemic infection.

Longer-term hepatotoxic effects can be seen with 6-mercaptopurine, azathioprine, and methotrexate. Jaundice secondary to cholestasis is seen with 6-mercaptopurine and azathioprine. Rarer, long-term effects of azathioprine include veno-occlusive disease and peliosis hepatis. Hepatic steatosis, fibrosis, and cirrhosis are known consequences of methotrexate therapy, are not detectable by routine liver chemistries, and require routine percutaneous liver biopsy after a 1- to 1.5-gm cumulative methotrexate dose.

PEARLS AND PITFALLS

1. Corticosteroid sparing is a known benefit of 6-mercaptopurine.
2. A trial of 6-mercaptopurine cannot be called a failure until the end of a trial period of at least 3 months.
3. There is little or no benefit to pushing the daily dose higher than 1.5 mg/kg body weight.
4. Pancreatitis from 6-mercaptopurine usually occurs within 30 days of initiation of therapy, usually is uncomplicated, and precludes future use of 6-mercaptopurine in that patient.
5. The signing of a "contract" by the patient minimizes the risk of misunderstandings in the use of this drug.

Suggested Reading

Alstead EM, et al. Safety of azathioprine in pregnancy in inflammatory bowel disease. Gastroenterology 1990; 99:443–446.
Although not recommended, azathioprine use was without complication in this retrospective review of 16 pregnancies in 14 women receiving azathioprine for inflammatory bowel disease (12 Crohn's disease, 2 UC).

Brooke BN, Hoffman DC, Swarbrick ET. Azathioprine for Crohn's disease. Lancet 1969; 2:612–614.
These initial six cases are the basis for the subsequent trials of immunosuppressive agents for treatment of inflammatory bowel disease.

Ewe K, et al. Azathioprine combined with prednisolone or mono therapy with prednisolone in active Crohn's disease. Gastroenterology 1993; 105:367–372.
Steroid-sparing is seen with azathioprine use. More patients were in remission on lower doses of prednisolone in the azathioprine-treated group. Immunosuppressive therapy should be reserved for patients with steroid-dependent disease.

Haber CJ, et al. Nature and course of pancreatitis caused by 6-mercaptopurine in the treatment of inflammatory bowel disease. Gastroenterology 1986; 91:982–986.
The authors report the clinical course of 13 cases of pancreatitis attributable to 6-mercaptopurine (6-MP) in 400 (3.25%) patients with inflammatory bowel disease. The pancreatitis tends to occur early (within 30 days), is usually mild, and recurs with rechallenge.

Korelitz BI, Present DH. Favorable effect of 6-mercaptopurine on fistulae of Crohn's disease. Dig Dis Sci 1985; 30:58–64.

The authors present the data from the original New England Journal of Medicine *report and add interesting long-term follow-up data supporting the claim that 6-MP is efficacious in the maintenance of fistulae closure for up to 5 years.*

Kozarek RA, et al. Methotrexate induces clinical and histologic remission in patients with refractory inflammatory bowel disease. Ann Intern Med 1989; 110:353–356.

Disease activity and steroid dose decreased in this group of 21 patients with inflammatory bowel disease (IBD). Unfortunately, four of seven UC patients required surgery.

Lennard-Jones JE. Inflammatory bowel disease: medical therapy revisited. Scand J Gastro Supple 1992; 192:110–116.

A review by the leading world expert of the different drugs available for treatment of IBD.

Markowitz J, et al. 6-Mercaptopurine in adolescents. Gastroenterology 1990; 99:1347–1351.

Compared with the year preceding 6-mercaptopurine therapy, the first year of 6-MP treatment resulted in decreased disease activity, cessation of prednisone in 80 percent of cases, and improved nutrition.

Present DH, et al. Treatment of Crohn's disease with 6-mercaptopurine. N Engl J Med 1980; 302:981–987.

The landmark article showing benefit of 6-MP. Reduction of steroid dosages, closure of fistulae, and clinical improvement in cases refractory to sulfasalazine and corticosteroids were demonstrated. The onset of response was often delayed as long as 3 months.

Present DH, et al. 6-Mercaptopurine in the management of inflammatory bowel disease: Short and long-term toxicity. Ann Intern Med 1989; 111:641–649.

Although toxicity is seen in about 10 percent of patients who received 6-mercaptopurine for inflammatory bowel disease (33% pancreatitis, 2% bone marrow depression, 2% allergic reactions, 0.3% drug-induced hepatitis in 120 UC patients and 276 patients with Crohn's disease), the authors conclude that the overall benefit of this agent outweighs these reversible effects, especially in patients with disease that is refractory to other therapies.

Singleton JW. Azathioprine has a very limited role in the treatment of Crohn's disease. Dig Dis Sci 1981; 26:368–371.

The author reviews the National Cooperative Crohn's Disease Study (NCCDS) and concludes that azathioprine has no role as initial therapy for active Crohn's disease. Although he concedes that it may be useful as an adjunct to prednisone in disease that is unresponsive to sulfasalazine and prednisone, he notes that the excess risk of cancer, as defined by Kinlen in patients given azathioprine for nontransplant, noncancer indications, is increased 1.6-fold.

Metronidazole

J. Thomas Dorsey III

Metronidazole is an antimicrobial agent with antibacterial, antiprotozoal, and anti-inflammatory actions that is useful in the treatment of a variety of infectious diseases of the gastrointestinal tract and in specific forms of Crohn's disease.

The parent compound, azomysin, was discovered by Nakamura in 1955 and was shown to have antitrichomonal activity in 1956. In 1959, Cosar showed the azomysin derivative, metronidazole, to have both in vitro and in vivo antitrichomonal activity. Metronidazole was the first and remains the most widely used derivative. Its effectiveness against anaerobes was demonstrated in 1963 and it was subsequently shown to be highly effective in parasitic diseases of the gut, most notably against *Entamoeba histolytica* and *Giardia lamblia*. The first evidence of activity in inflammatory bowel disease was shown in 1975; since that time it has been actively studied. Recently, metronidazole has been shown effective in combination therapy directed at *Helicobacter pylori*.

PHARMACOLOGY

1-(β-Hydroxyethyl)-2-methyl-5-nitroimidazole is a pale yellow, crystalline substance slightly soluble in water and alcohol. An oral dose is exceptionally well absorbed, yielding plasma levels similar to those achieved with an equal intravenous dose. It is also well absorbed rectally, although more variably and at a slower rate. Peak blood levels occur 1 to 2 hours after an oral dose. The drug circulates in the plasma less than 20 percent protein-bound. Serum half-life is 8 hours. It diffuses freely into total body water with levels in cerebrospinal fluid, saliva, bile, bone, and breast milk equivalent to serum levels. It appears rapidly on all mucosal surfaces, and bactericidal concentrations have been documented in pus from hepatic abscesses.

Nonhepatic metabolism in humans is negligible. The primary metabolic site is the liver via oxidation of side chains and glucuronide formation. Urinary excretion accounts for 60 to 80 percent of a given dose, with 80 percent as metabolites and 20 percent as unchanged drug. Stool excretion accounts for 6 to 15 percent. Metabolites may impart a reddish-brown discoloration to the urine but this has no clinical significance. Renal failure does not alter the distribution or metabolism of the drug and there is no need for dose reduction except in severe renal insufficiency. Hemodialysis removes 50 percent of a given dose. Patients with hepatic insufficiency as manifested by ascites, encephalopathy, low albumin levels, or a prolonged prothrombin time have decreased metabolism and require dose reduction.

MECHANISM OF ACTION, INDICATIONS, AND ADMINISTRATION

Anaerobic Bacteria and Protozoa

The drug is taken up by passive diffusion and rapidly metabolized, -reasing the intracellular concentration of unchanged drug and thus increasing the transmembrane concentration gradient leading to continuous uptake. Metabolism in bacteria is via reduction of the nitro group by nitroreductases, which play a major role in anaerobic energy metabolism. Metronidazole acts as an electron sink depriving the cells of reducing equivalent. In addition, the reduction of metronidazole yields free radicals, short-lived cytotoxic intermediates that interact with deoxyribonucleic acid (DNA) and other intracellular macromolecules. These metabolites disrupt the helical structure of DNA and cause single- and double-stranded breaks.

Inflammatory Bowel Disease

The mode of action in inflammatory bowel disease is unknown. Possible mechanisms include its antimicrobial effect in eliminating bacterial overgrowth and reducing the load of bacterial antigens. In an animal model metronidazole has been shown to inhibit some parameters of cell-mediated immunity, specifically granuloma formation. Finally, metronidazole may have a direct tissue effect.

Ulcerative Colitis

There have been two prospective, randomized, double-blind controlled trials of metronidazole in ulcerative colitis. In 1977, Davies and associates studied the effect of metronidazole suppositories in mild chronic proctitis. There was no evidence of benefit on clinical, endoscopic, or histologic parameters after 28 days of therapy. In the second study, a 5-day course of intravenous metronidazole failed to improve remission rate, need for urgent surgery, or late mortality in hospitalized patients with severe colitis requiring intravenous and topical steroids and total parenteral nutrition. Current evidence does not support the use of metronidazole in ulcerative colitis with several exceptions.

In patients with ulcerative colitis and incipient toxic megacolon (fever, leukocytosis, distention) broad-spectrum antibiotic therapy is indicated. A combination of gentamicin and metronidazole provides excellent coverage of anaerobes, but also covers *Clostridium difficile* and amebic infections that can complicate ulcerative colitis. Secondly, in patients who have had a colectomy and ileal pouch procedure, metronidazole has shown benefit in therapy of pouchitis. Finally, in some studies, metronidazole has shown benefit as a maintenance therapy for ulcerative colitis.

Crohn's Disease

Ursing and Kamme reported their experience with metronidazole in five patients with Crohn's disease in 1975. Four of the five improved clinically and biochemically within 4 weeks, and three of these were able to discontinue sulfasalazine and steroids. One patient had a more gradual response over 4 months.

Blichfeldt and associates treated 22 patients with Crohn's disease requiring sulfasalazine and steroids with metronidazole for 2 months in a double-blind crossover trial compared with placebo. Patients with small-bowel Crohn's disease showed no response, but those with colitis demonstrated a striking improvement in symptoms (diarrhea, abdominal pain, and sense of well-being) and biochemical markers (hematocrit and erythrocyte sedimentation rate).

Bernstein and associates studied the effect of metronidazole in 21 patients with chronic, unremitting perianal Crohn's disease. Twenty improved on a dose of 20 mg/kg/day and 10 healed completely

chronic therapy. In a follow-up study, Brandt confirmed the beneficial effects and showed that (1) therapy could be discontinued in only 28 percent of patients without recurrence, (2) recurrences were fewer if the drug was tapered rather than stopped abruptly, (3) all recurrences responded to reinstitution of therapy at full dose, and (4) remissions were maintained for the duration of the study (36 months) on therapy.

Ursing and associates compared metronidazole, 0.8 gm/day, to sulfasalazine, 3 gm/day, in a randomized, double-blind controlled trial and found no difference in efficacy. However, the metronidazole group had greater biochemical improvement. In addition, sulfasalazine nonresponders showed clinical response to metronidazole but metronidazole nonresponders demonstrated no clinical or biochemical response to sulfasalazine. It was concluded that both are efficacious in Crohn's disease of the colon, with metronidazole demonstrating slightly more efficacy.

Current indications for metronidazole in Crohn's disease include (1) perianal disease (abscesses, ulcerations, and fistulae, including retrovaginal fistulae) that requires higher doses, 1 to 2 gm/day; (2) Crohn's ileocolitis and colitis, in which it is as effective as sulfasalazine for mild to moderate disease at doses of 10 to 20 mg/kg/day; (3) metastatic skin ulcerations of Crohn's disease; and (4) sulfasalazine intolerance or allergy. There may be a role for metronidazole in therapy of enterocutaneous fistulae and recalcitrant small bowel disease, but these indications have not been studied in clinical trials.

The drug should be continued until either healing occurs, no additional benefits are seen, or side effects occur. The dose should be tapered in those who respond and if disease recurs the full dose should be reinstituted.

Bacterial Infections: Anaerobes

Metronidazole has little activity against gram-positive and gram-negative aerobic bacteria. It demonstrates activity against a wide variety of anaerobic organisms, including gram-negative rods (*Bacteroides* species such as *B. fragilis* and *Fusobacterium*), gram-positive rods (*Clostridium* species including *C. difficile* and *Eubacteriales*), and gram-positive cocci (*Peptococcus* and *Peptostreptococcus*). *Bifidobacterium, Actinomyces, Arachnida,* and *Propionibacterium* are resistant. *Bacteroides fragilis* is a common anaerobe that causes life-threatening infections. It is often multiply resistant to other antibiotics. It may manifest a relative resistance to metronidazole that is mediated by a decreased nitroreductase activity. In practice, this resistance can be overcome by increasing the dose.

Metronidazole has been effective in meningitis, brain abscess, osteomyelitis, septic arthritis, and endocarditis caused by these organisms. It is also quite effective in pelvic and intra-abdominal abscesses, including diverticular abscesses, biliary sepsis, hepatic abscess, and necrotizing enterocolitis.

A loading dose of 15 mg/kg is given over a period of 1 hour, followed by 7.5 mg/kg every 6 hours infused over 1 hour. When the patient is responding, therapy can be completed by oral administration of 7.5 mg/kg orally every 6 hours.

Clostridium Difficile–Associated Colitis

Teasley and associates demonstrated in a prospective, randomized clinical trial that metronidazole has equivalent efficacy, relapse rates, and patient tolerance to oral vancomycin therapy in treatment of *C. difficile*–associated colitis. Metronidazole has the advantage of being much less expensive. Dosage is 500 mg orally twice a day for 10 days. It should be noted that in rare instances metronidazole has apparently caused *C. difficile*–associated colitis. The oral route is preferred at dosages of 250 mg 4 times a day to 750 mg 3 times a day for 7 to 10 days. Although less effective, it can be given parenterally at 500 mg intravenously every 6 to 8 hours in patients who are unable to take oral medications.

Helicobacter pylori

Although not effective as a single agent, metronidazole used in combination with tetracycline and bismuth subsalicylate can eradicate 90 percent of infections after 2 weeks of therapy. This combination has been shown to accelerate ulcer healing and decrease ulcer recurrence at 2 years from 95 percent in ranitidine-healed ulcers to 12 percent in the study group. Resistance to metronidazole has been reported and approaches 40 to 50 percent in developing countries. Other combinations with efficacy against *H. pylori* include metronidazole with amoxicillin and ranitidine and omeprazole with amoxicillin.

Surgical Prophylaxis

Metronidazole has also been used perioperatively in colon surgery, appendectomy, and hysterectomy to decrease the incidence of intraabdominal and wound infections. It is as effective as other drugs in this setting.

Protozoal Infections

Amebiasis

Metronidazole is exceedingly active against *E. histolytica*. In culture, drug concentrations of 1 to 2 μg/ml kill 100 percent of organisms at 24 hours, and concentrations of 0.2 μg/ml kill 100 percent of organisms at 72 hours. There have been no reports of resistance, but asymptomatic cyst carriers are not adequately treated by metronidazole. The drug is active against dysenteric and hepatic forms of infection. Most hepatic abscesses respond dramatically with prompt reduction in size. Failure to respond after 48 hours may indicate the need for percutaneous or surgical drainage. In both dysentery and hepatic abscess, therapy must be followed by a luminacidal agent (iodoquinol) to ensure that no organisms persist. Adult dosage in dysentery and hepatic amebiasis is 750 mg orally or intravenously 3 times a day for 10 days, followed by iodoquinol, 650 mg orally 3 times a day for 20 days. In children, the correct dosage is 35 to 50 mg/kg/day in three doses for 10 days, followed by iodoquinol, 40 mg/kg/day (maximum 2 gm) in three divided doses for 20 days.

Balantidium coli

Balantidium coli is a parasite of hogs that can cause dysentery in humans and mimics *E. histolytica*. Metronidazole (500 mg orally 4 times a day for 10 days), followed by iodoquinol (650 mg orally 3 times a day for 20 days) is effective. In children, the dosage of metronidazole is 10 mg/kg 4 times a day for 10 days (maximum dose 2 gm/day), followed by iodoquinol, 40 mg/kg/day (maximum 2 gm) in three divided doses for 20 days.

Entamoeba polecki

Entamoeba polecki is another porcine parasite, seen in immigrants from southeast Asia. It may be mistaken for *E. histolytica.* Therapy consists of metronidazole in doses used for *E. histolytica* followed by diloxanide furoate, 500 mg orally 3 times a day for 10 days in adults, and 20 mg/kg/day in three doses for 10 days in children.

Giardiasis

Metronidazole has not been approved by the Food and Drug Administration (FDA) for the therapy of *G. lamblia,* but it is an effective and well-tolerated alternative to quinacrine. The recommended dosage is 250 mg orally 3 times a day for 5 to 7 days in adults and 5 mg/kg 3 times a day for 7 days in children. Asymptomatic cyst passers should be treated.

Blastocystis hominis

Blastocystis hominis is a protozoan that causes mild to moderate abdominal cramping and nonfebrile, nonbloody diarrhea that may be recurrent. Metronidazole, 750 mg orally 3 times a day for 10 days in adults and 35 to 50 mg/kg/day in three divided doses for 10 days in children, results in 60 to 70 percent cure rates.

Dracunculiasis

Infestation by the guinea worm, *Dracunculus medinensis,* is seen worldwide in the tropics. Metronidazole, 250 mg orally 3 times a day for 7 days, is an effective alternative to thiabendazole or niridazole.

SIDE EFFECTS AND CONTRAINDICATIONS

Metronidazole is generally well tolerated and only rarely are side effects sufficiently severe to cause discontinuation. Most side effects are self-limited.

Contraindications to use include hypersensitivity to metronidazole or other imidazoles. Relative contraindications are pregnancy (first trimester), a history of a blood dyscrasia, or active neurologic disease (neuropathy or seizure disorder).

The most common side effects are gastrointestinal. A metallic taste occurs in 92 percent of patients. Glossitis, stomatitis, furry tongue, and dry mouth are not uncommon. Anorexia, nausea, vomiting, epigastric pain and discomfort, and cramps are also seen. Therapy can cause an exacerbation of candidiasis. As mentioned previously, it has rarely been implicated in causing *C. difficile* colitis.

Neurologic side effects, including headache, ataxia, mood swings, vertigo, encephalopathy, and seizures, are not uncommon and warrant discontinuation of therapy. Peripheral neuropathy is common with prolonged use. It is commonly sensory with paresthesias involving lower extremities and is more prominent in the winter months. It is associated with higher doses and longer duration of therapy, with 50 percent of patients affected after 6 months of therapy. It is reversible if recognized early and the dose decreased or stopped. It can persist for a prolonged period after cessation of the drug.

Dermatologic side effects include urticaria, flushing, and pruritus. Genitourinary complaints include vaginal dryness and burning, cystitis, urethritis, pelvic pressure, and discoloration of urine.

Hematologic manifestations include reversible neutropenia and thrombocytopenia seen after long-term use. Complete blood counts are recommended during prolonged therapy. Phlebitis at the site of infusion has been reported.

Metronidazole causes an artifactual depression of serum glutamic oxaloacetic transaminase (SGOT) levels.

Metronidazole and its metabolites are mutagenic in bacterial culture. It is oncogenic in mice and rats but not in hamsters. Its mechanism of action in bacteria and protozoa involves direct damage to cellular DNA. Despite these findings, no chromosomal abnormalities were demonstrated in humans receiving 20 mg/kg/day for prolonged periods. No teratogenicity has been demonstrated in human fetuses.

Several retrospective human studies have shown no increased incidence of malignancies in patients receiving metronidazole. The most recent study showed no increased cancer in a group of 771 women followed for 15 to 25 years after exposure.

Used in pregnancy, metronidazole crosses the placenta and rapidly enters the fetal circulation. Although no teratogenic effect has been noted in several small series of human pregnancies or in rodents, the use of metronidazole is relatively contraindicated in pregnancy because of the possibility of carcinogenic potential with a long latent period.

In nursing mothers, metronidazole achieves breast milk concentrations similar to plasma levels. Although there are no known ill effects, the potential for carcinogenesis with a long latent period must be considered such that metronidazole's use in nursing mothers is relatively contraindicated.

Metronidazole is currently being investigated as a radiosensitizer to potentiate the effect of radiation on certain malignancies.

DRUG INTERACTIONS

Alcohol

Metronidazole can cause a disulfiramlike reaction, with cramps, headache, flushing, nausea, and vomiting. Alcohol should be strictly avoided until at least 24 hours after the last dose.

Sulfasalazine

Concern over metronidazole elimination of the bacterial population required for activation of sulfasalazine was dismissed by a study showing no change in blood sulfapyridine levels in 10 patients treated with both drugs over a 2-week period. Metronidazole does not decrease the bioavailability of sulfasalazine.

Warfarin

Metronidazole potentiates warfarin prolongation of prothrombin time. Prothrombin times should be monitored and doses adjusted accordingly when these two drugs are used together.

Cimetidine

Cimetidine decreases clearance of metronidazole. This drug interaction is of no significance in patients with intact liver and kidney function.

Anticonvulsants

Metronidazole decreases the clearance of phenytoin (Dilantin), causing elevated serum Dilantin levels. Both Dilantin and phenobarbital increase metronidazole clearance.

PEARLS AND PITFALLS

1. Human metabolism of metronidazole is almost exclusively hepatic. Dose reduction is required only in severe renal insufficienc

Table 10-1. Metronidazole: Pregnancy and breast-feeding

Agent	FDA pregnancy category	Risk vs benefit (by trimester)			Breast-feeding category
		1st	2nd	3rd	
Metronidazole	C1	$R \gg B$	$R \gg B$	$R \gg B$	IV

Food and Drug Administration (FDA) pregnancy categories:
A = Well-controlled studies fail to demonstrate risk to the fetus.
B1 = Animal studies fail to demonstrate risk to the fetus but no human studies are available.
B2 = Animal studies show some risk to the fetus but this is not confirmed in human studies.
C1 = Animal studies show risk to the fetus but no human studies are available.
C2 = Animal and human studies are unavailable.
D = Drugs associated with birth defects but with potential benefits that may outweigh known risks.
X = Drugs associated with birth defects and with potential risk that clearly outweighs potential benefit.
Risk vs benefit: $R \gg B$ = Proven or potential risk outweighs potential benefits.
$B > R$ = Potential benefits outweigh potential risks.
$R \gg B?$ = Risks may be outweighed by benefits in some circumstances.
? = Risk-to-benefit ratio is unknown.

Breast-feeding categories:
I = Drug does not enter breast milk.
II = Drug enters breast milk but is not known to be harmful in therapeutic doses.
IIIA = Drug may or may not enter breast milk but no adverse effects are expected.
IIIB = Drug may or may not enter breast milk but drug is systemically absorbed.
IV = Drug enters breast milk and poses a potential risk to the neonate.

2. Metronidazole has shown no benefit in the therapy of ulcerative colitis.
3. Indications for use of metronidazole in Crohn's disease include perineal disease, Crohn's colitis, and sulfasalazine intolerance or allergy. The drug should be continued until healing occurs, benefit plateaus, or side effects occur. Dose reduction should be gradual in those patients who respond and full-dose therapy should be reinstituted for relapse.
4. Metronidazole is effective in a variety of bacterial and protozoal infections, including *B. fragilis* infections and *C. difficile*–associated colitis, and as surgical prophylaxis. Amebiasis responds to metronidazole but a lumbricidal agent (iodoquinol) is necessary to ensure eradication.
5. Side effects are uncommon and well tolerated. A metallic taste is common and harmless. Neurologic side effects are serious and warrant discontinuation of the drug.
6. Laboratory abnormalities include a reversible neutropenia after long-term use and artifactual depression of SGOT levels.
7. Drug interactions of significance include a disulfiramlike reaction with alcohol use. Metronidazole potentiates the effects of warfarin and Dilantin. Concomitant use with sulfasalazine does not diminish bioavailability of sulfasalazine.
8. Although there is no evidence of carcinogenicity or teratogenicity in humans, the use of metronidazole in pregnant and nursing mothers is relatively contraindicated.
9. Metronidazole is active against *H. pylori* in a variety of regimens, but not as a single agent.

Suggested Reading

Beard CM, et al. Cancer after exposure to metronidazole. Mayo Clin Proc 1988; 63:147–153.

A follow-up study of 771 women exposed to metronidazole from 1960 to 1969 showing no increased risk of cancer.

Bernstein LH, et al. Healing of perineal Crohn's disease with metronidazole. Gastroenterology 1980; 79:357–365.

A study demonstrating the effectiveness of metronidazole in patients with chronic, unremitting perineal Crohn's disease.

Blichfeldt P, et al. Metronidazole in Crohn's disease. Scand J Gastroenterol 1978; 13:123–127.

A beneficial effect of metronidazole was noted on the clinical and biochemical markers in patients with Crohn's colitis.

Brandt LJ, et al. Metronidazole therapy for perineal Crohn's disease. Gastroenterology 1982; 83:383–387.

A follow-up study further defining the activity of metronidazole in perineal disease.

Chapman RW, Selby WS, Jewell DP. Controlled trial of intravenous metronidazole as an adjunct to corticosteroids in severe ulcerative colitis. Gut 1986; 27:1210–1212.

No benefit of intravenous metronidazole was seen after 5 days of therapy.

Davies PS, et al. Metronidazole in the treatment of chronic proctitis. Gut 1977; 18:680–681.

No benefit with metronidazole suppositories after 28 days of therapy.

Goldman P. Metronidazole. N Engl J Med 1980; 303:1212–1218.
A comprehensive review of the indications and adverse effects of metronidazole.

Graham DY, et al. Effect of triple therapy on duodenal ulcer healing. Ann Intern Med 1991;U115:266–269.
Eradication of H. pylori *speeds ulcer healing.*

Grove DI, Mahmoud AAF, Warren KS. Suppression of cell-mediated immunity by metronidazole. Int Arch Allerg Immunol 1977; 54:422–427.
Metronidazole inhibits granuloma formation in mice.

Rissing JP, Newman C, Moore WL. Artifactual depression of serum glutamic oxaloacetic transaminase by metronidazole. Antimicrob Agents Chemother 1978; 14:636–638.
Falsely low SGOT values in patients on metronidazole were noted.

Rosenblatt JE, Edson RS. Metronidazole. Mayo Clin Proc 1987; 62:1013–1017.
A concise review of metronidazole as an antibacterial agent.

Saginur R, Hawley DR, Bartlett JG. Colitis associated with metronidazole therapy. J Infect Dis 1980; 141:772–774.
A case report of C. difficile *colitis in a patient receiving metronidazole.*

Scully BE. Metronidazole. Med Clin North Am 1988; 72:613–621.
A comprehensive review emphasizing that surgical drainage of intraabdominal abscesses is the key to successful treatment, that metronidazole's role in Crohn's disease has not stood up in controlled trials, and that the true mechanism of action of metronidazole is unknown but presumed to be binding of toxic metronidazole intermediates to bacterial intracellular DNA.

Tanowitz HB, Weiss LM, Wittner M. Diagnosis and treatment of protozoan diarrhea. Am J Gastroenterol 1988; 83:339–350.
A clinical review of amebiasis and giardiasis with specific recommendations on therapy.

Teasley DG, et al. Prospective randomized trial of metronidazole versus vancomycin for *Clostridium difficile*–associated diarrhea and colitis. Lancet 1983; 2:1043–1046.
Metronidazole is as effective as vancomycin in the treatment of pseudomembranous enterocolitis.

Ursing B, Kamme C. Metronidazole for Crohn's disease. Lancet 1975; 1:775–777.
The first report of efficacy of metronidazole in inflammatory bowel disease.

Ursing B, et al. A comparative study of metronidazole and sulfasalazine for active Crohn's disease. Gastroenterology 1982; 83:550–562.
A follow-up study to the initial case report demonstrating benefit in a larger cohort.

Urtasun RC, Rabin HR, Partington J. Human pharmacokinetics and toxicity of high-dose metronidazole administered orally and intravenously. Surgery 1983; 93:145–148.
The first of five articles covering pharmacokinetics, toxicity, and mode of action in normal subjects and patients with renal insufficiency.

5-ASA and 4-ASA

David J. Roberts and D. Michael Jones

5-ASA

Sulfasalazine is the drug most commonly prescribed for inflammatory bowel disease. Despite its efficacy in the management of ulcerative colitis and Crohn's colitis, its high frequency of side effects has limited its use in up to 30 percent of patients. Sulfasalazine consists of 5–aminosalicylic acid (5-ASA) linked to a carrier molecule of sulfapyridine by an azo bond. It is well established that the active component of sulfasalazine is the 5-ASA moiety while the sulfapyridine carrier compound has no significant intrinsic effect on inflammatory bowel disease. Both subunits of the parent drug are liberated in the colon by the action of colonic bacteria on the azo bond. The systemically well-absorbed sulfa compound of sulfasalazine is responsible for the majority of the side effects of the parent drug. In contrast, 5-ASA is poorly absorbed through the colonic mucosa and exerts its effects locally. However, 5-ASA given orally is completely absorbed in the proximal small bowel, thus preventing it from working topically on the colonic inflammation. Efforts to sidestep the problem of sulfapyridine toxicity have led to novel methods of delivering 5-ASA unaltered to the colon and, more recently, to the distal small bowel in the treatment of Crohn's disease. Several new carriers orally deliver intact 5-ASA, and many studies have demonstrated the utility of 5-ASA given as a retention enema.

PHARMACOLOGY

The generic name for 5-ASA in the United States is mesalamine, while the compound is called mesalazine in Europe. 5-ASA is a salicylate analogue that can be readily bound to other moieties, including itself. Eight oral preparations have demonstrated effectiveness in clinical trials. Each differs in its carrier delivery system, but the drugs may be grouped into three main classes.

The first delivery method patterns itself on sulfasalazine and requires metabolism of the azo bond to release active mesalamine throughout the colon. Olsalazine (Dipentum) is a mesalamine dimer containing an azo bond. The two 5-ASA molecules remain linked and inactive until the colonic aerobic and anaerobic bacteria liberate the active ingredient. Balsalazide is a similar drug under investigation. This pro-drug consists of mesalamine bound through an azo linkage to an inert carrier (para-aminobenzyl-beta-alanine). Only Dipentum is commercially available in the United States.

The second delayed-release mechanism of mesalamine involves coating the compound with acrylic-based resins or other pH-sensitive binding substances. This method does not require metabolic conversion and allows the pharmacologist to target drug delivery based on the pH dependent dissolution of the coating substance. The only commercially available representative of this class in the United States is Asacol. This formulation utilizes mesalamine coated with Eudragit-S and releases the drug at a pH greater than 7.0. Other formulations either under investigation or available outside the United States include Claversal, Salofak, and RowasalI coated with Eudragit-L, and RowasalI embedded in coteric opadry.

The third formulation allows pH-independent release of mesalamine without reliance on colonic bacteria. Pentasa employs microspheres with an insoluble, semipermeable ethylcellulose membrane to allow diffusion-dependent delivery of the drug throughout the gastrointestinal tract. The promise of controlled delivery of 5-ASA to the distal small bowel has made this formulation a popular one with recent studies on the effect of 5-ASA on Crohn's disease.

All of these compounds are effective in delivering most of the aminosalicylic acid to the colon, where it is poorly absorbed and excreted in the feces. The fraction of 5-ASA that is absorbed (approximately 10%) is rapidly acetylated by the liver and excreted in the urine. A significant percentage of 5-ASA is also acetylated by the colonic mucosa and excreted in that form in the feces; this acetylated form may also have significant therapeutic effect topically.

Retention enemas (Rowasa) have also been studied as a method of delivering mesalamine to the colon. The 5-ASA is suspended in 60 ml of a neutral base solution and instilled in the rectum, usually overnight. Preliminary studies have shown that 100-ml enemas distribute consistently from the rectum to the splenic flexure. Local delivery to the proctorectum is available through a formulation of 500 mg mesalamine suppositories (Rowasa). Most of the 5-ASA is excreted unchanged in the feces.

MECHANISM OF ACTION

Despite the use of aminosalicylates (including sulfasalazine) for over 60 years, the mechanism of action of these drugs is still not certain. Their effects on the acute inflammatory response may be mediated by their action on leukotriene production and their ability to inhibit the intracellular release of interleukin-1. These drugs may have a different mechanism for maintaining remission in inflammatory bowel disease involving leukocyte recruitment. The 5-ASA preparations inhibit the chemotactic response to leukotriene B_4, reduce levels of platelet activating factor, and inhibit leukocyte adhesion. Recent ^{3}H-thymidine incorporation studies suggest that 5-ASA may have an effect on protein production, including antibody production and receptor expression, by directly interfering with deoxyribonucleic acid (DNA) synthesis.

INDICATIONS

Proctosigmoiditis

Mesalamine in the form of retention enemas (Rowasa) is often the drug of first choice for patients with proctitis or limited proctosigmoiditis. The Food and Drug Administration (FDA) has approved 5-ASA enemas for the treatment of mild to moderate left-sided proctocolitis. Controlled studies have shown 5-ASA to be superior to both placebo and sulfasalazine enemas, effecting remission in 60 to 70 percent of acute flares. Recurrence rates are similar to those of sulfasalazine. For patients with disease limited to the rectal vault, mesalamine suppositories (Rowasa 500 mg) may be more convenient.

Ulcerative Colitis, Active Disease

Mesalamine in the form of Asacol and Pentasa is approved for the treatment of mild to moderately active ulcerative colitis. The efficacy of the delayed-release mesalamine preparations has recently been documented in three double-blind, placebo-controlled randomized trials. The doses studied were Asacol in two 400-mg tablets 3 times a day and Pentasa administered as 4 gm/day.

Ulcerative Colitis, Maintenance Therapy

Olsalazine (Dipentum) was shown to be effective in prolonging remission in ulcerative colitis in two placebo-controlled trials. Despite the similarity of formulations, only Dipentum carries FDA approval for maintenance therapy of ulcerative colitis in patients intolerant of sulfasalazine. By gradually titrating up to a dose of 1 gm/day, some of the dose-dependent diarrhea associated with this drug may be avoided (see Pearls and Pitfalls).

Crohn's Disease, Active

There is a considerable body of data available on the use of mesalamine preparations in the treatment of Crohn's disease. Four recent studies failed to show any effect of mesalamine in several different formulations over placebo. A recent multicenter, double-blind placebo-controlled dose-response study has suggested that Pentasa at 4 gm/day is safe and effective in active Crohn's disease. The topical distribution of Pentasa to the small bowel may explain its apparent efficacy. As yet, no 5-ASA compound has FDA approval for the treatment of Crohn's disease.

Crohn's Disease, Maintenance Therapy

Several recent studies suggest a role for 5-ASA in maintenance therapy for Crohn's disease, but the trials are plagued by the underlying capricious nature of Crohn's. While no 5-ASA drug carries FDA approval for this indication, both Asacol and Pentasa appear superior to placebo in preventing or delaying clinical relapses in Crohn's disease after a follow-up period of 3 years. See Table 11-1, clinical studies involving formulations available in the U.S.

DOSAGE

The dosages of the mesalamine formulations available in the United States vary widely and parallel the clinical trials that established their efficacy. Asacol is manufactured as 400-mg tablets, and the recommended dosage for mild to moderately active ulcerative colitis is 800 mg 3 times a day. Pentasa is approved for the same indica-

Table 11-1. Clinical studies involving formulations available in the US

Disease entity	Rowasa enemas	Dipentum	Asacol	Pentasa
Proctosigmoiditis	Yes	NS	NS	NS
UC: Maintenance	NS	Yes	NS	NS
UC: Active disease	NS	NS	Yes	Yes
Crohn's: Maintenance	NS	NS	No	Yes
Crohn's: Active disease	NS	NS	Yes	Yes

Key: Yes: Demonstrated efficacy in clinical trials
No: No demonstrated effect in clinical trials
NS: Not studied
UC: Ulcerative colitis

tion and is available in 250-mg pills with a recommended dosage of 4 gm/day (4 tablets qid).

Dipentum is the only olsalazine preparation and is indicated for maintenance of remission in patients with ulcerative colitis who are intolerant of sulfasalazine. It is manufactured in 250-mg units; the recommended dosage is 500 mg twice a day.

5–Aminosalicylic acid enemas (Rowasa) consist of 4 gm of ASA in 100 ml buffered solution given as an overnight retention enema. Despite strong evidence that smaller doses of enemas as low as 1 gm may be equally effective, no lower-dose enema formulations are commercially available. For disease limited to the distal rectum, a 500-mg suppository is also available (Rowasa). Tapering the dose when stopping the drug may alleviate the acute flares that are occasionally associated with abrupt cessation of therapy.

SIDE EFFECTS

Oral 5-ASA compounds have been relatively free of side effects, with an incidence of 3 to 5 percent in drug company–generated surveys. The 5-ASA formulations have been tolerated by over 80 percent of those patients labeled as sulfasalazine intolerant. Infrequently reported complaints have included headache, nausea, and indigestion. In controlled clinical trials, mesalamine has a side effect frequency at or below that of placebo (15%), while sulfasalazine carries a 25 to 30 percent incidence of adverse effects.

A small percentage of patients taking mesalamine report a side effect that occurs with sulfasalazine, the so-called toxic colitis reaction. Nearly all patients with paradoxical worsening of diarrhea due to sulfasalazine will experience a similar effect with the 5-ASA drugs. Additionally, olsalazine has a relatively high incidence of dose-dependent secretory diarrhea, which characteristically appears at the initiation of therapy and may be confused with the "toxic colitis" reaction.

To date few side effects have been attributed to the 5-ASA enemas. The most notable is local anal trauma associated with repeated insertion of the enema tube. 5-ASA enemas in the dosages recommended appear safe. In one study, the placebo group reported more side effects than did the treatment group.

PEARLS AND PITFALLS

1. 5–Aminosalicylic acid in the oral or enema form is not indicated for severe flares of ulcerative colitis.
2. Evidence is emerging to support a role for certain 5-ASA preparations for chronic suppressive therapy of Crohn's disease, or for small-bowel Crohn's disease. However, these early studies need confirmation and long-term follow-up. To date, no 5-ASA drug has FDA approval for this indication.
3. Mesalamine has been detected in breast milk and minute quantities cross the placenta. The FDA has listed the drug as category B and advises that the drug be used in pregnancy only if clearly needed. However, recent reports on use in pregnancy suggest that these compounds have the same relative safety as sulfasalazine in pregnant patients (Table 11-2).
4. 5-ASA enemas are effective when retained for as little as 30 minutes. The patient who experiences difficulty with overnight retention may achieve benefit despite reduced enema retention time.

Table 11-2. 5-ASA and 4-ASA: Pregnancy and breast-feeding

Agent	FDA pregnancy category	Risk vs benefit (by trimester)			Breast-feeding category
		1st	2nd	3rd	
4-ASA, 5-ASA	B1	B > R	B > R	B > R	II

Food and Drug Administration (FDA) pregnancy categories:
A = Well-controlled studies fail to demonstrate risk to the fetus.
B1 = Animal studies fail to demonstrate risk to the fetus but no human studies are available.
B2 = Animal studies show some risk to the fetus but this is not confirmed in human studies.
C1 = Animal studies show risk to the fetus but no human studies are available.
C2 = Animal and human studies are unavailable.
D = Drugs associated with birth defects but with potential benefits that may outweigh known risks.
X = Drugs associated with birth defects and with potential risk that clearly outweighs potential benefit.
Risk vs benefit: R >> B = Proven or potential risk outweighs potential benefits.
B > R = Potential benefits outweigh potential risks.
R >> B? = Risks may be outweighed by benefits in some circumstances.
? = Risk-to-benefit ratio is unknown.
Breast-feeding categories:
I = Drug does not enter breast milk.
II = Drug enters breast milk but is not known to be harmful in therapeutic doses.
IIIA = Drug may or may not enter breast milk but no adverse effects are expected.
IIIB = Drug may or may not enter breast milk but drug is systemically absorbed.
IV = Drug enters breast milk and poses a potential risk to the neonate.

One-fourth of the commercially prepared enema dose may be equally effective.

5. 5-ASA does not appear to affect male fertility.
6. Because of the high incidence of a dose-dependent diarrhea associated with olsalazine preparations, most authorities recommend gradually increasing the dose of Dipentum.
7. Pharmacoscintigraphic studies have confirmed that the release and distribution of 5-ASA is not affected by food. Taking the medicine with meals may decrease some nonspecific adverse reactions.

4-ASA

An alternative to 5-ASA is para-aminosalicylic acid (PAS) or 4-ASA. This compound is an isomer of 5-ASA and has been used for years worldwide in large doses (8–12 gm) as a treatment for tuberculosis. PAS preparations offer the advantages of lower cost, equal efficacy when given topically, and better pharmacologic stability compared to the 5-ASA congeners. In addition, the good safety record from years of use as an antituberculous drug may make PAS an attractive alternative to 5-ASA in the treatment of inflammatory bowel disease. However, clinical research does not yet support the use of PAS in these diseases.

Clinical studies with 4-ASA have been limited to topical treatment of distal proctocolitis; only two studies have assessed oral PAS in the treatment of ulcerative colitis. 4-ASA retention enemas (formulated as 2 gm in 60-ml water) appear effective in the same clinical settings where 5-ASA enemas are indicated. No PAS enema preparations are currently available. Recent clinical studies were small using oral PAS as an alternative to sulfasalazine in the treatment of ulcerative colitis, and PAS compounds are not currently approved by the FDA for the treatment of inflammatory bowel disease. PAS is manufactured under the trade names of Teebacin and Parasal and dispensed as 500-mg tablets.

Suggested Reading

5-ASA AND ULCERATIVE COLITIS: ACUTE

Hanauer S, et al. Mesalamine capsules for the treatment of active ulcerative colitis: Results of a clinical trial. Am J Gastroenterol 1993; 88:1188–1197.

Pentasa is safe and effective monotherapy in doses of 2 to 4 gm in the treatment of mild to moderately active ulcerative colitis.

Schroeder KW, et al. Coated oral 5–aminosalicylic acid therapy for mild to moderately active ulcerative colitis. N Engl J Med 1987; 317:1625–1629.

Very early study on the use of 5-ASA in ulcerative colitis that compared placebo with 1.6 and 4.8 gm Asacol. Only the 4.8-gm dose was superior to placebo; the current recommended dose of Asacol is 2.4 gm.

Sninsky CA, et al. Oral mesalamine for mildly to moderately active ulcerative colitis. Ann Intern Med 1991; 115:350–355.

A placebo-controlled trial of Asacol demonstrating modest results at a dose of 1.6 and 2.4 gm / day. Improvement was seen in approximately 43 and 50 percent, respectively.

Sutherland LR, et al. Sulfasalazine revisited: A meta-analysis of 5-aminosalicylic acid in the treatment of ulcerative colitis. Ann Intern Med 1993; 118:540–549.

Useful article to temper enthusiasm over the more expensive 5-ASA as the first-line drug in ulcerative colitis. Sixteen trials met the criteria for review, and the authors report clear benefit of the 5-ASA formulations over placebo. However, they failed to substantiate the advantage of the drugs over sulfasalazine in the patients who were not intolerant to the sulfa preparation.

5-ASA AND ULCERATIVE COLITIS: REMISSION MAINTENANCE

Nakshabendi IM, et al. Is Asacol as effective as sulphasalazine in maintaining remission of Crohn's disease and ulcerative colitis? Postgrad Med J 1992; 68:189–191.

Retrospective study over a 4-year period comparing Asacol in varying doses with sulfasalazine for inflammatory bowel disease in remission. It suggests that, despite its limitations, Asacol is as effective as sulfasalazine in maintaining remission in ulcerative colitis and Crohn's disease limited to the colon. In the US only olsalazine is approved for this indication.

Rijk MC, et al. Relapse preventing effect and safety of sulfasalazine and olsalazine in patients with ulcerative colitis in remission. Am J Gastroenterol 1993; 87:438–442.

This is considered the definitive study with over one year follow-up. Sulfasalazine and olsalazine are equally effective in maintaining remission of ulcerative colitis. The two drugs have a similar incidence of adverse effects.

Wright JP, et al. Olsalazine in maintenance of clinical remission in patients with ulcerative colitis. Dig Dis Sci 1993; 38:1837–1842.

A double-blind, placebo-controlled study of 100 patients who had recently recovered from an attack of ulcerative colitis. The dose of olsalazine was higher than the currently recommended dose at 2 gm / day, and drug-induced diarrhea was a significant side effect in 16 percent (8 of 49) of the treated group. In those patients who tolerated the drug, rapid relapse was prevented, with the median time to relapse for placebo of 100 days prolonged to approximately 1 year with olsalazine.

5-ASA AND PROCTOSIGMOIDITIS

Biddle WL, et al. 5-Aminosalicylic acid enemas: Effective agent in maintaining remission in left-sided ulcerative colitis. Gastroenterology 1988; 94:1075–1079.

This randomized, double-blind, placebo-controlled trial demonstrates the efficacy of 5-ASA enemas in the maintenance of remission for 1 year in 75 percent of patients receiving drug, versus an 85 percent relapse rate within 16 weeks for patients receiving placebo.

Campieri M, et al. Mesalamine suppositories in the treatment of ulcerative proctitis or distal proctosigmoiditis. A randomized controlled trial. Scand J Gastroenterol 1990; 25:663–668.

Mesalamine suppositories given as 500 mg twice a day are safe, well tolerated, and effective in patients with active distal proctosigmoiditis.

Cobden I, et al. Is topical therapy necessary in acute distal colitis?

A double blind comparison of high dose oral mesalamine v. steroid enemas in the treatment of active distal ulcerative colitis. Aliment Pharmacol Ther 1991; 5:513–522.
Both treatments produced clinical improvement with decreases in stool frequency, rectal bleeding, urgency, and tenesmus. Oral therapy appears as effective as topical, twice-daily steroid enemas. Unfortunately, 5-ASA retention enemas, generally used for this indication, were not included in this study.

D'Arienzo A, et al. 5-Aminosalicylic acid suppositories in the maintenance of remission in idiopathic proctitis: A double blind placebo controlled clinical trial. Am J Gastroenterol 1992; 85:1079–1082.
5-ASA suppositories given as 800 mg/day for 1 year are safe and effective for distal ulcerative colitis in remission. The remission rate for the control group was 21 percent, while the 5-ASA–treated group's rate was 92 percent.

5-ASA AND CROHN'S DISEASE: ACUTE

Mahida YK, et al. Slow release 5-aminosalicylic acid (Pentasa) for the treatment of active Crohn's disease. Digestion 1990; 45:88–92.
Double-blind, placebo-controlled trial of Pentasa given at lower doses (1.5 gm/day) than the Singleton paper below. This group failed to show an effect greater than that of placebo.

Singleton JW, et al. Mesalamine capsules for the treatment of active Crohn's disease: Results of a 16-week trial. Pentasa Crohn's Disease Study Group. Gastroenterology 1993; 104:1293–1301.
This double-blind, randomized, multicenter, prospective trial demonstrated that Pentasa is safe and effective as a single agent in active Crohn's disease of the ileum and colon. The group chose 4 gm/day of the mesalamine preparation, a dose demonstrated to provide the greatest small-bowel release of the drug.

5-ASA AND CROHN'S DISEASE: REMISSION MAINTENANCE

Gendre JP, et al. Oral mesalamine (Pentasa®) as maintenance treatment in Crohn's disease: A multicenter placebo controlled study. Gastroenterology 1993; 104:435–439.
Over 160 patients with inactive disease were randomized to receive placebo or Pentasa (2 gm/day) for 2 years. Pentasa was safe and effective maintenance for Crohn's disease when given within 3 months of achieving remission. However, if treatment was begun beyond 3 months of remission induction, Pentasa was no better than placebo.

Prantera C, et al. Oral 5-aminosalicylic acid (Asacol) in the maintenance of Crohn's disease. The Italian IBD Study Group. Gastroenterology 1992; 103:363–368.
A randomized, placebo-controlled, multicenter trial of Asacol, 2.4 gm/day, in 125 patients with inactive Crohn's disease. The cumulative relapse rates for the treated and control groups were 12 percent versus 22 percent at 3 months and 34 percent versus 55 percent at 1 year. Asacol was safe and effective in preventing or delaying a clinical relapse in Crohn's disease.

4-ASA

Ginsberg AL, et al. Placebo controlled trial of ulcerative colitis with oral 4-aminosalicylic acid. Gastroenterology 1992; 102:448–452.
Forty patients were randomized to 4 gm/day 4-ASA or placebo for a 12-week trial. Oral 4-ASA therapy was safe and effective in the

treatment of ulcerative colitis. By both clinical and sigmoidoscopic parameters, a significant improvement was seen in the 4-ASA group. This study is one of the few to investigate the already available and less costly 4-ASA preparations in inflammatory bowel disease.

O'Donnel LJ, et al. Double blind, controlled trial of 4-aminosalicylic acid and prednisolone enemas in distal ulcerative colitis. Gut 1992; 33:947–949.

This study of 45 patients demonstrated that 2 gm 4-ASA enemas had similar efficacy as corticosteroid enemas. There was a trend in favor of 4-ASA for symptomatic improvement.

Sharma MP, et al. A prospective, randomized, double-blind trial comparing prednisolone and 4-aminosalicylic acid enemas in acute distal colitis. J Gastroenterol Hepatol 1992; 7:173–177.

Forty patients were randomized to steroid or 4-ASA enemas. Sigmoidoscopic and histologic improvement were better in the 4-ASA group. Clinical responses were similar, although 4 of 20 of the steroid-treated group had to withdraw because of worsening symptoms.

MISCELLANEOUS

Campieri M, et al. Optimum dosage of 5-aminosalicylic acid as rectal enema in patients with active ulcerative colitis. Gut 1991; 32: 929–931.

This study suggests that 1 gm of 5-ASA is a sufficient dose for mild to moderately active ulcerative colitis.

Habal FM, et al. Oral 5-aminosalicylic acid for inflammatory bowel disease in pregnancy: Safety and clinical course. Gastroenterology 1993; 105:1057–1060.

Oral 5-ASA appears safe for the management of inflammatory bowel disease during pregnancy (see Pearls and Pitfalls).

Total Parenteral Nutrition

Michael M. Van Ness

Intravenous hyperalimentation was first utilized by Sir Christopher Wren in 1656. Using goose quill connected to a pig's bladder, he was able to introduce ale, opium, and wine into dogs' veins. During the 1800s, this method was refined to treat diarrhea and shock. By the early 1900s, intravenous use of glucose was recognized for surgical patients. It was in the early 1950s that central venous infusion via the subclavian vein was started by the French surgeon Aubaniac as a means of administering blood rapidly to battle casualties in the French-Indochina war. In 1965, Dudrik and his colleagues applied this concept to total parenteral nutrition (TPN) to deliver essential nutrients and calories for nutritional support.

Enteral alimentation is the preferred method of nutritional support in clinically functioning gastrointestinal tracts. The advantages of enteral alimentation include physiologic maintenance of intestinal structure and function by the trophic effects of intraluminal nutrients, augmented insulin response to enterally administered carbohydrates, and delivery of more nutritionally complete feeding solutions than is possible by parenteral formulas. There are relative and absolute contraindications, however, to the use of enteral alimentation. As an alternative, total parenteral nutrition may be used.

INDICATIONS

Total parenteral nutrition provides varying amounts of carbohydrate, protein, fat, vitamins, and minerals intravenously to individuals who are unable to assimilate nutrients via the gastrointestinal tract because of gut dysfunction. TPN may be delivered via central or peripheral vein, and the decision to provide central versus peripheral TPN is related to several factors: (1) duration of the treatment plan, (2) the energy requirements of the patient, (3) the overall goal of treatment (i.e., to minimize weight loss, maintain weight, or gain weight), and (4) the availability of adequate routes of administration. Indications of each mode are the following.

Peripheral Vein Feedings

1. When enteral intake is interrupted, but is expected to resume within 5 to 7 days
2. As supplementation to enteral feedings or transitional phase until enteral feedings meet needs
3. In mild to moderate malnutrition, necessitating intervention in order to prevent further protein depletion
4. In normal or mildly elevated metabolic rate
5. When there is no organ failure
6. When a central vein cannot be accessed
7. Phlebitis appears to be less if a fat emulsion is used in combination with heparin (500 units/liter) and hydrocortisone (5 mg/liter) via a thin, longer catheter (23-gauge, 15-cm pediatric control line).

Central Vein Feedings

1. Patients are unable to tolerate enteral intake for greater than 7 days

2. In moderately to severely elevated metabolic rate
3. In moderate to severe malnutrition not correctable with enteral feedings
4. In cardiac, renal, or hepatic failure or other conditions that necessitate fluid restrictions
5. When there is limited access to peripheral veins

Curtailing the imbalance of metabolic homeostasis and loss of lean body mass is the major objective of adjunctive TPN in various gastrointestinal disorders. Specific clinical settings in which TPN should be a part of routine care include: (1) massive (> 70%) small-bowel resection; (2) impaired intestinal motility or absorption, as in scleroderma, systemic lupus erythematosus (SLE), sprue, and ischemia; (3) radiation enteritis; (4) severe intractable diarrhea, vomiting in chemotherapy patients, or severe pancreatitis; (5) severely catabolic patients (> 50% body surface area burns, multiple trauma, extensive surgery, and sepsis); and (6) severe inflammatory bowel disease.

Clinical settings where TPN would be helpful are (1) major surgery, (2) moderate stress (30–50% body surface area burns, trauma, moderately severe pancreatitis, neurologic trauma, and other similar stresses), (3) enterocutaneous fistulae, (4) hyperemesis gravidarum, (5) moderate malnutrition in patients who require medical and surgical intervention, and (6) inflammatory adhesions with small-bowel obstruction.

NUTRITION AND DIET THERAPY IN INFLAMMATORY BOWEL DISEASE

Malnutrition is a common complication of Crohn's disease and ulcerative colitis. The etiology is multifactorial and includes inadequate intake, excess intestinal losses, malabsorption, and increased requirements. The medical therapy of inflammatory bowel disease has long included bowel rest, either for therapeutic intent or because the severity of disease precludes oral intake. The efficacy of parenteral and enteral nutrition as primary therapy is unproven, but there are clear indications for employing nutritional therapy, which include use as supportive care, growth failure, and use as an adjunct to surgical intervention.

Nutritional support is a valuable tool for Crohn's patients with inflammatory strictures or for those with diffuse disease that is not surgically correctable, including those patients who are otherwise unable to sustain themselves due to anorexia, nausea, vomiting, or postprandial pain. There is no evidence that nutritional therapy obviates the ultimate need for surgery some time in a patient's course, but some patients sustain a prolonged remission on medical therapy alone, thus postponing surgical intervention. Supportive therapy has been most useful in patients with short-bowel syndrome, whether from Crohn's disease or other causes. These patients are able to be maintained long term on parenteral and enteral nutrition, allowing them mobility and survival previously not available.

Nutritional therapy is useful as an adjuvant to surgical intervention. Because of malnutrition, many patients with inflammatory bowel disease require preoperative and postoperative nutritional support. The routine use of parenteral nutrition has not decreased the need for surgery, but a decrease in postoperative complications has been documented in malnourished patients with ulcerative colitis who are receiving preoperative parenteral nutrition. Parenteral nutrition has historically been used with good success in the treatment of non-Crohn's enterocutaneous fistulae, but this efficacy has not carried over to Crohn's fistulae except when combined with surgical excision. Wound healing and general recovery are enhanced by the maintenance of good nutritional status.

The least controversial use of nutritional support is in the reversal of growth arrest in children with inflammatory bowel disease. Twenty to 40 percent of children with inflammatory bowel disease suffer from growth retardation or delayed puberty. It is well documented that this growth retardation can be reversed if they are provided with adequate calorie, protein, mineral, and vitamin intake. The supplementation does not provide long-term remission of disease, but the caloric boost provides for weight gain and linear growth while it is maintained. These improvements have been noted despite concurrent medical therapy, including steroids, and have been unrelated to the activity of the disease.

Several recent reports have documented remission of uncomplicated Crohn's disease using elemental diets as the primary therapy. They have compared favorably to steroids in a controlled trial. The patients were treated with Vivonex orally to provide 40 to 60 kcal/kg/day and 8 to 12 gm/day protein. After 4 weeks, food was slowly reintroduced into the diet. The decreased morbidity of diet therapy as compared to steroid therapy with the same results makes it an attractive alternative, but it needs to be confirmed by other investigators before it is applied more widely.

The mechanisms by which nutritional therapy is of benefit in these patients include correction of inadequate intake of nutrients, reversal of loss of enteral protein, and enhanced absorption of all nutrients after restitution of adequate oral intake. Even utilizing enteral nutrition, protein losses in the stool are shown to stabilize or decrease during therapy. Elemental feedings cause little stimulation of digestive hormones as compared to whole proteins. Other benefits of enteral and parenteral diets are postulated but less well documented. These include decreased mucosal exposure to antigens, decreased mechanical irritation, altered bowel flora, and alterations of microbial metabolism.

The administration of nutritional supplements has by no means been standardized. Generally, enteral nutrition is preferable to parenteral because of fewer complications. Several commercial elemental diets are available and as yet none has been definitively shown to be more efficacious than the others. Elemental feedings are absorbed high in the intestinal tract and thus are often suitable even in patients with tight strictures secondary to Crohn's disease. Most patients can be maintained on elemental diets either orally or by nasogastric tube. Potential complications limiting their use include unpalatability, bloating, dumping syndrome, and abdominal pain. These problems can sometimes be avoided by advancing from one-third-strength to full-strength feedings over 3 days to allow the gut to adapt to the hyperosmolar fluid. Enteral supplementation can be utilized in the hospital and at home and can be administered during sleeping hours through a nasogastric tube to allow for more normal daytime activity.

Parenteral nutrition has not been shown to have any therapeutic benefit over enteral nutrition in the treatment of patients with inflammatory bowel disease. It is extremely useful, however, in patients who are unable to tolerate enteral nutrition or who must be maintained NPO. Some patients with short-bowel syndrome can be maintained on parenteral nutrition until they recover enough gut function to tolerate enteral feedings.

The drawback of parenteral nutrition is that it must be administered through a central venous catheter, with all the attendant complications of placing and maintaining the catheter. Despite the increased difficulty, home parenteral nutrition has been successful utilizing subcutaneously tunneled indwelling catheters in patients who require long-term therapy. To be successful, these programs require the support of a coordinated nutrition team that works to supply, maintain, and monitor these patients. This multidisciplinary or team approach requires members to serve a distinct role in the management of the TPN patient. The members of the team should include a physician, a registered nurse, a dietitian, and a pharmacist dedicated to optimizing nutritional support of patients during hospitalization and rehabilitation. This team can best ensure a smooth transition from hospital to home care, if necessary. One major advantage of this concerted effort is the significant reduction of complications of catheter sepsis, thrombosis, and metabolic derangements. Adhering strictly to protocols with firm guidelines also lessens risk and rate of complications.

ADMINISTRATION

Total parenteral nutrition solutions generally contain calories (concentrated dextrose), a nitrogen source, electrolytes, vitamins, minerals, and an essential fatty acid source.

1. *Calories*—The caloric requirement should be met mainly as glucose and protein supplemented by fat. Traditionally, using formulas such as the Harris-Benedict equation, the basal metabolic rate (BMR) is calculated, with the total caloric requirement being a multiple of the BMR, depending on the clinical condition of the patient. The baseline caloric requirements in the adult range from 40 to 45 kcal/kg/day. In hypermetabolic states, energy requirements are increased. For example, in febrile states, there is a 12 percent increase with each degree above 37°, a 20 to 30 percent increase with major surgery, a 40 to 50 percent increase with severe sepsis, and a 100 percent or greater increase with major burns. Alternate caloric sources not frequently used are fructose, sorbitol, and xylitol.
2. *Proteins*—The recommended daily requirement for adults with normal liver and kidney function is 1.0 to 1.5 gm/kg/day. Crystalline amino acid solutions are given to provide 42.5 gm protein (e.g., Aminosyn, 8.5% in 500 ml) and 25 gm protein (Aminosyn, 5% in 500 ml) via the central route and peripheral route, respectively. These solutions provide essential and nonessential amino acids. Branched-chain amino acids are usually in higher concentration than the rest of the essential amino acids, as some studies suggest benefit in the treatment of patients with hepatic encephalopathy. In contrast, the aromatic amino acids phenylalanine and tryptophan are in lower concentration, as they are thought to aggravate hepatic coma.
3. *Dextrose*—Dextrose is the major source of calories and by far the least expensive. Usually a 50 percent solution is employed in central venous hyperalimentation while a 10 percent solution is appropriate for peripheral use. A concomitant infusion of fat emulsion or slowing the rate of infusion can decrease peripheral

vein irritation. Patients with diabetes mellitus or resistance to insulin require a lower dextrose concentration. In contrast, a higher concentration (70%) can be used in patients whose total volume intake must be restricted. Each gram of dextrose has 3.4 kcal.

4. *Electrolytes*—The electrolyte ranges in Table 12-1 are recommended in each bottle of solution on a daily basis unless contraindicated.
5. *Vitamins*—Parenterally administered vitamin doses should meet the American Medical Association guidelines for vitamin therapy except for vitamin K. Because of its allergic and cardiac effects (palpitations and blood pressure changes), vitamin K is frequently left out of the solution unless specifically ordered. Vitamin supplements are given as needed in single doses of separate vitamins. Biotin and vitamin B_{12} may need to be specifically ordered.
6. *Trace elements*—Trace elements include zinc, copper, manganese, and chromium and are usually added to solutions by the pharmacy. Individual minerals can be added in suspected deficiencies.
7. *Lipid emulsions*—The two major indications for fat emulsions are the treatment and prevention of essential fatty acid deficiency and the provision of calories. Fat emulsions are increasingly used to deliver concentrated calories. Solutions are composed of fat (soybean and safflower), an emulsified (1.2% egg yolk) phospholipid, and glycerol (2.5%). All three compounds provide calories. Available preparations provide a caloric density of 1.1 to 2.0 kcal/ml and obviate the need for excessive intravenous volume in patients.
8. *Other additives*—Heparin in a concentration of 1 unit/ml parenteral nutrition solution should be given to prevent fibrin sheath formation on the catheter (which can lead to venous thrombosis). Regular insulin can be added to the solution to prevent glucosuria

Table 12-1. Electrolyte ranges

Calcium	10–15 mEq/day (5 mEq/liter)
Magnesium	8–24 mEq/day (8 mEq/liter)
Potassium[a]	90–240 mEq/day (20–50 mEq/liter)
Sodium	60–150 mEq/day (20–50 mEq/liter)
Acetate[a]	80–120 mEq/day (30–50 mEq/liter)
Chloride[a]	60–150 mEq/day (20–50 mEq/liter)
Phosphorus[b]	30–50 mM/day (10–15 mM/liter)

[a]Amino acid solution 5% (Aminosyn 5%–500 ml) provides 43 mEq acetate and 2.7 mEq potassium.
Amino acid solution 8.5% (Aminosyn 8.5%–500 ml) provides 45 mEq acetate, 17.5 mEq chloride, and 2.7 mEq potassium.
Amino acid solution 10% (Aminosyn 10%–500 ml) provides 74 mEq acetate and 2.7 mEq potassium.
Essential amino acid solution 5.2% (Aminosyn RF 5.2%–300 ml) provides 31.5 mEq acetate and 1.5 mEq potassium.
[b]When ordered as potassium phosphate, each prescribed millimole of phosphorus will contribute 1.47 mEq potassium. Likewise, 1 mM sodium phosphate will contribute 1.3 mEq sodium.
Reprinted from *The University of Michigan Hospitals Parenteral and Enteral Nutrition Manual*, 1980, The Regents of the University of Michigan, p. 24.

and hyperglycemia. Glutamine, 0.57 gm/kg body weight per day, has been shown to be of real benefit.

9. *Albumin*—Supplemental albumin infusions are expensive, are of no independent benefit beyond providing calories, and are *not recommended.*

How to Order TPN Solutions

Most patients' protein and calorie requirements are met with standard solutions containing 25% dextrose, 4% crystalline amino acids, electrolytes, minerals, trace elements, and vitamins. The total caloric value is approximately 1000 kcal/liter or 1 kcal/ml. The nonprotein calorie per gram of nitrogen ratio is 127:1. A sample of TPN formulation is shown in Table 12-2.

Most hospitals and institutions have their own standard orders and administration forms. TPN solution should be given in sequential order as long as the patient is on parenteral nutrition. Orders to increase or decrease any ingredient should be filled 24 hours in advance of the change in order to minimize the economic burden of TPN therapy.

Generally therapy is instituted slowly by administering 1 liter for the first 24 hours. The rate of delivery can be subsequently increased by a liter per day until the volume that satisfies the patient's protein and caloric needs is achieved.

Alterations of TPN solutions for specific diseases require knowledge of their pathophysiology and tailoring solutions to nutrient requirements and tolerances. For example, in patients with pancreatitis, hypertriglyceridemia is contradicted and lipid infusion should be omitted. The severe malabsorption or diarrhea seen in inflammatory bowel disease often results in electrolyte and mineral losses, especially potassium, magnesium, zinc, and bicarbonate. Repletion of these essential elements requires electrolyte supplementation. As another example, calcium, lipid, and fat soluble vitamins are often deficient in patients with inflammatory disease, who thus require

Table 12-2. Mixed amino acid formulation

Amino acids (4.25%)	42.5 gm	**Approximate volume**
Dextrose (25%)	250.0 gm	1050 ml
Calcium	4.5 mEq	**Approximate osmolarity**
Magnesium	5.0 mEq	1825 mOsm
Potassium	40.0 mEq	**Total caloric value**
Sodium	35.0 mEq	1020 kcal (approx. 1 kcal/ml)
Acetate	74.5 mEq	**Nitrogen content**
Chloride	52.5 mEq	6.7 gm
Phosphorus	12.0 mM	**Nonprotein calorie/gm nitrogen**
Heparin sodium	1000 units	127 : 1
Multivitamins with biotin, B_{12}, and folic acid	10 ml	
Trace elements	5 ml	

Reprinted from *The University of Michigan Hospitals Parenteral and Enteral Nutrition Manual,* 1980, The Regents of the University of Michigan.

Table 12-3. Potential modulation of standard TPN (4.25% AA/25% dextrose) with standard electrolytes, multivitamins, and trace minerals in various diseases*

Disease	Dextrose	Amino acids	Fat	Electrolyte	Vitamins	Trace minerals
Pancreatitis	NM	↑ (5%)	Daily if glucose intolerance Omit if ↑ TG	↑ NaCl if NG losses are excessive	↑ B vit, folate if ETOH ↑ A,D,E,K if steatorrhea	NM
Renal failure	↑ (35%) if fluid restriction	↓ (2.1% mixed EAA and non-EAA) or (EAA only 1.35–2.7%) ↑ (5%) if dialysis	Daily if glucose intolerance Omit if ↑ TG	↓ Na+ ↓ Other electrolytes per labs and renal function	Provide ↑ B vits if dialysis	Omit
Cardiac disease	↑ (35%) if fluid restriction	NM	Omit if ↑ TG	↓ Na ↑ K^+, Mg^{2+}, Ca^{2+} if diuretic therapy ↑ $PO_4^{=}$	NM	Se supplementation ↑ Zinc if diuresis
Pulmonary disease	↑ (35%) if fluid restriction Carb should provide no > 50% calories	NM	Daily → fat should provide 50% kcal	↓ Na^+ if fluid balance is + ↑ $PO_4^{=}$	NM	NM

Liver disease	↑ (35%) if fluid restriction	↑ (5%) If encephalopathy ↓ (2.1%) or ↓ (4%–↑ BCAA/↓ AAA)	Daily if glucose intolerance √ TG level	↓ Na^+ ↑ K^+, Mg^{2+}, Ca^{2+} if lactulose therapy ↑ Bicarb if lactulose therapy	↑ A, D, E, K if steatorrhea ↑ B_1 ↑ Folate	Omit Cu and Mn if cholestasis
Stress	In ebb/complicated stress ↓ (15–20%)	↑ (5–7%) or provide ↑ BCAA solution ↑ (5%)	Daily if glucose intolerance Omit if ↑ TG	↑ Mg, K^+, $PO_4^=$	NM	↑ Zn
Gastrointestinal disease	NM	↑ (5%)	NM	↑ NaCl if ↑ NG losses ↑ Bicarb, K^+, Mg^{2+} if lower GI losses are excessive	↑ Biotin, vit K ↑ Vitamin C	↑ Zn with high fistula/ileostomy output/diarrhea

↑ ( ), increase concentration to; ↓ ( ), decrease concentration to; NM, no modulation necessary; ↑, increase; ↓, decrease; TG, triglyceride; EAA, essential amino acids; NEAA, nonessential amino acids.

*Standard electrolytes, multivitamins, and trace minerals: Na, 45 mEq/liter; Ca, 4.5 mEq/liter; Cl, 35 mEq/liter; PO_4, 10 mEq/liter; K, 20 mEq/liter; Mg, 5 mEq/liter; acetate, 29.5 mEq/liter; MVI-12, 1 amp; trace minerals, 1 amp providing the 4 following minerals: zinc, 3 mg; copper, 1 mg; manganese, 0.4 mg; chromium, 0.001 mg.

Reprinted from SH Krey, RL Murray (eds), *Dynamics of Nutrition Support: Assessment, Implementation, Evaluation.* New York: Appleton-Century-Crofts, 1986. P 430.

parenteral supplementation to normalize calcium, essential fatty acid, and fat-soluble vitamin levels. Other potential modifications of standard TPN solutions are shown in Table 12-3.

Catheter maintenance requires meticulous aseptic techniques and dry, sterile, and air-occlusive dressings that are applied to the catheter insertion site and changed every 48 hours. Administration sets and tubings are changed every 24 hours to prevent contamination and infection.

Monitoring

Before parenteral nutrition is begun, several parameters are assessed:*

Baseline laboratory evaluation:
SMA-20: serum electrolytes and pH
Serum Ca^2+, inorganic phosphorus
Blood urea nitrogen (BUN)
Serum creatinine
Liver function tests
Total protein/albumin
Serum glucose
Carbon dioxide
Prothrombin time (PT), partial thromboplastin time (PTT)
Serum magnesium
Complete blood count (CBC) with differential
Serum iron, total iron-binding capacity
Serum triglycerides (if fat emulsion is used)
Urine analysis
Serum and urine osmolarity
Additional tests for central vein infusions: serum levels of B_{12}, folate, trace elements (Mn, Cu, Zn)

These parameters allow assessment of the appropriateness and adequacy of nutrient regimes.

The ultimate goal of monitoring during parenteral nutrition is the avoidance of complications. Once TPN has begun, the following ongoing monitoring procedures are indicated:*

Every 4 to 6 hours: vital signs, urine glucose and ketones
Daily: serum electrolytes, BUN, carbon dioxide, serum glucose, pH, fluid intake and output, weight
Twice per week: SMA-20, CBC with differential (when the patient's condition is stable, these may be ordered weekly)
Weekly: serum magnesium, serum and urine osmolarity, urine analysis, serum triglycerides (until fat emulsion is discontinued), other serum vitamin and mineral levels as needed

The length of therapy is variable and mainly dependent on the clinical situation. As an adjunct to medical care, it should be continued until the patient is able to take adequate nutrition orally. One or 2 weeks of therapy preoperatively replaces nutrients and enables body stores to be replenished. Growth failure in children requires 6 weeks or more of therapy, depending on disease activity and treatment goals. Elemental diet therapy for Crohn's disease has been used for 4 weeks with the gradual introduction of oral intake after that.

*Reprinted from SH Krey, RL Murray (eds), *Dynamics of Nutrition Support: Assessment, Implementation, Evaluation.* New York: Appleton-Century-Crofts, 1986. 287.

Growth failure in children has been treated with 60 to 80 kcal/kg/day and 2 to 3 gm/kg/day protein. Adults in all groups are usually given 40 to 60 kcal/kg/day and 1 to 2 gm/kg/day protein. These should be accompanied by vitamins and minerals to meet the daily requirements. Therapy can be monitored by weight gain, growth, standard nutritional indicators (albumin, transferring, absolute lymphocyte count), anthropometric measurements, or clinical response.

COMPLICATIONS

Catheter-Related Complications

Mechanical

1. Pneumothorax—The most prevalent complication of subclavian venipuncture, occurring in up to 5 percent of attempted catheterizations
2. Subclavian artery puncture—The second most frequent complication
3. Carotid artery puncture—The most common complication of percutaneous internal jugular catheterization; a resulting hematoma may lead to tracheal compression and respiratory compromise
4. Air embolism
5. Brachial plexus injury

Septic

The catheter may become contaminated due to improper care (improper handling of solutions) or seeding from a distant site of infection.

Metabolic Complications

1. Hyperglycemia—Usually self-correcting; treat only if 4+ glucosuria or significant osmotic diuresis is present. Ten units of regular insulin per liter may be added. If untreated, hyperosmolar hyperglycemic nonketotic coma may develop.
2. Hypoglycemia—Due to sudden decrease or cessation of solution infusion secondary to iatrogenic or mechanical problems. Substitution of 10% dextrose as a temporizing measure can be lifesaving.
3. Hyperkalemia—Secondary to underutilization of administered potassium in the inadequately anabolic patient.
4. Hypokalemia—Requirement increases as patient begins to synthesize protein and becomes anabolic.
5. Hypercalcemia, hypermagnesemia, or hyperphosphatemia—These are due to underutilization.
6. Hypocalcemia—Secondary to decreased total serum albumin; asymptomatic because of normal ionized calcium level.
7. Hypomagnesemia—Increased requirement during increased anabolism and protein synthesis.
8. Hypophosphatemia—Needed for synthesis of intracellular high-energy phosphate compounds, metabolic structure, and bone formation; thus, increased requirement in anabolic state.
9. Hyperlipidemia—Secondary to rapid infusion of lipid emulsion.
10. Essential fatty acid deficiency—Increased needs during anabolic states that cannot be met by limited stores of linoleic acid.
11. Mineral deficiency—Well documented; should be repleted on a daily basis.

Organ-Related Complications

1. Lungs—Increased oxygen consumption and carbon dioxide production in hypermetabolic patients are associated with high glucose loads of TPN.
2. Liver—Fatty liver, cholestasis, and nonspecific triaditis.

Suggested Reading

American Society for Parenteral and Enteral Nutrition Board of Directors. Guidelines for use of total parenteral nutrition in the hospitalized adult patient. JPEN 1986; 10:441–445.
Guidelines for the role of TPN in different clinical settings.

Askanazi J, et al. Respiratory changes induced by the large glucose loads of total parenteral nutrition. JAMA 1980; 243:1444–1447.
A study of the adverse effects of high glucose loads of TPN on oxygen consumption and carbon dioxide production.

Baker AL, Rosenberg IH. Hepatic complications of total parenteral nutrition: Need for prospective investigation. Am J Med 1987; 82:489–497.
A summary of the current understanding of the pathogenesis and management of liver injury during short-term TPN.

Howard L, et al. National trends in the use of home parenteral and enteral nutrition therapy. JPEN 1994; 18:225.
There is increased use of home nutritional therapy.

Keohane PP, et al. Effect of catheter tunneling and a nutrition nurse on catheter sepsis during parenteral nutrition. Lancet 1983; 2: 1388–1390.
The importance of the role of nursing care and catheter tunneling in the reduction of TPN catheter sepsis.

Mehta PL, et al. Comparison of enteral versus parenteral nutritional support in post-operative liver transplant recipients. JPEN 1994; 18:265.
Early postoperative jejunostomy feeding is safe and preferred to TPN.

Muggia-Sullam M, et al. Postoperative enteral versus parenteral nutritional support in gastrointestinal surgery. Am J Surg 1985; 149:106–112.
This study does not lend support to the commonly held belief that enteral nutrition is superior to TPN.

Nehme AE. Nutritional support of the hospitalized patient: The team concept. JAMA 1980; 243:1906–1908.
A comparison of two groups of patients undergoing TPN. The first group was managed by a nutrition support team and the second by a variety of physicians. The complication rate was significantly higher in the second group.

Shanbhogue LKR, et al. Parenteral nutrition in the surgical patient. Br J Surg 1987; 74:172–180.
A discussion of all aspects of parenteral nutrition in the surgical patient.

The Veteran Affairs Total Parenteral Nutrition Cooperative Study Group: Perioperative total parenteral nutrition in surgical patients. N Engl J Med 1991; 725:525–532.
Preoperative total parenteral nutrition does *improve outcome in severely malnourished patients.*

Winters C. Parenteral nutrition. In SJ Chobanian, MM Van Ness (eds), *Manual of Clinical Problems in Gastroenterology*. Boston: Little, Brown, 1993.

A quick review of parenteral nutrition.

Ziegler TR, et al. Clinical and metabolic efficacy of glutamine-supplemented parenteral nutrition after bone marrow transplantation. Ann Intern Med 1992; 116:821–828.

The addition of glutamine, 0.57 gm/kg body weight per day, improves clinical outcome. Glutamine enhances nitrogen balance, ameliorates intestinal mucosal damage, decreases hepatic steatosis, and decreases bacteremia.

Acute Infectious Gastrointestinal Disease Drugs

There is a general belief in Western society that infectious illness is not a significant concern or, that if an infection occurs, it can easily be managed with any number of modern pharmaceuticals. The rise of multidrug-resistant tuberculosis, the outbreaks of *Escherichia coli* 0157:H7, and the saga of the human immunodeficiency virus should be enough to dispel such a notion of invincibility. The human gastrointestinal tract, essentially an organ in continual contact with the environment throughout its course, is particularly vulnerable to infection. That fact is not lost on the 20 to 50 percent of travelers to high-risk areas in whom an acute infectious gastroenteritis will develop at some time during their trip.

Bacterial infections of the gastrointestinal tract are on the rise, even in developed countries. The average citizen is estimated to suffer an infection 1 to 6 times a year. Worldwide, there are estimated to be more cases of parasitic infection than there are people in the world. To make matters worse, there are legitimate fears that the eighth pandemic of cholera may be beginning. All of this supports the need for health care workers to be informed about treatment of gastrointestinal infections, no matter where their practices are or from where their patients come.

In the patient with acute infectious diarrhea, the history is important. A good differential diagnosis can be made by the presence or absence of associated cases, the timing of onset, relation to particular meals, and the presence of fever, vomiting, or dysentery. Questions of particular importance that should be asked of all patients are the possibility of recent travel, recent antibiotic use, rectal intercourse, or exposure to day care or institutionalized populations. Affirmative answers to these questions significantly alter the differential diagnosis and thus the clinical approach.

The patient with mild diarrhea generally needs little more than a clinical assessment, symptomatic relief, and reassurance. In moderate or more severe diarrhea, some laboratory testing is indicated. The most valuable is a fecal leukocyte test, which, if positive, confirms the presence of diffuse inflammation of the colonic mucosa. Negative results do not rule out the presence of a bacterial pathogen. *Shigella,* for instance, often has no fecal leukocytes during the early, small-bowel phase.

A stool culture need not be submitted in every case of diarrhea. Rather, only those patients with moderate or severe diarrhea, fever, dysentery, fecal leukocyte-positive stools, or symptoms for more than a week need to be cultured. This approach significantly reduces cost and allows the laboratory to give more attention to those cultures that are clinically important.

The most important initial decision facing the clinician is whether to hospitalize the patient. The presence of significant dehydration, intractable vomiting, serious underlying medical problems, severe toxicity, or extremes of age are all indications for hospitalization.

Most patients with infectious diarrhea heal themselves without antibiosis if adequate attention is paid to fluid and electrolyte management. Oral rehydration is best accomplished with a glucose and electrolyte solution, and is reasonable and time-tested. It relies on the principle of solvent drag, the passive absorption of water and sodium following active transport of glucose. A recipe for homemade solution is in the section on cholera in Chap. 13. Good commercial solutions are Pedialyte, Gatorade, and Exceed.

Viral and fungal diseases have become important clinical entities because of the more frequent use of immunosuppressive drugs and the acquired immunodeficiency syndrome (AIDS) epidemic. Both of those classes of pathogens primarily cause esophageal disease. Infections of the esophagus are readily localized to that organ because the usual symptoms, dysphagia and odynophagia, are fortunately relatively specific. Detection of the actual pathogen is a more difficult task. It requires isolation of the particular virus or fungus, or demonstration of the appropriate morphologic change. Fiberoptic endoscopy is the best study to provide this information since it affords the opportunity to observe the morphology as well as to obtain specimens for culture, histology, and microscopy.

The treatment of protozoal and parasitic infections is well covered in the chapters to follow. The parasitic infections are not commonly encountered in the United States, but in the homosexual, institutionalized individual, world traveler, and military population, these are important causes of disease. In these cases, the clinical suspicion of the physician and the technical ability of the laboratory are the cornerstones of diagnosis. It must be remembered that barium studies, antacids, antidiarrheal drugs, and even antimicrobials can hinder the laboratory diagnosis of protozoal and parasitic infections. The clinician must rely on perseverance and serology or biopsy in such cases to reach a diagnosis.

Many chapters in this section are necessarily more disease-oriented than in the other parts of the book. In the management of infectious gastrointestinal illness, the identification of the actual pathogen is the critical step in the treatment regimen. The ability to expeditiously arrive at the correct diagnosis is thus the first step in drug therapy for these diseases. Nevertheless, every attempt has been made to help the reader with the newest aspects and the basic pharmacology of drug therapy for these infections.

Michael S. Gurney

Suggested Reading

Cook GC. The clinical significance of gastrointestinal helminths—a review. Trans R Soc Trop Med Hyg 1986; 80:675.
This is an outstanding review of human helminthic infections.

Cuckler AC. Estimated incidence of worldwide helminthic infections. J Parasitol 1976; 61:55.
A time-honored discussion of the problem of parasitic infections. Unfortunately, most of Cuckler's calculations are still accurate today.

Drugs for parasitic infections. Med Lett Drugs Ther 1988; 30:15.
The Medical Letter *is famed for its concise, dispassionate discus-*

sions of therapeutic agents. This article is a comprehensive listing of these infrequently used drugs.

DuPont HL, Ericsson CD. Prevention and treatment of traveler's diarrhea. N Engl J Med 1993; 328:1821–1827.

A state-of-the-art discussion from the world's authority on the problem.

Fry RD. Infectious enteritis: A collective review. Dis Colon Rectum 1990; 33:520–527.

This a fine review of the problem in America.

Rao GG, Fuller M. A review of hospitalized patients with gastroenteritis. J Hosp Infect 1992; 20:105–111.

Rao and Fuller do a fine job of investigating and estimating the hospital morbidity of gastrointestinal infections.

Rubinoff MJ, Field M. Infectious diarrhea. Annu Rev Med 1991; 42:403–410.

This is a fine discussion about new developments with many intestinal pathogens.

Bacterial Infections

Michael S. Gurney and John D. Malone

Salmonella

Salmonella are gram-negative bacilli of the Enterobacteriaceae tribe that can cause four separate clinical entities: gastroenteritis, bacteremia, typhoid fever (enteric fever), and a chronic carrier state. Gastroenteritis, the most common, is characterized by several days of diarrhea with polymorphonuclear leuckocytes present on fecal smear and positive stool cultures. The *Salmonella enteritidis* group is the usual pathogen in gastroenteritis. This group, the largest, contains 1400 biotypes such as *typhimurium, catertitis,* and *heidelberg*. Antibiotics may prolong illness and result in persistent positive stool cultures. Bacteremia related to *S. choleraesuis* presents with fever and chills without gastrointestinal symptoms and accounts for 8 to 15 percent of all *Salmonella* infections. Localized infections are common, causing infected aortic aneurysms or osteomyelitis. Typhoid fever (usually due to *S. typhi* or *paratyphi*) is a systemic illness characterized by high intermittent fevers and prostration. Antecedent diarrhea is infrequent. Constipation and hepatosplenomegaly may be important clinical clues. Untreated, mortality is 15 to 20 percent. Approximately 400 cases per year occur in the United States, with hundreds of thousands in underdeveloped countries. The fourth clinical entity is an asymptomatic chronic carrier state, defined when stools are positive for *S. typhi* or *paratyphi* for 1 year. This is due to colonization of the liver and biliary tract.

TRANSMISSION

In the US, contaminated poultry and meat processing are major sources. Chickens and turkeys acquire *Salmonella* early in life. Eggs are infected before the shell calcifies; therefore, heating in the shell for 3 minutes may not kill organisms. Water contaminated with fecal waste is common in the underdeveloped world and a risk in flood situations. Since humans are the only reservoir of *Salmonella typhi*, chronic carriers pose a public health risk, especially in food workers with poor handwashing habits after defecation.

An inoculum of 10^5 organisms results in a 30 percent infection rate, in contrast to *Shigella,* where only 100 organisms are necessary. *Salmonella* is destroyed by a pH of 2.0 and unaffected by a pH greater than 5. Individuals with partial gastrectomies are at increased risk because of absent acid and rapid gastric emptying time. Normal bacterial flora are also partially protective since they compete for metabolic growth requirements. A slow bowel transit time (as occurs with antimotility agents) may also increase infection potential by allowing for increased mucosal barrier penetration.

Besides those with low gastric acid production, typhoid fever–susceptible individuals include those with sickle cell disease (decreased phagocytic opsonizing capacity), leukemia or lymphoma (impaired cellular prevention mechanisms), and schistosomiasis (adherence of *Salmonella* to fluke tegument). Bartonellosis- and malaria-infected individuals are also prone.

TREATMENT

As compelling as it is to treat an ill patient, it must be remembered that antibiosis has not been shown to shorten the course of symptoms in nontyphoidal salmonellosis, yet it increases the risk of formation of a chronic carrier state. Typhoid fever is an exception, however. Antibiotics clearly are indicated and have been shown to improve outcome. Fluoroquinones are the initial drug of choice. Ceftriaxone, cefoperazone, and trimethoprim-sulfamethoxazole are alternatives. Chloramphenicol was often prescribed in the past, but is used infrequently now because of drug resistance and fears of toxicity.

Single-dose dexamethasone in high doses (3 mg/kg body weight) intravenously has been shown to improve survival in severe typhoid fever manifested by delirium, obtundation, stupors, coma, or shock.

Ciprofloxacin

Ciprofloxacin, 500 to 750 mg, should be given orally twice a day for 10 days. The intravenous dosage is 400 mg twice a day. The advantages are low resistance rates, excellent tolerance, and ease of administration. Disadvantages include high cost and unestablished safety profile in pregnant women and children.

Cefoperazone

Cefoperazone, 100 mg/kg/day body weight, should be administered twice a day for 14 days. A trial in children with severe typhoidal shock showed good efficacy.

Ceftriaxone

Ceftriaxone, 1.5 to 2.0 gm twice a day, should be given for 5 days.

Trimethoprim and Sulfamethoxazole

The adult dosage is 160 mg trimethoprim (TMP) and 800 mg sulfamethoxazole (SXT; one double-strength tablet) twice a day for 14 days. The dosage for children is 185 mg/mole TMP and 925 mg/mole SXT each 24 hours.

Choramphenicol plasmid-mediated resistance also codes for SXT and, therefore, TMP may be the only active component. If a patient shows no response in 72 hours, antibiotics should be changed. Ineffective drugs (even if in vitro sensitive) include aminoglycosides and tetracycline; the effectiveness of first-generation cephalosporins is questionable.

PEARLS AND PITFALLS

1. *Salmonella* gastroenteritis is usually due to the *S. enteritidis* group (1400 biotypes). Antibiotics are contraindicated in most settings, and adequate hydration is recommended.
2. New alternatives for enteric (typhoid) fever include cefoperazone, ceftriaxone, and ciprofloxacin. These drugs have proved exceedingly effective in clinical trials. Steroids in high doses improve survival in severe cases. Enteric isolation is necessary. Bone marrow and liver biopsy have a higher yield than blood culture.
3. Chronic carriers of *Salmonella typhi* or *paratyphi* are defined when stool cultures are positive for 1 year. Cholelithiasis is a possible underlying cause, and cholecystectomy may be indicated. Ciprofloxacin, 750 mg twice a day for 30 days, may be an alternative.

4. Differential diagnostic points
   a. Pulse-temperature deficit may occur with typhoid fever.
   b. Other diseases with possible pulse-temperature deficit include brucellosis, tularemia, rheumatic fever, infectious mononucleosis, leptospirosis, tuberculosis, Hodgkin's lymphoma, and rickettsial infections (Rocky Mountain spotted fever).
5. Clinical clues to enteral infection
   a. Salmonellosis: Group outbreak following a certain meal; incubation approximately 24 hours
   b. Staphylococcal: Exotoxic induction; severe vomiting and diarrhea within 20 to 60 minutes of ingestion
   c. *Shigella*: Toxicity greater than *Salmonella,* fever higher, stools bloody, increased number of fecal leukocytes compared to other bacterial infections
   d. *Vibrio parahemolyticus*: Shellfish-associated, with mild watery diarrhea
   e. *Bacillus cereus*: Watery diarrhea after ingesting contaminated food (rice)
   f. Calicivirus: Involves teenage children in clusters; fever lasts 1.5 to 3.0 days
   g. Rotavirus: Involves children 4 to 5 years old
   h. Enterotoxigenic *Escherichia coli*: Occurs in travelers to underdeveloped countries; 3-day illness with cramps and diarrhea (nonbloody), low-grade fever, and nausea
   i. *Giardia*: Onset 10 days after exposure to water from mountain streams; malodorous stools
   j. *Campylobacter*: Bloody diarrhea lasting 3 days; puppy in household with diarrhea
6. Table 13-1 lists antibiotics and their appropriateness for use in pregnancy and breast-feeding.

Shigellosis

Shigellosis is due to a gram-negative, nonmotile rod of the tribe Escherichieae, genus *Shigella,* and is the common cause of bacillary dysentery. The term *dysentery* describes the condition of frequent stools containing blood and mucus. Transmission is through fecal and oral routes involving contaminated food, water, hands, and flies. Outbreaks associated with poor sanitation have occurred in day care centers, American Indian reservations, and military campaigns, and in institutionalized mentally retarded individuals and travelers to underdeveloped countries. Infection may occur with inoculums as small as 100 viable cells, as compared with *S. typhi,* which requires 10^5 for infection, or enterotoxigenic *E. coli* and *Vibrio cholerae,* with 10^7 organisms needed for infection.

Four species of *Shigella* exist: *S. dysenteriae, S. flexneri, S. boydii,* and *S. sonnei. Shigella,* along with *Salmonella,* is differentiated from other common nonpathogenic gram-negative rods such as *E. coli* by the inability to ferment lactose and produce acid. Because dye indicators are not changed by a lowered pH on the MacConkey bacterial screening agar, colonies appear clear and colorless. More selective media such as *Salmonella*/*Shigella* agar containing a high bile salt content that inhibits the growth of most other coliforms can also be utilized. Currently *S. sonnei* is isolated 60 percent of the time and *S. flexneri* is isolated in 36 percent of cases. *Shigella*

Table 13-1. Bacterial infections: Pregnancy and breast-feeding

Agent	FDA pregnancy category	Risk vs benefit (by trimester)			Breast-feeding category
		1st	2nd	3rd	
Amoxicillin	C2	?	?	?	IIIB
Ampicillin	C2	?	?	?	IIIB
Colestipol	C2	?	?	?	IIIA
Cefoperazone	B1	B > R	B > R	B > R	IIIA
Ceftriaxone	B1	B > R	B > R	B > R	IIIA
Chloramphenicol	C2	R >> B	R >> B	R >> B	IV
Cholestyramine	C1	B > R	B > R	B > R	IIIA
Ciprofloxacin	C1	R >> B?	R >> B?	R >> B?	IV
Erythromycin	B1	B > R	B > R	B > R	IIIA
Fluoroquinolones	?	?	?	?	?
Furazolidone	?	?	?	?	?
Gentamicin	C2	?	?	?	IV

Sulfamethoxazole	C1	R > B	R > B	R > B	IV
Tetracycline	C1	R > B	R > B	R > B	IV
Trimethoprim	C1	R > B	R > B	R > B	IV
Vancomycin	C2	?	?	?	IV

Food and Drug Administration (FDA) pregnancy categories:
A = Well-controlled studies fail to demonstrate risk to the fetus.
B1 = Animal studies fail to demonstrate risk to the fetus but no human studies are available.
B2 = Animal studies show some risk to the fetus but this is not confirmed in human studies.
C1 = Animal studies show risk to the fetus but no human studies are available.
C2 = Animal and human studies are unavailable.
D = Drugs associated with birth defects but with potential benefits that may outweigh known risks.
X = Drugs associated with birth defects and with potential risk that clearly outweighs potential benefit.
Risk vs benefit: R >> B = Proven or potential risk outweighs potential benefits.
B > R = Potential benefits outweigh potential risks.
R >> B? = Risks may be outweighed by benefits in some circumstances.
? = Risk-to-benefit ratio is unknown.
Breast-feeding categories:
I = Drug does not enter breast milk.
II = Drug enters breast milk but is not known to be harmful in therapeutic doses.
IIIA = Drug may or may not enter breast milk but no adverse effects are expected.
IIIB = Drug may or may not enter breast milk but drug is systemically absorbed.
IV = Drug enters breast milk and poses a potential risk to the neonate.

dysenteriae was the most common species in the early 1900s. Changing patterns probably reflect building immunity.

Pathogenesis involves the ability of a small inoculum to resist gastric acidity and multiply in the small bowel causing upper abdominal distress and watery stools. Individuals with low gastric acid production (vagotomy and pyloroplasty, H_2-blockers, antacids) or those receiving steroid suppression are more susceptible. Bacteria pass to the colon where mucosal cell invasion results in acute onset of dysentery. Incubation ranges from 1 to 3 days for *S. dysenteriae,* to 3 to 7 days for *S. sonnei* and *S. flexneri.* Shiga toxin produced by *S. dysenteriae* is cytotoxic in tissue culture and also causes transudation of fluid in tissue cells through adenylate cyclase activation. Prostaglandin stimulation may also contribute to secretory activity.

Disease may be self-limited over a 7- to 10-day period. However, attention to fluid and electrolytes (especially in children) is stressed since dehydration is a major cause of mortality. Antibiotic treatment definitely shortens the length and severity of disease. In contrast to *Salmonella* infections, development of a chronic carrier state is very infrequent and not related to treatment. Therefore, antibiotic treatment of all shigellosis is generally recommended.

TREATMENT

With respect to drug therapy, antibacterial plasmid-mediated resistance to sulfas, tetracycline, ampicillin, and trimethoprim-sulfamethoxazole has developed through the decades. Individuals with foreign-travel exposure have a high rate of resistant *Shigella,* including multidrug resistance. In the United States, resistance patterns on 252 *Shigella* isolates randomly collected by the Centers for Disease Control in 1985 and 1986 were as follows: tetracycline, 43 percent resistant; ampicillin, 32 percent; TMP-SXT, 7 percent; chloramphenicol, 5 percent; and gentamicin, 4 percent. A rapid rise in the resistance to nalidixic acid has been reported from an American Indian reservation.

Treatment recommendations are as follows:

Fluoroquinones

Ciprofloxacin: 500 mg twice a day for 3 to 5 days is standard therapy, and is quite effective. One gram orally per day for 2 days is effective for species other than *S. dysenteriae.* Addition of an antimotility agent such as loperamide or Imodium is safe and will shorten the period of diarrhea.

Norfloxacin: 400 mg twice a day for 5 days.

Fluoroquinones have caused cartilage damage in immature animals, and should not be used in children and pregnant women if possible.

Trimethoprim and Sulfamethoxazole

The adult dosage is 160 mg TMP and 800 mg SXT (one double-strength tablet) orally twice a day for 5 days. The dosage for children is 10 mg/kg body weight TMP and 50 mg/kg SXT per day orally twice a day for 5 days.

TMP-SMX is the best choice if medication allergy is not a problem.

PEARLS AND PITFALLS

1. Resistance to ampicillin is common, and resistance to trimethoprim-sulfamethoxazole is increasing, especially in foreign countries (Africa and the Far East particularly).

2. Bloody diarrhea of sudden onset containing fecal leukocytes may also characterize other pathogens, such as *Campylobacter* (most common), enteropathogenic *E. coli, Salmonella, Yersinia,* and *Entamoeba histolytica.* Inflammatory bowel disease (ulcerative colitis or regional enteritis) is also a possibility.
3. For the laboratory, fresh stools (preferably less than 4 hours old) should be submitted. The laboratory should be alerted with a differential diagnosis of pathogens written on the laboratory slip to ensure appropriate evaluation—not just "diarrhea" or "stool culture."
4. Transmission is by the fecal-oral route. Humans are the only reservoir. High transmission rates occur in families, especially among young siblings. For hospitalized individuals, appropriate precautions would include thorough handwashing. Centers for Disease Control Guidelines of Enteric Precautions are indicated.
5. The rare chronic carrier is difficult to treat. Antibiotics are seldom effective. Lactulose may be of assistance. Ciprofloxacin, 750 mg twice a day for 30 days, has been found to be effective in *Salmonella typhi* carriers.

Vibrio Cholera

Vibrio cholera has been epidemic in India since the beginning of recorded history, and has been responsible for seven pandemics since 1817. Although it is an important cause of morbidity and mortality in Asia and Africa, it is uncommon in the United States and is limited to the Gulf Coast area. Nevertheless, it has great potential for epidemics, and the last pandemic in 1961 did extend to the United States. A new strain of cholera has recently been recognized in Bangladesh and may be the beginning of the eighth pandemic.

Cholera produces a classic secretory diarrhea by production of a toxin that binds irreversibly to the small-intestinal mucosa and stimulates cyclic AMP production. The increased intracellular cyclic AMP leads to secretion of water and electrolytes into the gut. The volume of fluid produced can be most impressive; well-hydrated patients with severe cholera have been known to produce an amount of diarrheal fluid equal to their own weight. Inability to replace the gut fluid losses in severe cases leads to the traditional outcome of cholera before rehydration therapy: dehydration, shock, and death (70–80% of cases). Cholera is virtually the only infectious diarrhea able to cause circulatory collapse in adults.

In reality, most cases of cholera are subclinical or indistinguishable from other infectious diarrheas. Seven to 25 percent (depending on biotype) require medical attention and 2 to 11 percent require hospitalization. The usual case of cholera begins abruptly and the first few stools contain fecal material. However, the stools rapidly become clear and liquid, with flecks of mucus (rice-water stools). Vomiting may occur initially but usually ceases as the infection progresses. If the patient is not rehydrated, the consequences of dehydration rapidly ensue. Dehydration is the most devastating consequence of cholera, but metabolic acidosis and hypokalemia may occur as a result of loss of bicarbonate and potassium in the stool.

Diagnosis is made by the clinical setting, by dark-field microscopy revealing the characteristic motility pattern, by stool culture, and by serology, which becomes positive four days after the onset of symptoms.

Rapid rehydration with fluid and electrolytes is the critical element in cholera treatment. Patients who are severely dehydrated or unable to take fluids orally need rapid intravenous fluid replacement. Most other patients can be successfully treated with oral rehydration solutions. The rate of intravenous replacement for severely dehydrated adults is 2 liters over the first 30 minutes. If improvement is noted, the rate can be slowed to 110 ml/kg body weight over the next 4 hours. Children in shock need 30 mg/kg in the first hour and an additional 40 ml/kg in the next 2 hours. Ringer's lactate with 10 mEq/liter added potassium is the proper intravenous solution. In both children and adults, oral rehydration solution can then be ingested if the patient's condition is stable.

The formula for oral rehydration solution recommended by the World Health Organization is sodium, 90 mmole/liter; potassium, 20 mmole/liter; chloride, 80 mmole/liter; bicarbonate, 30 mmole/liter; and glucose, 111 mmole/liter. A number of clinical trials have shown that this solution is safe and clinically useful in the treatment of all types of diarrhea in all groups of patients. For mild dehydration, the solution should be given at the rate of 50 mg/kg body weight within the first 4 hours. For moderate dehydration, 100 ml/kg should be given in the same time period. Vomiting rarely prevents successful use of oral rehydration solution. Occasionally the diarrhea is so severe that both intravenous and oral routes must be utilized.

Antibiotics are not a substitute for rehydration therapy, but reduce the volume and duration of diarrhea and shorten the period of *Vibrio* excretion. Doxycycline, given as a single 300-mg dose, is the drug of choice for adults. Trimethoprim-sulfamethoxazole is preferable for children, in a dose of 25 mg/kg for SMX, twice a day for 3 days. Furazolidone (5–7 mg/kg), a nonabsorbable antibiotic, may be preferable in children and pregnant women but requires a longer course of treatment. Antibiotic resistance has not been a problem except in outbreaks in Bangladesh and Kenya. The recent outbreak in Bangladesh and Pakistan is resistant to TMP-SMX and furazolidone.

Atropine and steroids are unnecessary and may be harmful. Kaolin and antispasmodics are of no clinical value. Chlorpromazine and nicotinic acid inhibit intestinal secretion and may be of small benefit.

In recent years, several noncholera vibrios have become clinically important. *Vibrio parahemolyticus* has been identified as a food-borne cause of gastroenteritis. It is usually caused by mishandling of seafood after cooking. Clinical manifestations include diarrhea (98%), nausea (71%), vomiting (52%), headache (42%), and low-grade fever (27%). The incubation period is from 4 to 96 hours, and the illness usually subsides within 3 days. Therapy is primarily supportive, with replacement of fluid and electrolyte losses. There are no good data on antibiotic efficacy but tetracycline would be a reasonable choice if antimicrobials are needed.

Vibrio vulnificus has been identified as a cause of wound infections and primary septicemia, particularly in patients with chronic illnesses. Patients with chronic liver disease seem to be the group at greatest risk. *Vibrio vulnificus* infections are most remarkable for their virulence: A recent study showed a 55 percent mortality for septicemia, and a 24 percent mortality for wound infections. Almost all septicemia cases occurred after ingestion of raw oysters. The wound infections occurred after exposure of preexisting wounds to sea water. Tetracycline is the most effective agent but early treatment is mandatory. Since this organism is so devastating, prevention by avoidance of raw seafood and protection of wounds from warm sea water (particularly estuaries) represent the prudent course to follow.

PEARLS AND PITFALLS

1. Patients with low gastric acid output, either from medications (H_2-blockers), surgery, or gastric atrophy, are much more vulnerable to cholera infection. If a patient is receiving chronic acid suppression and is traveling to an endemic area, it would be prudent to temporarily stop the medication or change to a medication such as sucralfate (Carafate).
2. Cholera is virtually the only infectious diarrhea that can cause shock in a healthy adult.
3. Hypotension from cholera should *not* be treated with vasopressors or cardiac stimulants. The proper therapy is fluid, fluid, fluid.
4. Existing vaccines are only 60 percent effective in preventing cholera. Since the efficacy of vaccines is low, the side effects are significant, and the usual traveler is at low risk, routine cholera immunization for travel to an endemic area is not recommended.
5. If oral rehydration solution is not available, a homemade recipe for temporary oral rehydration solution is 1 tsp salt, 1 tsp bicarbonate, and 4 tsp table sugar dissolved in 1 liter of water. Commercial electrolyte and sugar solutions such as Pedialyte, Gatorade, and Exceed are also good substitutes.

Campylobacter

Campylobacter's name is derived from the Greek terms for curved (campylo) and rod (bacter), and it describes these motile, nonsporeforming, comma-shaped gram-negative rods, which are some of the most common bacterial pathogens in humans. The most common species causing enteritis in humans are *C. fetus* subspecies *fetus* and *C. jejuni*.

Campylobacter comprises a worldwide zoonosis with reservoirs in cattle, sheep, swine, fowl, dogs, cats, and rodents. Human infection frequently occurs after slaughterhouse contamination of undercooked meats, particularly poultry products. Consumption of raw (unpasteurized) milk and untreated water (as by backpackers and campers) and contamination of municipal water systems have resulted in outbreaks. Raw clams, cake icing, and salads have been reported to cause infection. Contact with household pets, especially young dogs and cats with diarrhea, has been implicated. Some cases of traveler's diarrhea are also caused by *C. jejuni*.

CAMPYLOBACTER JEJUNI

Campylobacter jejuni is isolated more often from diarrhea stool specimens than are *Salmonella* or *Shigella*. Intestinal infection results in enteritis, with fever, malaise, crampy abdominal pain, and diarrhea ranging from loose stools to voluminous movements of water and gross blood. Disease is self-limited in a majority of patients; however, 10 to 20 percent have symptoms that last longer than 1 week. The relapse rate is 5 to 10 percent. Severe infections may occur, with large amounts of blood in the stool, tenesmus, high fevers, and toxic megacolon. In *C. jejuni,* bacteremia occurs in fewer than 1 percent, usually in infants and the elderly. Complications such as meningitis endocarditis, pancreatitis, and cholecystitis are extremely rare. A reactive arthritis can occur in individuals who are HLA-B27 positive.

CAMPYLOBACTER FETUS

In contrast, *Campylobacter fetus* is frequently associated with bacteremia. Intermittent diarrhea and nonspecific abdominal pain occur in 35 percent of patients. However, more systemic signs of relapsing fevers, chills, myalgias, and night sweats are more typical. A predilection for seeding of vascular sites results in mycotic aneurysms of the abdominal aorta, thrombophlebitis, and endocarditis. Other localized infections from bacteremia include septic arthritis, lung abscess, cholecystitis, and meningoencephalitis. Most patients recover with necessary antibiotic therapy. Self-limiting bacteremias have also been observed.

THERAPY

Many *Campylobacter* intestinal infections are self-limited, with resolution of bloody diarrhea, cramps, and fevers by the time cultures return. Several studies have not shown any benefit of antibiotics over placebo; however, patient numbers were small and treatment started late. Individuals who need treatment include those with high fever and bloody diarrhea, and those with worsening or unimproved symptoms at the time of bacterial culture confirmation. Erythromycin eliminates *Campylobacter* in 72 hours and has few serious side effects. A chronic carrier state does not occur. In children, early treatment may diminish spread in households, day care settings, or nursery schools.

Treatment

Enteritis:

1. Ciprofloxacin: Adults, 500 mg twice a day orally for 5 days. Exceedingly effective but expensive. It has a broad spectrum against bacterial enteric pathogens. Use in adults only.
2. Erythromycin: Adults, 250 mg 4 times a day orally for 5 to 7 days. Children, 40 mg/kg/24 hours for 5 to 7 days. Resistance from 1 to 8 percent in Southeast Asia and Sweden.
3. Tetracycline: Adults, 250 to 500 mg 4 times a day orally for 5 days. Children greater than 10 years old, 50 mg/kg/24 hours for 5 days. Plasmid-mediated resistance 15 percent in Canada.
4. Furazolidone: 5 mg/kg/24 hours. Useful in children due to oral preparation.

Septicemia: Imipenem, 500 mg every 6 hours.

PEARLS AND PITFALLS

1. Symptoms of abdominal cramps and bloody diarrhea may represent *Shigella* or *Salmonella*; however, *Campylobacter* is more common. Ciprofloxacin is effective with all these pathogens.
2. Stool cultures need to be labeled for *Campylobacter* since special medium and lowered oxygen are required for growth.
3. Historical aspects indicating possible *Campylobacter* enteritis would include exposure to young dogs or cats with diarrhea and consumption of unpasteurized milk, poorly cooked meats, or fresh surface water.
4. Ineffective medications in *Campylobacter* enteritis include
   a. Trimethoprim-sulfamethoxazole

b. Vancomycin
c. Metronidazole
d. Unprotected beta-lactam rings (ampicillin, penicillin, cephalosporins, ticarcillin)

Clostridium difficile

Pseudomembranous colitis from *C. difficile* is a distinct clinical entity characterized by inflammatory plaques and pseudomembranes in the large intestine, associated with diarrhea. It was first described in 1893 and was occasionally reported over the next 70 years as a rare complication of surgery, uremia, malignancy, and other conditions. The incidence of pseudomembranous colitis rose dramatically in the 1970s as a result of increased sensitivity to it by physicians and the advent of clindamycin and lincomycin as antimicrobials. In the late 1970s, the association with *C. difficile* was shown conclusively by Bartlett and others.

Pseudomembranous colitis should be suspected in any patient in whom diarrhea develops within 10 weeks of antibiotic therapy. Specific findings include nonbloody, watery diarrhea (90–95%), bloody diarrhea (5–10%), fever (80%), leukocytosis (80%), fecal leukocytes (50%), and rebound tenderness (10–20%). The diagnosis is based on the clinical setting, the endoscopic appearance (85–90% have pseudomembranes on flexible sigmoidoscopy; 10% have pseudomembranes only in the right colon), a positive toxin assay (90% have toxin; false-positive rate 5%), or a positive culture. The culture is more difficult to perform, requires more time, and is less sensitive and less specific.

TREATMENT

The natural course of pseudomembranous colitis is usually self-limited if the offending antibiotic is discontinued. However, one-third of patients require hospitalization or extension of their hospital stay for this complication. The first step in therapy is to stop the antibiotic. If an infection exists that requires further treatment, a different antimicrobial agent should be given. For mild cases of colitis, a resin that binds the toxin such as colestipol (5 gm tid) or cholestyramine (4 gm tid) can be used. Colestipol is more palatable and binds 4 times more toxin per gram in vitro, but the two have not been compared clinically. Moderate to severe colitis does not improve with a binding resin, and antibiotics should be used.

The usual initial drug is oral metronidazole, 250 mg 4 times a day for 10 days. Metronidazole is as effective as the primary alternative, vancomycin, but is much less expensive. However, pseudomembranous colitis has occurred after metronidazole, and resistant strains are reported, albeit rarely. Therefore, vancomycin is generally preferred for critically ill patients.

Vancomycin has extensive clinical experience in pseudomembranous colitis, but is generally reserved for special circumstances because of the considerable expense (weight-for-weight it is 4 times the price of gold). The dose is 125 mg every 6 hours for 1 to 2 weeks. Critically ill patients may be given 500 mg every 6 hours, with a reduction in dose after clinical improvement. The clinical response is usually within 2 to 3 days. Disadvantages include bad taste, expense (up to $500 for a 10-day course), and a relapse rate of approximately 20 percent. Vancomycin is only minimally absorbed when given orally; therefore, systemic toxicity is not usually a problem. However, with prolonged therapy in patients with renal failure, elevated serum levels have occurred and toxicity has been reported. Such patients should have drug levels monitored.

For patients too ill or too soon postsurgery to take oral medication, metronidazole may be given intravenously, 500 mg every 6 hours. There is good evidence that parenteral metronidazole is secreted into the bowel and achieves intraluminal concentrations adequate to inhibit *C. difficile*. Another approach recently shown to be effective is to place a pigtail catheter endoscopically, and to flush with an initial 2000-mg bolus of vancomycin, followed by 100 mg every 6 hours and after each stool. Occasionally patients are unresponsive to therapy and progress to toxic megacolon or perforation. The only recourse in such patients is surgery.

A significant problem is recurrence of the infection. This may be due to persistence of *C. difficile* spores in the colon or because of impaired immune response. Recurrence usually responds to another course of treatment but multiple relapses can occur. In such cases, Tedesco and associates have shown that the following schedule is effective: vancomycin, 125 mg every 6 hours for 1 week; then 125 mg every 12 hours for 1 week; then 125 mg/day for 1 week; then 125 mg every other day for 1 week; then, finally, 125 mg every third day for 2 weeks. This regimen was designed to deal with the possibility of *C. difficile* spores in the colon. None of Tedesco's 22 patients had another relapse after this course. Another recent regimen to deal with relapses used combined vancomycin, 125 mg 4 times a day, and rifampin, 600 mg twice a day for 1 week. Clinical outcome was good in the seven patients treated, but stool cultures in all seven became positive again 1 month after therapy. Other alternatives include use of a binding resin, administration of microorganisms such as *Lactobacillus* strains or *Saccharomyces boulardii,* or administration of intravenous immunoglobulin.

PEARLS AND PITFALLS

1. Never give antimotility agents to patients with documented or suspected pseudomembranous colitis. Such drugs are associated with the development of toxic megacolon.
2. Do not give steroids (if possible) to patients with pseudomembranous colitis. Steroids are associated with a high perforation rate in animal models.
3. If patients do not respond to a resin-binding agent, do not simply add an antibiotic. The resin must be discontinued since it binds the antibiotic in the gut lumen.
4. A new antimicrobial, Teicoplanin, is structurally related to vancomycin, and may have a lower relapse rate. Clinical experience is still very limited.
5. Pseudomembranes observed by sigmoidoscopy are not specific for *C. difficile* infection. They can also be seen in shigellosis, amebiasis, ischemic colitis, and *Yersinia* infections. Conversely, a sigmoidoscopy negative for pseudomembranes does not mean the absence of infection. The pseudomembranes may be right-sided only in 10 percent of cases, or they may be microscopic.
6. Normal patients can have both a positive *C. difficile* toxin (1–5%) or culture (up to 20%).

Suggested Reading

SALMONELLA

Asperilla MO, et al. Quinolone antibiotics in the treatment of salmonella infections. Rev Infect Dis 1990; 12:873–889.
A thorough review article discussing the clinical experience with salmonellosis and the quinolones.

DuPont HL. Quinolones in *Salmonella typhi* infection. Drugs 1993; 45 (suppl 3):119–124.
DuPont reviews the worldwide experience in treatment of typhoid fever with quinolones.

Eng RHK, et al. Eradication of non-typhi salmonella infection by ciprofloxacin. Am J Med 1990; 89:386–388.
Four chronic carriers of salmonella were treated successfully with ciprofloxacin and the carrier state was eradicated.

Mishu B, et al. *Salmonella enteritidis* gastroenteritis transmitted by intact chicken eggs. Ann Intern Med 1991; 115:190–194.
An outbreak of salmonella infections in Knoxville, Tennessee, was traced to infected eggs used in hollandaise and bernaise sauces. Salmonella can survive even in fully cooked eggs.

Neill MA, et al. Failure of ciprofloxacin to eradicate convalescent fecal excretion after acute salmonellosis: Experience during an outbreak in health care workers. Ann Intern Med 1991; 114: 195–199.
A sobering note about the possibility of prolonged fecal excretion in salmonella infections. Even in health care workers, who may need to be isolated from patients, conservative therapy is still perhaps the wisest.

Pope JW, Gerde H. Typhoid fever: Successful therapy with cefoperazone. J Infect Dis 1986; 153:272.
A randomized trial involving 25 Haitian children with severe typhoid fever found cefoperazone as effective as chloramphenicol.

SHIGELLA

Bandres JA, et al. Trimethoprim/sulfamethoxazole remains active against enterotoxigenic *Escherichia coli* and *Shigella* species in Guadalajara, Mexico. Am J Med Sci 1992; 303:289–291.
TMP-SMX remains effective against isolates from Mexico. One caveat: In vitro sensitivity does not always translate into in vivo efficacy.

Bennish ML, Azad AK, Yousefzadeh D. Intestinal obstruction during shigellosis: Incidence, clinical features, risk factors, and outcome. Gastroenterology 1991; 101:626–634.
Shigellosis in the Third World is associated with a 9 percent mortality. However, if signs of obstruction occur, the risk rises to 33 percent. The authors reviewed over 1200 patients in Bangladesh to study this complication of the infection.

Bennish ML, et al. Treatment of shigellosis: Comparison of one- or two-dose ciprofloxacin with standard five-day therapy. Ann Intern Med 1992; 117:727–734.
An excellent trial of various short courses of treatment for shigellosis. The 1- or 2-day regimens were fine for all infections except those with Shigella dysenteriae *type 1, for which the 5-day therapy was best.*

Bhattacharya SK, et al. Randomized clinical trial of norfloxacin for shigellosis. Am J Trop Med 1991; 45:683–687.
Norfloxacin showed fine efficacy in a large trial.
Lee LA, et al. Hyperendemic shigellosis in the United States: A review of surveillance data for 1967–1988. J Infect Dis 1991; 164:894–900.
The United States experience with shigellosis over two decades is reviewed. Surprisingly, in 1988 over 22,000 cases were reported.
Mathan VI, Mathan MM. Intestinal manifestations of invasive diarrheas and their diagnosis. Rev Infect Dis 1991; 13 (suppl 4): s311–s313.
The clinical presentation in Shigella *infections is reviewed.*
Murphy GS, et al. Ciprofloxacin and loperamide in the treatment of bacillary dysentery. Ann Intern Med 1993; 118:582–586.
It formerly was thought that antimotility agents were contraindicated in all infectious enteritis. This study clearly shows that loperamide is not only safe, but significantly reduces the duration of symptoms.
Zajdowitz T. Epidemiologic and clinical aspects of shigellosis in American forces deployed to Saudi Arabia. South Med J 1993; 86:647–650.
The clinical presentation of nine cases in Saudi Arabia is described. Only one of the patients presented with classic dysentery, and two had "pseudomeningitis."

CHOLERA

Blake PA. *Vibrios* on the half-shell: What the walrus and the carpenter didn't know. Ann Intern Med 1983; 99:558.
A short but pertinent warning about the dangers of raw seafood ingestion. This is even more important today.
Bonner JR, et al. Spectrum of *Vibrio* infections in a Gulf Coast community. Ann Intern Med 1983; 99:464.
An excellent article on the various manifestations of Vibrio *infection.*
Holmberg SD. *Vibrios* and *Aeromonas.* Infect Dis Clin North Am 1988; 2:655.
An excellent review of the various species of Vibrio *and their illnesses. Holmberg also discusses the nonvibrio Vibrionaceae such as* Aeromonas hydrophila *and* Plesiomonas shigelloides.
Johnston JM, et al. Cholera on a Gulf Coast oil rig. N Engl J Med 1983; 309:523.
A description of the various manifestations of a cholera "epidemic" on an oil rig.
Klontz KC, et al. Syndromes of *Vibrio vulnificus* infections. Ann Intern Med 1988; 109:318.
A compilation of 62 cases of V. vulnificus *infections from Florida is reported. The virulence of the organism is stressed.*
Morris JG Jr. *Vibrio* and *Aeromonas.* In SL Gorbach (ed), *Infectious Diarrhea.* Boston: Blackwell, 1986.
A well-written review by one of the leading authorities in the field.
Morris JG Jr. *Vibrio vulnificus:* A new monster of the deep? Ann Intern Med 1988; 109:261.
An editorial in the same issue as Klontz's article. Morris stresses the need for prevention.

CAMPYLOBACTER

Blaser MT, Reller LB. *Campylobacter* enteritis. N Engl J Med 1981; 305:1444.

A complete review of Campylobacter jejuni, *including historical background, epidemiology, pathogenesis, clinical features, and treatment.*

Klein BS, Vergeront JM. *Campylobacter* infection associated with raw milk: An outbreak of gastroenteritis due to *Campylobacter jejuni* and thermotolerant *Campylobacter fetus* subspecies *fetus.* JAMA 1986; 225:361.

Unpasteurized milk and heat-tolerant strains were identified in source outbreaks.

Saeed AM, Harris NV, DiGiacomo RF. The role of exposure to animals in the etiology of *Campylobacter jejuni/coli* enteritis. Am J Epidemiol 1993; 137:108–113.

Possible transmission of Campylobacter *from household pets was studied. Simply having a pet did not confer any risk. However, exposure to a pet with diarrhea—especially dogs—apparently caused nearly 10 percent of the cases.*

Shandera WX, Tormey MP, Blaser MJ. An outbreak of bacteremic *Campylobacter jejuni* infection. Mt Sinai J Med 1992; 59:53–56.

Campylobacter jejuni *usually causes an enteritis, but in this unusual outbreak, bacteremia/sepsis occurred without diarrhea. The source was eventually traced to processed turkey.*

Southern JP, Smith RMM, Palmer SR. Bird attack on milk bottles: Possible mode of transmission of *Campylobacter jejuni* to man. Lancet 1990; 336:1425–1432.

For all of us who have always suspected that those bird droppings on our windshields were more than chance occurrences, here is proof: A careful epidemiologic study traced an outbreak of C. jejuni *in South Wales to bird attacks on milk bottle tops as they rested peacefully on porches in the morning. Perhaps Hitchcock was right.*

Skirrow MB. *Campylobacter.* Lancet 1990; 336:921–923.

A fine review of Campylobacter *from the public health perspective.*

CLOSTRIDIUM DIFFICILE

Bartlett JG. *Clostridium difficile*: Clinical considerations. Rev Infect Dis 1990; 12 (suppl 2):S243–S251.

A fine review of the history and current clinical thought on pseudomembranous colitis.

Johnson S, et al. Nosocomial *Clostridium difficile* colonisation and disease. Lancet 1990; 336:97–100.

Clostridium difficile *is now recognized as a leading cause of nosocomial infections. In this study, 21 percent of all ward patients who were hospitalized for more than one week became colonized with the organism.*

Kelly CP, et al. *Clostridium difficile* colitis. N Engl J Med 1994; 330:257–262.

A fine review of the clinical problem.

Kleinfeld DI, Sharpe RJ, Donta ST. Parenteral therapy for antibiotic-associated pseudomembranous colitis. J Infect Dis 1988; 157:389.

Kleinfeld and associates report success using intravenous metronidazole in one patient and review the pertinent literature.

Leung DYM, et al. Treatment with intravenously administered gamma globulin of chronic relapsing colitis induced by *Clostridium difficile* toxin. J Pediatr 1991; 118:633–637.
Leung and associates had the interesting hypothesis that relapses were due to impaired production of immunoglobulins G and A to C. difficile *toxin A. They did indeed find low immunoglobulin levels in five children with relapsing pseudomembranous colitis. All five had resolution of their infection with intravenous gamma globulin.*
Morris JB, Zollinger RM, Stellato TA. Role of surgery in antibiotic-induced pseudomembranous colitis. Am J Surg 1990; 160: 535–539.
Occasionally pseudomembranous colitis will be so fulminant that the colon may perforate before therapy can take hold. This article discusses the surgical experience with the complications of C. difficile.
Tedesco FJ, Gordon D, Fortson WC. Approach to patients with multiple relapses of antibiotic-associated pseudomembranous colitis. Am J Gastroenterol 1985; 80:867.
The best study of treatment for relapse. A tapering 21-day course of vancomycin followed by 21 days of pulse vancomycin cured 22 patients with prior multiple relapses.

Antifungal Agents

M.R. Chowdhury and D. Michael Jones

Candida species are commensal organisms in the gastrointestinal tract. The most prevalent site of colonization is the mouth, and various oral structures may be sites for candidal proliferation. *Candida albicans* is the species most frequently isolated from all sites in both healthy individuals and those who are immunocompromised. A disruption of host defense mechanisms facilitates candidal colonization and invasion of the gut. Table 14-1 lists the factors that predispose to gastrointestinal candidiasis. Pathogenesis of candidal (and other fungal) infections involves both the mechanisms by which the organisms cause the local manifestations of disease and the mechanisms by which the organisms gain access to the circulation, resulting in systemic disease. Symptoms caused by *C. albicans* in the gastrointestinal tract are related primarily to tissue invasion. The gut is the most important portal of entry of *Candida* species into the circulation. The process by which the yeast transmigrates the wall of the digestive tract gaining access to the circulation is known as persorption and has been demonstrated in animals and humans.

Several antifungal agents are available for the treatment of oral or esophageal candidiasis. Nystatin and clotrimazole are commonly used as first line agents, especially in patients who are presumed to be immunocompetent. If these topical agents fail, oral systemic therapy is initiated. Parenteral compounds are reserved for patients who have severe dysphagia or do not respond to simpler measures.

Nystatin

Nystatin is a polyene antibiotic derived from cultures of *Streptomyces noursei.* It acts by binding to sterols in the cell membrane of the fungus, resulting in altered cell membrane permeability and leakage of intracellular components. Nystatin is commonly used in the treatment of mild oral and esophageal candidiasis.

PHARMACOKINETICS

Nystatin is poorly absorbed from the gastrointestinal tract and almost entirely excreted unchanged in the feces. Detectable blood levels are obtained only after massive doses.

DOSAGE AND ADMINISTRATION

Nystatin is available in oral suspension and tablet forms. Uncomplicated oral candidiasis may respond well to topical agents alone, and Nystatin Suspension, 100,000 units/ml, may be effective at a dose of 5 ml used 4 to 5 times a day for 2 weeks. The suspension should be swished in the mouth for at least 30 seconds before swallowing. A flavored nystatin pastille with equivalent clinical benefit has been introduced. Each nystatin pastille contains 200,000 units of nystatin, and the recommended dosage is one pastille dissolved in the mouth 5 times a day for 2 weeks. A 10-mg nystatin vaginal tablet may also be used as a troche 5 times a day for 2 weeks.

Table 14-1. Factors that predispose to gastrointestinal candidiasis

Host factors
- Age: Infancy, elderly
- Immunological
  - Mucocutaneous candidiasis
  - Acquired immunodeficiency syndrome
- Depressed phagocytic function
  - Quantitative (neutropenia)
  - Qualitative (myeloperoxidase deficiency, chronic granulomatous disease)
- Diabetes mellitus
- Endocrinopathies
- Disruption of mucosa
  - Chemotherapy
  - Radiation
  - Surgical trauma
  - Ischemia
- Debilitation

Exogenous factors
- Antimicrobial agents
- Dietary (high refined sugar; avitaminosis)
- Steroid and other immunosuppressive drugs
- Antacids
- Microbial synergy
- Duration of hospitalization

SIDE EFFECTS AND CONTRAINDICATIONS

Adverse reactions to nystatin are rare, even with prolonged administration. High doses may produce diarrhea, nausea, and vomiting. Hypersensitivity reactions are extremely rare. Adverse effects for pregnancy and breast-feeding are listed in Table 14-2.

Azole Antifungal Agents

The discovery of the antifungal activity of azole compounds represented an important advance in the management of superficial and systemic fungal infections. The first agent that exhibited a potential systemic effect was clotrimazole. Azoles are classified as imidazoles (miconazole and ketoconazole) or triazoles (itraconazole and fluconazole), determined by the number of nitrogen atoms (2 or 3, respectively) in the five-member azole ring.

The antifungal effects of the azoles are targeted primarily at ergosterol, the main sterol in the fungal cell membrane. The azoles inhibit ergosterol synthesis through an interaction with c-14 alpha-demethylase, an enzyme dependent on cytochrome P-450, necessary for conversion of lanosterol to ergosterol.

PHARMACOKINETICS

The azole antifungal compounds differ substantially in their pharmacokinetic properties. Miconazole was the first azole introduced for systemic therapy. About 50 percent of the orally administered dose is absorbed from the gastrointestinal tract; only the intravenous form of the drug is available in the United States. The usual dose is 0.6 to 1.8 gm. The drug is 90 percent protein bound and predominantly metabolized in the liver.

Ketoconazole is available only as an oral preparation. Its absorption depends on acid in the stomach because it must be converted to the hydrochloride salt. Administration of antacids or H_2-antagonists greatly reduces absorption. Other situations that may reduce gastric acidity and impair absorption include the gastropathy of acquired immunodeficiency syndrome (AIDS), gastric surgery, and the relative hypochlorhydria of aging. Administration of ketoconazole with food enhances absorption. The usual dose is 200 to 400 mg. Ketoconazole is 85 percent bound to plasma proteins and 15 percent bound to blood cell membranes and hemoglobin. About 70 percent of a dose is excreted over 4 days, 57 percent in feces and 13 percent in urine.

Fluconazole is available as both an oral and intravenous preparation. The drug is rapidly and completely absorbed from the gastrointestinal tract; therefore, serum concentrations are similar following either route of administration. Gastrointestinal absorption is not

Table 14-2. Antifungal agents: Pregnancy and breast-feeding

Agent	FDA pregnancy category	Risk vs benefit (by trimester)			Breast-feeding category
		1st	2nd	3rd	
Amphotericin	B2	?	?	?	IV
Clotrimazole	B1	R >> B	?	?	IIIA
Fluconazole	C	?	?	?	IV
Itraconazole	C	?	?	?	IV
Ketoconazole	C	?	?	?	IV
Miconazole	B1	B > R	?	?	IIIA
Nystatin	C	?	?	?	IIIA

Food and Drug Administration (FDA) pregnancy categories:
A = Well-controlled studies fail to demonstrate risk to the fetus.
B1 = Animal studies fail to demonstrate risk to the fetus but no human studies are available.
B2 = Animal studies show some risk to the fetus but this is not confirmed in human studies.
C1 = Animal studies show risk to the fetus but no human studies are available.
C2 = Animal and human studies are unavailable.
D = Drugs associated with birth defects but with potential benefits that may outweigh known risks.
X = Drugs associated with birth defects and with potential risk that clearly outweighs potential benefit.
Risk vs benefit: R >> B = Proven or potential risk outweighs potential benefits.
B > R = Potential benefits outweigh potential risks.
R >> B? = Risks may be outweighed by benefits in some circumstances.
? = Risk-to-benefit ratio is unknown.
Breast-feeding categories:
I = Drug does not enter breast milk.
II = Drug enters breast milk but is not known to be harmful in therapeutic doses.
IIIA = Drug may or may not enter breast milk but no adverse effects are expected.
IIIB = Drug may or may not enter breast milk but drug is systemically absorbed.
IV = Drug enters breast milk and poses a potential risk to the neonate.

greatly affected by gastric acidity, and the presence of food does not impact substantially on absorption. Because 5 to 10 days are required for steady-state concentrations to be achieved in the serum, an initial loading dose (twice the usual daily dose) is recommended. The usual daily dose is 100 to 400 mg. The drug is evenly distributed in body tissues, crosses the blood-brain barrier, and penetrates into the vitreous and aqueous humors of the eye. Fluconazole is minimally metabolized by the liver and excreted largely unchanged in the urine; dosage adjustment is necessary in patients with renal impairment.

Itraconazole is a highly lipophilic compound that is almost insoluble in water and dilute acids. It is ionized only at low pH (i.e., gastric juice). The bioavailability of itraconazole after a single oral dose is about 55 percent and varies depending on the formulation. Absorption is enhanced by the presence of food in the stomach and reduced by antacids but not by H_2-antagonists. Itraconazole is available in oral form; usual dose is 200 mg. The serum half-life increases with dose, achieving steady state after 2 weeks. Itraconazole plasma concentrations are quite low, but tissue concentrations are 2 to 3 times higher. The drug is highly metabolized in the liver with 54 percent excretion in the feces and 35 percent in the urine as metabolites. Pharmacokinetics of itraconazole are not affected by renal impairment.

INDICATIONS

Although miconazole was the first azole available for parenteral administration, it has limited activity against candidal infections. Ketoconazole is indicated with oral or esophageal candidiasis in patients who fail to respond to nystatin or clotrimazole. Ketoconazole has generally been more effective than nonabsorbable agents in the therapy for oropharyngeal and esophageal candidiasis. It is also effective in the treatment of many superificial dermatophyte and yeast infections of the skin and mucous membranes. At least one prospective, randomized trial has compared ketoconazole to amphotericin B in the treatment of candidal infections in immunocompromised patients; both drugs were equally effective for esophagitis.

Fluconazole has been studied extensively for treatment of oropharyngeal and esophageal candidiasis, mostly in patients with AIDS or cancer. It was found superior to topical agents such as nystatin or clotrimazole in this population. Several studies reported responses to fluconazole among patients who failed to respond or relapsed while receiving therapy with ketoconazole. Fluconazole is effective in chronic hepatosplenic candidiasis, which occurs predominantly in patients with chronic leukemia; the drug appears to be useful in cases that have not resolved when treated with amphotericin B and flucytosine. Fluconazole is effective for prophylaxis of candidal infections in neutropenic patients. A randomized, double-blind study demonstrated that fluconazole was more effective than ketoconazole in the treatment of oral thrush among patients with AIDS and AIDS-related complex (ARC).

ADVERSE EFFECTS OF AZOLE COMPOUNDS

The potential toxicities of azole compounds are gastrointestinal, hepatic, endocrinologic, metabolic, and hematologic. Hepatic toxicity has been the major concern with azole compounds. Transient elevations of hepatic aminotransferase and alkaline phosphatase levels during the first 2 weeks of treatment occur in 10 percent of patients who receive ketoconazole. The enzymes usually return to normal with continued treatment. When hepatotoxicity occurs, it is usually hepatocellular, although a cholestatic or mixed pattern may be seen. Hepatotoxicity is usually reversible when the drug is discontinued.

Endocrinologic toxicity has been reported primarily with ketoconazole and is dose and duration dependent. Serum testosterone levels are reduced and may result in decreased libido and potency in patients who take ketoconazole. Gynecomastia occurs occasionally in men receiving prolonged therapy; this may abate with continued therapy. Miconazole causes normocytic or microcytic anemia in 45 percent of patients and thrombocytosis in 30 percent.

A major concern with use of azole compounds has been potential for drug-drug interactions. This occurs because the same cytochrome P-450 enzyme involved in metabolism of the azoles is also involved in the metabolism of other drugs. The potential for drug-drug interactions occurs most frequently with ketoconazole. Rifampin reduces the serum concentrations of ketoconazole. Ketoconazole enhances the anticoagulation effect of warfarin (Coumadin), and increases serum concentrations of cyclosporine, sulfonylureas, and phenytoin. Ketoconazole decreases serum concentrations of theophylline. Fluconazole absorption is reduced about 15 percent when it is administered with cimetidine. At daily doses of more than 200 mg, fluconazole interacts with warfarin, phenytoin, and cyclosporine.

Amphotericin B

Amphotericin B is a polyene antibiotic derived from a strain of the actinomycete *Streptomyces nodosus*. Both its therapeutic effect and its attendant toxicity are related to its affinity for sterols in cell membranes. Fortunately, its affinity for ergosterol, the sterol in fungal membranes, is 500 times greater than its affinity for cholesterol, the major sterol in mammalian cell membranes. Binding of amphotericin B to cell membrane sterol increases cellular permeability, resulting in leakage of essential cellular components and damage to the cell.

Amphotericin B is indicated in those patients with candidiasis who are unresponsive to nystatin or the azoles, are unable to swallow, or demonstrate evidence of dissemination or deep infection.

PHARMACOKINETICS

Because amphotericin B is highly insoluble, it is marketed as a colloidal suspension with deoxycholate and buffer. It is absorbed poorly from the gastrointestinal tract and must be administered intravenously. The plasma half-life is 24 hours. Amphotericin B binds rapidly to tissue sites, and only about 10 percent of the drug is retained in plasma, where it is tightly bound to plasma proteins. There is poor penetration of the blood-brain barrier. After multiple doses, approximately 2 to 5 percent of the drug can be detected in the urine. The primary pathway for excretion of amphotericin B is not known.

DOSAGE AND ADMINISTRATION

Amphotericin B given at a dosage of 0.3 to 0.5 mg/kg/day for 7 to 10 days is effective for the treatment of candidal esophagitis. For clinical use, amphotericin B should be prepared in preservative-free sterile water added to 5% dextrose in water to attain a final concentration of less than 0.1 mg/ml. An initial test dose of 1 mg amphotericin B should be given intravenously over 20 minutes, with monitoring of temperature and blood pressure every 30 minutes for 4 hours. If the test dose is tolerated, an initial dose of 0.25 mg/kg intravenously should be administered over 4 to 6 hours. To avoid disturbing the colloidal suspension, no other materials should be placed in the intravenous fluid or tubing, with the possible exceptions of small amounts of heparin or hydrocortisone to decrease phlebitis.

SIDE EFFECTS AND CONTRAINDICATIONS

Adverse reactions to amphotericin B are many. The toxic reactions can be divided into three groups: immediate systemic reactions, renal reactions, and hematologic and other reactions. Chills, fever, malaise, and hypotension will develop in many patients within the first several hours during which the drug is administered. The symptoms can usually be minimized by decreasing the concentration of the drug and its rate of administration and by pretreatment with antipyretic agents, diphenhydramine, and, if needed, small doses of corticosteroids (hydrocortisone 10–25 mg) before each dose.

During the course of amphotericin B therapy, renal toxicity usually presents a more serious problem than do systemic reactions. Often renal toxicity is the limiting factor in determining the extent and efficacy of treatment. A decreased glomerular filtration rate is universal. An attempt is usually made to keep blood urea nitrogen (BUN) less than 50 mg/dl and serum creatinine less than 3 mg/dl by temporarily discontinuing therapy. Renal tubular acidosis, cylindruria, and hypokalemia are not uncommon, and potassium replacement is usually required. Nephrotoxicity is increased when amphotericin B is administered with aminoglycosides; the drug also potentiates digitalis toxicity. In patients who receive 4 gm or more of the drug, loss of renal function is significant and irreversible; nephrocalcinosis may ensue.

Hematologic toxicity is only slightly less common than renal toxicity. Significant anemia is very common. True allergic and hepatic reactions to amphotericin B probably do not occur.

PEARLS AND PITFALLS

1. The addition of 5 to 50 mg heparin to the infusion of amphotericin B helps diminish local phlebitis. Fever and chills can be reduced by giving 25 mg hydrocortisone intravenously. Meperidine may also be effective in controlling amphotericin B–induced chills.
2. Advanced esophageal candidiasis can affect nerve endings, and occasionally patients notice a reduction in pain as the disease progresses.
3. If a patient presents with unexplained candidiasis, a search must be undertaken for predisposing diseases or drugs.
4. The absence of oral thrush does not rule out esophageal candidiasis; however, 20 to 80 percent of patients with *Candida* esophagitis also have oral thrush.

Suggested Reading

Blum RA, et al. Increased gastric pH and bioavailability of fluconazole and ketoconazole. Ann Intern Med 1991; 114:755–757.

Bodey GP. Azole antifungal agents. Clin Infect Dis 1992; 14 (suppl 1):s161–s169.

Danesmend TK, Warnonock DW. Clinical pharmacokinetics of ketoconazole. Clin Pharmacokinetics 1988; 14:13–34.

Dewit S, et al. Comparison of fluconazole and ketoconazole for oropharyngeal candidiasis in AIDS. Lancet I 1989; 764–767.

Dismukes WE, et al. Oral azole drugs as systemic antifungal therapy. N Engl J Med 1994; 330:263–272.

Drutz DJ. Newer antifungal agents and their use, including an update on amphotericin B and flucytosine. Curr Clin Top Infect Dis 1982; 3:97.

An excellent review of amphotericin B.

Huang YC, et al. Pharmacokinetics and dose proportionality of ketoconazole in normal volunteers. Antimicrob Agents Chemother 1986; 30:206.

A comprehensive review of pharmacokinetics and bioavailability of ketoconazole.

Kauffman CA, et al. Hepatosplenic candidiasis: Successful treatment with fluconazole. Am Jnl Med 1991; 91(2); 137–141.

Rubin RH. Mycotic infections. Sci Am Med 1988; Vol 2, 7 Infect Dis IX;12–13.

Schentag JJ. Drug interaction studies and safety profile of fluconazole. Hosp Formulary 1991; 26:16–20.

Viral Infections

Brooks D. Cash and D. Michael Jones

Viral infections of the gastrointestinal system account for 30 to 40 percent of cases of infectious diarrhea in the United States. Five major classes of human gastrointestinal viruses have been identified: rotavirus, enteric adenovirus, Norwalk virus, calcivirus, and astrovirus. The treatment of these viruses remains largely symptomatic.

With the emergence of the acquired immunodeficiency syndrome (AIDS) epidemic, increasing numbers of gastrointestinal infections with anorectal herpes simplex virus and cytomegalovirus are encountered. Antiviral drugs, such as acyclovir, ganciclovir, and foscarnet, are used with increasing frequency to treat these infections.

In addition, the treatment of chronic viral hepatitis with recombinant interferon alpha-2b is widely used and under extensive investigation.

Acyclovir

MECHANISM OF ACTION

Acyclovir, or 9-[2-hydroxyethoxymethyl]guanine, an acyclic guanine analogue, is highly effective against herpes simplex virus replication. It enters infected cells and is phosphorylated by virus-specific thymidine kinase to a monophosphate form that inhibits viral deoxyribonucleic acid (DNA) polymerase and acts as a terminator of the viral DNA strand.

PHARMACOKINETICS

Acyclovir is excreted unchanged by the kidneys, and clearance is dependent on renal function. In adults without renal impairment the half-life is 2.5 hours, while in the anuric patient it approaches 19.5 hours.

Oral acyclovir has a bioavailability of 20 percent, and steady state is reached after one day. Acyclovir penetrates most tissues and body fluids, including vaginal secretions and herpetic vesicular fluid. Concentrations in cerebrospinal fluid are 50 percent of plasma levels.

INDICATIONS

Acyclovir reduces the severity and duration of primary and recurrent mucocutaneous herpes infections, including herpes proctitis.

SIDE EFFECTS

Acyclovir is well tolerated and has a large safety margin. Oral use has been associated with nausea and vomiting in 2 to 3 percent and headache in fewer than 1 percent of patients. Intravenous therapy has been associated with nephrotoxicity caused by crystallization of the drug in the renal tubules, which may be avoidable with adequate pretreatment hydration and is usually reversible with interruption of therapy or dosage adjustment. Neurologic side effects (<1%), such as lethargy, confusion, seizure, and delirium, can occur after intravenous administration when the serum concentration exceeds

Table 15-1. Viral infections: Pregnancy and breast-feeding

Agent	FDA pregnancy category	Risk vs benefit (by trimester)			Breast-feeding category
		1st	2nd	3rd	
Acyclovir	C1	R >> B	R >> B	R >> B	IV
Ganciclovir	C1	R >> B	R >> B	R >> B	IV

Food and Drug Administration (FDA) pregnancy categories:
A = Well-controlled studies fail to demonstrate risk to the fetus.
B1 = Animal studies fail to demonstrate risk to the fetus but no human studies are available.
B2 = Animal studies show some risk to the fetus but this is not confirmed in human studies.
C1 = Animal studies show risk to the fetus but no human studies are available.
C2 = Animal and human studies are unavailable.
D = Drugs associated with birth defects but with potential benefits that may outweigh known risks.
X = Drugs associated with birth defects and with potential risk that clearly outweighs potential benefit.
Risk vs benefit: R >> B = Proven or potential risk outweighs potential benefits.
B > R = Potential benefits outweigh potential risks.
R >> B? = Risks may be outweighed by benefits in some circumstances.
? = Risk-to-benefit ratio is unknown.
Breast-feeding categories:
I = Drug does not enter breast milk.
II = Drug enters breast milk but is not known to be harmful in therapeutic doses.
IIIA = Drug may or may not enter breast milk but no adverse effects are expected.
IIIB = Drug may or may not enter breast milk but drug is systemically absorbed.
IV = Drug enters breast milk and poses a potential risk to the neonate.

25 μg/ml. The drug should be used with caution in patients who are receiving intrathecal methotrexate or interferon. Acyclovir should not be used during pregnancy (see Table 15-1).

ADMINISTRATION

Oral acyclovir in a dosage of 400 mg 5 times a day for 10 days is given for treatment of herpes proctitis. Intravenous therapy may be used, depending on the severity of disease.

Ganciclovir

MECHANISM OF ACTION

Ganciclovir, 9-[1,3-dihydroxy-2-propoxymethyl] guanine, is a synthetic purine nucleoside analogue of guanine and differs from acyclovir by the addition of a hydroxymethyl group. This makes the drug more active than acyclovir against cytomegalovirus. Ganciclovir enters the cell and is transformed into ganciclovir triphosphate by nonspecific viral phosphorylating enzymes and cellular kinases. It inhibits viral DNA polymerase and is incorporated into viral DNA causing chain termination. The level of triphosphorylated form is 10 to 100 times higher in infected cells than in noninfected cells.

PHARMAKOKINETICS

Ganciclovir has a half-life of 3.3 hours. It is cleared unchanged by the kidney, and dosage adjustments are needed with renal impairment.

INDICATIONS

Cytomegalovirus usually manifests as disease only in individuals with diminished T-cell immunity. It is the most common cause of viral infectious diarrhea in patients with AIDS and is found at some point in 5 to 10 percent of all patients. Dieterich and associates showed that ganciclovir maintenance therapy resulted in a clinical improvement in 75 percent of AIDS patients and clinical stabilization in another 13 percent. Clinical end points included maintenance of weight, diminished pain, reduction of ulcer size, and/or normalization of elevated liver-associated enzymes.

SIDE EFFECTS

The most common side effects associated with ganciclovir are granulocytopenia and thrombocytopenia. Granulocytopenia occurs in 13 to 67 percent of patients and usually resolves with interruption of therapy. Thrombocytopenia occurs in 10 to 19 percent of patients. Severe hematologic toxicity is common in patients receiving ganciclovir and zidovudine. Other reactions include rash, fever, nausea, vomiting, confusion, and seizures.

ADMINISTRATION

Ganciclovir is initiated at 2.5 mg/kg intravenously infused over 1 hour every 12 hours for 10 to 14 days. Maintenance therapy consists of 5.0 to 7.5 mg/kg/day given 5 to 7 days per week.

Foscarnet

MECHANISM OF ACTION

Foscarnet (trisodium phosphonoformate hexahydrate), an inorganic pyrophosphate analogue, acts by selectively inhibiting viral DNA polymerases and reverse transcriptases without appreciable effects on host cell enzymes. Activity has been demonstrated against ganciclovir-resistant cytomegalovirus.

PHARMACOKINETICS

Foscarnet is a polar acidic compound that is cleared unchanged by the kidneys. It has a serum half-life of 3.4 hours.

INDICATIONS

Foscarnet inhibits replication of all known herpesviruses in vitro. Dieterich and associates recently showed that foscarnet induces remission of cytomegalovirus gastrointestinal disease that is resistant to ganciclovir in 67 percent of patients.

SIDE EFFECTS

Renal toxicity is the major side effect of foscarnet, and has been reported in approximately 33 percent of patients. Nephrotoxicity is minimized with dosage adjustment, intermittent dosing, and aggressive hydration. Other adverse reactions include anemia, granulocytopenia, nausea, vomiting, and electrolyte disturbances.

ADMINISTRATION

Foscarnet is initiated at a dose of 60 mg/kg body weight intravenously over 1 hour 3 times a day for 2 to 3 weeks. Maintenance therapy consists of 90 to 120 mg/kg over 2 hours daily. Increased toxicity has been reported with more rapid infusion rates. Dose adjustment is necessary with renal disease.

Interferon Alpha-2b

MECHANISM OF ACTION

Interferon alpha-2b is a 17,000-kilodalton protein available in recombinant form for use in certain viral infections. The drug acts like a hormone by binding to specific cell membrane receptors and becoming internalized, where it induces cellular enzymatic activities to promote an antiviral state. These include activation of ribonucleases (RNases), decreasing protein phosphorylation and production, and decreasing virion release from the infected cell. The interferons are neither virucidal nor virustatic.

PHARMACOKINETICS

The pharmacokinetic properties of the interferons are not well understood. After intramuscular injection the peak level is reached within 1 to 6 hours. Clearance is primarily renal. Oral administration is not practical due to proteolysis of the molecule.

INDICATIONS

Interferon alpha-2b produces aminotransferase and histologic normalization in about 50 percent of selected cases of chronic hepatitis C. Promising results have also been seen in the treatment of chronic hepatitis B. Relapse of hepatitis after cessation of treatment remains problematic. The indications, dose, and duration of treatment in chronic viral hepatitis B and C are controversial. Further studies involving short- and long-term administration are under way.

SIDE EFFECTS

Interferon alpha-2b is generally well tolerated. Reported common side effects include fever, chills, myalgias, nausea, vomiting, and headaches. More serious but less frequent side effects include hematopoietic toxicity and depression.

Suggested Reading

Bridgen D, Whiteman P. The clinical pharmacology of acyclovir and its prodrugs. Scand J Infect Dis 1985; 47 (suppl):33–39. *Thorough review of clinical pharmacology of acyclovir.*

Davis G, et al. Treatment of chronic hepatitis C with recombinant interferon alpha. N Engl J Med 1989; 321:1501–1510.

Dieterich D, et al. Ganciclovir treatment of gastrointestinal infections caused by cytomegalovirus in patients with AIDS. Rev Infect Dis 1988; 10 (suppl 3):S532–S537.

Dieterich D, et al. Foscarnet treatment of cytomegalovirus gastrointestinal infections in acquired immunodeficiency syndrome patients who have failed ganciclovir induction. Am J Gastroenterol 1993; 88:542–548.

Greenberg S. Human interferon in viral diseases. Infect Dis Clin North Am 1987; 1:383–423.

Levinson M, Jacobson P. Treatment and prophylaxis of cytomegalovirus disease. Pharmacotherapy 1992; 12:300–318.

Smith P, et al. Intestinal infections in patients with the acquired immunodeficiency syndrome (AIDS). Ann Intern Med 1988; 108: 328–333.

Taburet A, et al. Pharmacokinetics of foscarnet after twice daily administrations for treatment of cytomegalovirus disease in AIDS patients. Antimicrob Agents Chemother 1992; 36:1821–1824.

Protozoal Infections

Walter J. Coyle and D. Michael Jones

Giardiasis

Giardia lamblia is the most commonly diagnosed pathogenic intestinal parasite in the United States and the most frequent cause of waterborne epidemic diarrheal disease. The spectrum of infection ranges from asymptomatic cyst carrier, to mild self-limited diarrhea, to chronic diarrhea associated with weight loss, steatorrhea, abdominal bloating, and flatulence. Three drugs are available in the United States for the treatment of *G. lamblia*. Metronidazole has become the drug of choice even though it is not approved by the Food and Drug Administration (FDA) for the treatment of giardiasis. Cure rates with this drug are 85 to 90 percent. Furazolidone is available in suspension form and may be useful in the treatment of young children; cure rates range from 75 to 90 percent. Paromomycin, approved for intestinal amebiasis, is less effective than the other choices but may be useful in pregnant patients because it is not absorbed (Table 16-1). Quinacrine (Atabrine) was once the drug of choice but is no longer available in this country and is unlikely to return to the market. Tinidazole, related to metronidazole, is only available in Europe but has a similar efficacy to metronidazole.

METRONIDAZOLE (FLAGYL)

Recommended dosage of metronidazole for giardiasis in adults is 250 mg twice a day for 5 days. In children 15 mg/kg body weight is given twice a day for 5 days. (Metronidazole is reviewed more extensively in Chap. 17, Amebiasis.)

FURAZOLIDONE (FUROXONE)

Furazolidone is a nitrofuran derivative that interferes with various parasitic enzyme systems. It is active against *G. lamblia* as well as *Salmonella, Shigella,* and *Vibrio cholerae.* It is the only drug against *Giardia* formulated as an oral suspension, making it particularly useful in young children. Side effects are common and include nausea, vomiting, hypersensitivity reactions, and headache. Mild hemolysis may occur in the patient who is glucose 6-phosphate dehydrogenase (G-6-PD) deficient. When combined with alcohol, furazolidone may cause a disulfiramlike reaction. It is a monoamine oxidase (MAO) inhibitor, and caution should be used when it is given with other MAO inhibitors, tyramine-containing foods, and sympathomimetic amines. Metabolic degradation products of furazolidone may turn the urine brown. Animal studies have demonstrated increased incidence of lung tumors in mice and mammary neoplasia in rats. The recommended dosage for adults is 100 mg 4 times a day for 7 to 10 days. For children, 1.25 mg/kg is given 4 times a day for 7 to 10 days.

PAROMOMYCIN (HUMATIN)

Paromomycin is a poorly absorbed oral aminoglycoside antibiotic. Nearly 100 percent of the drug can be recovered intact from the sto-

Table 16-1. Protozoal infections: Pregnancy and breast-feeding

Agent	FDA pregnancy category	Risk vs benefit (by trimester)			Breast-feeding category
		1st	2nd	3rd	
Azithromycin	B2	R >> B	R >> B	R >> B	IIIB
Furazolidone	C1	R >> B	R >> B	R >> B	IV
Metronidazole	C1	R >> B	R >> B	R >> B	IV
Octreotide	B1	?	?	?	IIIA
Paromomycin	?	?	?	?	?
Spiramycin	C1	R >> B	R >> B	R >> B	IV

Food and Drug Administration (FDA) pregnancy categories:
A = Well-controlled studies fail to demonstrate risk to the fetus.
B1 = Animal studies fail to demonstrate risk to the fetus but no human studies are available.
B2 = Animal studies show some risk to the fetus but this is not confirmed in human studies.
C1 = Animal studies show risk to the fetus but no human studies are available.
C2 = Animal and human studies are unavailable.
D = Drugs associated with birth defects but with potential benefits that may outweigh known risks.
X = Drugs associated with birth defects and with potential risk that clearly outweighs potential benefit.
Risk vs benefit: R >> B = Proven or potential risk outweighs potential benefits.
B > R = Potential benefits outweigh potential risks.
R >> B? = Risks may be outweighed by benefits in some circumstances.
? = Risk-to-benefit ratio is unknown.

Breast-feeding categories:
I = Drug does not enter breast milk.
II = Drug enters breast milk but is not known to be harmful in therapeutic doses.
IIIA = Drug may or may not enter breast milk but no adverse effects are expected.
IIIB = Drug may or may not enter breast milk but drug is systemically absorbed.
IV = Drug enters breast milk and poses a potential risk to the neonate.

making it an ideal choice in pregnancy (see Table 16-1). Reported side effects include nausea, abdominal cramps, and diarrhea. The recommended dosage for adults is 25 to 30 mg/kg/day in three divided doses for 7 days. It is available as 250-mg capsules.

SUMMARY

There is no ideal drug available for the treatment of giardiasis. Metronidazole is not approved in the United States for the treatment of this infection. It is well tolerated; however, there is concern for potential mutagenicity. Furazolidone is well tolerated, especially in the pediatric population; however, it is less effective than metronidazole and has potential carcinogenicity. The only safe choice for pregnancy is paromomycin, but it is not as effective as the other agents and does not have FDA approval for giardiasis. Treatment of the pregnant patient should be reserved for the situation in which symptoms from infection are severe and benefit outweighs potential risk.

PEARLS AND PITFALLS

1. Giardiasis is rarely associated with fever and bloody diarrhea, helping to distinguish it from bacterial dysentery and amebiasis.
2. Disaccharidase deficiency is commonly caused by *Giardia* and may persist for several weeks after treatment. Consider lactose intolerance in patients who continue to have excessive flatus, bloating, and foul stools after treatment for giardiasis.
3. *Giardia* cysts require stomach acid to excyst and become trophozoites.

Cryptosporidiosis

Cryptosporidium is a protozoan that originally was a well-recognized cause of enteritis only in domestic animals. In 1976, the first reported infection in humans occurred in an immunocompromised patient. Since the advent of acquired immunodeficiency syndrome (AIDS), *Cryptosporidium* has become a well-recognized cause of enteritis. It is estimated that approximately 4 percent of patients with AIDS have *Cryptosporidium* enteritis. In the immunocompromised patient, cryptosporidiosis is characterized by prolonged, severe, watery diarrhea that may be associated with abdominal cramping, weight loss, anorexia, nausea, and myalgias. It is estimated that 15 to 20 percent of AIDS diarrhea is caused by *Cryptosporidium*. The biliary tree can also be involved with this infection; sclerosing cholangitis and gangrenous cholecystitis have been reported. Conversely, in the immunocompetent patient, cryptosporidiosis presents as an acute, self-limited enteritis manifested by nausea, vomiting, abdominal cramping, anorexia, and watery, frothy bowel movements. Worldwide, cryptosporidiosis may be the third most common enteropathy in humans. Symptoms resolve within 10 to 14 days without therapy.

Trials with spiramycin have been disappointing, and it is not effective for this disease. Paromomycin has proved effective in several small trials and case studies. Its efficacy in controlling symptoms is greater than 90 percent, with one study reporting eradication in 3 of 7 patients. Most trials exhibit high relapse rates, and maintenance therapy is recommended. A few reports of the use of azithromycin, 1.25 gm/day for 2 weeks, have shown efficacy, but further study is required. Control of diarrhea but not infection can frequently be achieved by using octreotide.

PAROMOMYCIN (HUMATIN)

In clinical trials and case reports, *Cryptosporidium* has been treated with a paromomycin dosage of 500 mg every 6 hours orally for 2 weeks. Maintenance therapy has been 250 mg orally twice a day.

OCTREOTIDE (SANDOSTATIN)

Octreotide is a stable cyclic octapeptide that has activity similar to that of somatostatin. It inhibits gastrin, vasoactive intestinal polypeptide (VIP), glucagon, secretin, motilin, and pancreatic peptide. In diarrheal illness due to cryptosporidiosis, response rates of 30 to 50 percent have been described. Presently, it is available only for subcutaneous or intravenous use. Side effects occurring in 3 to 10 percent of patients include nausea, vomiting, and abdominal discomfort. Pain at the site of injection is not uncommon. Less common problems include headache, altered glucose metabolism, and fatigue. Fifteen to 20 percent of patients receiving long-term therapy may develop cholelithiasis or biliary sludge, and periodic ultrasound examination of the gallbladder is recommended by the manufacturer. The recommended dosage of octreotide is 300 to 500 μg 3 times a day given subcutaneously.

Isosporiasis

Isospora belli is a coccidian protozoal parasite that has been found to cause chronic diarrhea in 1 to 3 percent of patients with AIDS. Like cryptosporidiosis it is self-limited in normal hosts but may be life-threatening in the immunocompromised patient. It is particularly common in the tropical and subtropical zones and is passed by fecal-oral transmission. It can be diagnosed by small-bowel biopsy or examination of the stool using the Ziehl-Neelson method or Kenyoun (acid-fast) stain. Prompt response to treatment has been reported using trimethoprim (TMP)-sulfamethoxazole (SMX). Dosages have been 160 mg TMP/800 mg SMX 4 times a day for 10 days. Relapse is common and daily dosing may be necessary for an indefinite period. Pyrimethamine-sulfadoxine (Fansidar) has been given successfully as maintenance therapy using a weekly dosing regimen. Pyrimethamine alone has been successful in sulfa-allergic patients in doses of 50 to 75 mg/day. Initial reports of efficacy with metronidazole and furazolidone were not confirmed in subsequent studies.

Microsporidiosis

The Microsporidia are obligate, intracellular, protozoal parasites. They are ubiquitous in the environment. Several species exist but *Enterocytozoan bieneusi* and *Septata intestinalis* have received the most attention as possible human pathogens. *Enterocytozoan bieneusi* has been shown to infect the enterocytes of the villous tips of the small intestine in patients with AIDS. It may cause chronic diarrhea and cholangitis in the immunocompromised host. Recently, the association with chronic diarrhea has been questioned since many AIDS patients have microsporidiosis without symptoms. Diagnosis is made by small-bowel biopsy or detection of the spores in stools. In the largest trial to date, 10 of 13 patients responded to metronidazole treatment. Trials of various agents are presently under way. Octreotide has been used for symptomatic relief of diarrhea.

Suggested Reading

GIARDIASIS

Abramowicz M (ed). Drugs for parasitic infections. Med Lett Drugs Ther 1993; 911:111–112.
Recommended drugs and dosages for most parasitic infections.

Bassily S, et al. The treatment of *Giardia lamblia* infection with mepacrine, metronidazole, and furazolidone. J Trop Med Hyg 1970; 73:15–18.
A comparative study of drug therapy for giardiasis in 80 Egyptian adults. Quinacrine cured 100 percent, metronidazole 95 percent, and furazolidone 80 percent.

Craft JC, Murphy T, Nelson JD. Furazolidone and quinacrine. Am J Dis Child 1981; 135:164–168.
A comparative study of therapy for giardiasis in children.

Farthing MJ. *Giardia* comes of age: Progress in epidemiology, immunology, and chemotherapy. J Antimicrob Chemother 1992; 30: 563–566.
Complete review of most current concepts.

Flanagan PA. Giardia: Diagnosis, clinical course and epidemiology. A review. Epidemiol Infect 1992; 109:1–22.
Thorough review of natural history of the infection.

Jones JE. Giardiasis. Primary Care 1991; 18:43–52.
Practical review of giardiasis for the primary care provider.

Murphy TV, Nelson JD. Five versus ten days of therapy with furazolidone for giardiasis. Am J Dis Child 1983; 137:267–271.
A prospective, randomized trial of 22 children with giardiasis demonstrating that 5-day therapy for most children is inadequate.

Smith JW. Giardiasis. Ann Rev Med 1980; 31:373–380.
A review of giardiasis, with focus on diagnosis and treatment.

CRYPTOSPORIDIOSIS

Armitage K, et al. Treatment of cryptosporidiosis with paromomycin. Arch Intern Med 1992; 152:2497–2499.
One of the first prospective trials using paromomycin for treatment of cryptosporidiosis.

Cell JP, et al. Effect of octreotide on refractory AIDS-associated diarrhea. A prospective, multicenter clinical trial. Ann Intern Med 1991; 115:705–710.
Excellent trial showing benefits for some patients with octreotide along with side effects and limitations.

Dworkin BM. Gastrointestinal Manifestations of AIDS. In GP Wormser (ed), *AIDS and Other Manifestations of HIV Infection* (2nd ed). New York: Raven, 1992.
In-depth review of all protozoal infections encountered in the patient with AIDS.

Fichtenbaum CJ, Ritchie DJ. Use of paromomycin for treatment of cryptosporidiosis in patients with AIDS. Clinical Infect Dis 1993; 16:298–300.

Retrospective analysis of seven patients treated with paromomycin for cryptosporidiosis. One hundred percent response with eradication in three of seven patients.

Meisel JL, et al. Overwhelming watery diarrhea with a *Cryptosporidium* in an immunosuppressed patient. Gastroenterology 1976; 70:1156–1158.

The first reported case of cryptosporidiosis in humans.

Smith PD (mod.), NIH Conference. Gastrointestinal infection in AIDS. Ann Intern Med 1992; 116:63–77.

Good overview of the broad spectrum of infections in patients with AIDS. Reviews the use of octreotide.

Soave R. Cryptosporidiosis and isosporiasis in patients with AIDS. Infect Dis Clin North Am 1988; 2:485–494.

An excellent clinical review.

ISOSPORIASIS

DeHovitz JA. *Isospora belli* infections in patients with HIV disease. AIDS Reader 1991; 8:23–26.

Extensive review of the life cycle of this infection.

Pape JW, Vendier RI, Johnson WD. Treatment and prophylaxis of *Isospora belli* infections in patients with AIDS. N Engl J Med 1989; 320:1044–1047.

Excellent review of the treatment and prevention of relapses in isosporiasis.

Weiss LM, et al. *Isospora belli* infection: Treatment with pyrimethamine. Ann Intern Med 1988; 109:474–475.

One of the first articles citing pyrimethamine for sulfa-allergic patients with isosporiasis.

Wittner M, Tanowitz HB, Weiss LM. Parasitic infections in AIDS patients. Cryptosporidiosis, isosporiasis, microsporidiosis, and cyclosporiasis. Infect Dis Clin North Am 1993; 7:569–586.

Most current and thorough review of all protozoan infections in humans.

MICROSPORIDIOSIS

Curry A, Canning EU. Human microsporidiosis. J Infect Dis 1993; 27:229–236.

Complete and current review of infection in humans.

Pol S, et al. *Microsporidia* infection in patients with the human immunodeficiency virus and unexplained cholangitis. N Engl J Med 1993; 328:95–99.

Review of eight patients. Suggests role of Microsporidia as a cause of cholangitis.

Rabeneck L, et al. The role of *Microsporidium* in the pathogenesis of HIV-related chronic diarrhea. Ann Intern Med 1993; 119:895–899.

Suggests high asymptomatic carrier rate in patients with AIDS and questions this protozoan as a cause of chronic diarrhea.

Weber R, et al. Improved light microscopic detection of Microsporidia spores in stool and duodenal aspirates. N Engl J Med 1992; 326:161–166.

Prospective study presenting a practical and inexpensive way to detect spores.

Amebiasis

Barry E. Herman and D. Michael Jones

Approximately 10 percent of the world's population is infected with *Entamoeba histolytica*. In the United States the prevalence is about 5 percent. At greatest risk are those exposed to poor sanitary conditions, the institutionalized, and the homosexual population. The spectrum of infection ranges from asymptomatic cyst passers to disseminated amebiasis with liver or other abscesses. The choice of medication depends on the stage of infection. Drug selection is further dependent on cost, compliance, adverse reactions, and availability. Several amebicidal drugs are either unavailable in the United States or obtainable only from the Centers for Disease Control.

Most agree that in addition to metronidazole, treatment with an intraluminal agent should be considered after an episode of amebic colitis or liver abscess. Controversy exists as to whether treatment of asymptomatic carriers with an intraluminal agent should be considered. Much of the support for not treating the cyst carriers is that most harbor nonpathogenic zymodemes of *E. histolytica*.

The drug of choice is metronidazole for invasive disease, and although some controversy exists, iodoquinol for luminal disease. Both of these agents are readily available in the United States.

Metronidazole (Flagyl)

Metronidazole is a synthetic 5-nitroimidazole compound that is amebicidal at the mucosal level of the intestine and at extraintestinal sites. Its activity in the intestinal lumen is variable. The mechanism of action of metronidazole is not fully understood. Metronidazole enters the organism, where it undergoes reduction and activation. Short-lived toxic intermediate products are thought to bind to and damage deoxyribonucleic acid (see Chap. 10, Metronidazole).

PHARMACOKINETICS

Metronidazole achieves excellent absorption after oral administration, reaching peak plasma concentrations in 1 to 2 hours. Absorption is delayed when it is taken with food, but total bioavailability is unchanged. The serum half-life is 8 hours, and serum levels are proportionate to the dose administered. Metronidazole is lipid-soluble and has excellent tissue penetration, including cerebrospinal fluid. The liver metabolizes 50 percent of the absorbed drug. The kidneys excrete 60 to 80 percent of the dose given as metabolites or intact parent compound. The remainder is either excreted in the stool or metabolized extrahepatically.

INDICATIONS AND DOSAGE

Metronidazole is the drug of choice for mild to moderate intestinal amebiasis, severe amebic dysentery, and amebic abscesses. Therapy with metronidazole should always be followed by a luminally active drug such as iodoquinol to eradicate trophozoites and cysts thereby preventing relapse. Treatment regimens are summarized in Table 17-1 and should result in a greater than 90 percent cure rate

Table 17-1. Treatment of *Entamoeba histolytica*

Agent	Adult dosage
Intestinal amebiasis[a,b] *or hepatic abscesses*[a,c]	
Metronizadole[d]	750 mg po tid × 10 days
Dehydroemetine	1.0–1.5 mg/kg/day IM for 5 days
Emetine	1 mg/kg/day IM for 5 days
Asymptomatic cyst passers	
Iodoquinol	650 mg po tid × 20 days
Paromomycin	25–35 mg/kg tid for 7 days
Diloxanide furanoate	500 mg po tid for 7 days

[a]Should be followed by an intraluminal agent.
[b]Tetracycline and erythromycin have been used to treat invasive colitis.
[c]May require catheter or surgical drainage.
[d]IV 15 mg/kg over 1 hr followed by 7.5 mg/kg q6h.

For patients who are unable to take metronidazole orally, a parenteral preparation is available. It should be given as a loading dose of 15 mg/kg infused over 1 hour, followed by 7.5 mg/kg every 6 hours.

SIDE EFFECTS AND CONTRAINDICATIONS

The most common side effects of metronidazole are gastrointestinal (Table 17-2). Nausea, vomiting, and a metallic taste occur in 5 to 10 percent of patients. Other, less common reactions include burning of the tongue, rash, vaginal and urethral irritation, dark urine, and reversible neutropenia. Nervous system toxicity may occur with high doses given for prolonged periods. Peripheral neuropathy (characterized primarily by numbness or paresthesias), seizure, encephalopathy, and cerebellar dysfunction have been reported. If abnormal neurologic symptoms are observed, the medication should be discontinued immediately. Isolated cases of metronidazole-induced pancreatitis and gynecomastia have been published.

Metronidazole is structurally similar to disulfiram (Antabuse) and may cause a disulfiramlike reaction when alcohol is ingested. Additionally, metronidazole may potentiate the effect of warfarin by inhibiting its metabolism. When warfarin is given concomitantly, the dose should be reduced and the prothrombin time followed closely. Metronidazole is mutagenic in some bacteria, and lung cancer has occurred in mice with long-term use. The risk of cancer in patients receiving short courses of the agent is negligible. Further studies are needed to fully evaluate the potential teratogenicity of metronidazole in humans. Although it has been used without adverse outcome in pregnancy, routine use in gestational patients is discouraged, especially during the first trimester. In patients with chronic liver disease dosage reduction may be required, especially in the presence of concurrent renal insufficiency; under these circumstances, it is advisable to monitor serum drug levels.

Emetines

Alternative agents include emetine, 1 mg/kg/day, or dehydroeme-[illegible]e, 1.0 to 1.5 mg/kg/day, intramuscularly for 5 days. The emetines

Table 17-2. Adverse reactions of antiamebic agents

Agent	Adverse reactions
Extraluminal agents	
Metronidazole	Nausea, vomiting, metallic taste Disulfiram reaction Peripheral neuropathy Interferes with warfarin metabolism
Emetine and dehydroemetine	Myocardial depression Rhythm disturbance Neuromuscular complaints Gastrointestinal symptoms
Luminal agents[a]	
Iodoquinol	Avoid in those allergic to iodine, with hepatic failure or pregnant patients Optic atrophy (rare)
Paromomycin[b]	Diarrhea 15%
Diloxanide furanoate	Flatulence (15–80%) Diarrhea (0–3%)

[a]About 90% or greater effectiveness.
[b]> 80% effectiveness for mild to moderate intestinal disease.

have frequent adverse side effects such as neuromuscular symptoms, gastrointestinal complaints, myocardial depression, and rhythm disturbances. They should always be considered second-line drugs and used with great caution, including hospitalization for observation and cardiac monitoring.

Iodoquinol

Iodoquinol (diiodohydroxyquin) is a halogenated oxyquinole that is amebicidal for both trophozoites and cysts. The mechanism of action is unknown. It is poorly absorbed from the gastrointestinal tract and therefore is not effective in extraintestinal amebiasis. It is administered as 650 mg orally 3 times a day for 20 days. Side effects are uncommon and include diarrhea, abdominal pain, and rash. Iodoquinol contains 64 percent organically bound iodine and can interfere with thyroid function testing or cause iodine dermatitis. It is contraindicated in patients with iodine intolerance, hepatic disease, and pregnancy. Rare cases of optic atrophy have been reported with high doses for prolonged periods.

A related drug, iodochlorhydroxyquin, can lead to a syndrome of subacute myelo-optic neuropathy and is no longer available in the United States.

Paromomycin

Paromomycin is an aminoglycoside that is amebicidal against trophozoite and cyst forms. It is not absorbed when taken orally. It acts on the ribosome and inhibits protein synthesis. Paromomycin comes in 250-mg capsules and is administered in dosages of 25

Table 17-3. Amebiasis: Pregnancy and breast-feeding

Agent	FDA pregnancy category	Risk vs benefit (by trimester)			Breast-feeding category
		1st	2nd	3rd	
Diloxanide	C2	?	?	?	?
Iodoquinol (diiodohydroxyquin)	C2	R >> B?	R >> B?	R >> B?	IV
Metronidazole	C1	R >> B	R >> B	R >> B	IV
Paromomycin	C2	?	?	?	IIIB

Food and Drug Administration (FDA) pregnancy categories:
A = Well-controlled studies fail to demonstrate risk to the fetus.
B1 = Animal studies fail to demonstrate risk to the fetus but no human studies are available.
B2 = Animal studies show some risk to the fetus but this is not confirmed in human studies.
C1 = Animal studies show risk to the fetus but no human studies are available.
C2 = Animal and human studies are unavailable.
D = Drugs associated with birth defects but with potential benefits that may outweigh known risks.
X = Drugs associated with birth defects and with potential risk that clearly outweighs potential benefit.
Risk vs benefit: R >> B = Proven or potential risk outweighs potential benefits.
B > R = Potential benefits outweigh potential risks.
R >> B? = Risks may be outweighed by benefits in some circumstances.
? = Risk-to-benefit ratio is unknown.

Breast-feeding categories:
I = Drug does not enter breast milk.
II = Drug enters breast milk but is not known to be harmful in therapeutic doses.
IIIA = Drug may or may not enter breast milk but no adverse effects are expected.
IIIB = Drug may or may not enter breast milk but drug is systemically absorbed.
IV = Drug enters breast milk and poses a potential risk to the neonate.

35 mg/kg/day in three divided doses for 7 days. The major adverse reaction is diarrhea.

Diloxanide Furanoate

An alternative to iodoquinol is diloxanide furanoate, which is only available from the Centers for Disease Control. It is effective in eliminating intraluminal amebas in over 90 percent of patients. The dose regimen is 500 mg 3 times a day for 10 days. It is well tolerated; the primary complaint is increased flatulence.

PEARLS AND PITFALLS

1. Bismuth, barium, gallbladder dye, kaolin, nonabsorbable antacids, and antibiotics may interfere with stool examination for amebiasis.
2. Serologic testing for amebiasis may remain positive for up to 10 years after cure if the indirect hemagglutination assay is used. The enzyme-linked immunosorbent assay (ELISA), counter immunoelectrophoresis, and agar gel diffusion methods may revert to negative within 6 to 12 months.
3. Ulcerative colitis and amebiasis may appear identical on barium enema or proctosigmoidoscopy. Amebic serologic testing and stool examination are critical to distinguish between the two conditions before corticosteroid therapy.
4. A small percentage of amebic liver abscesses may be superinfected with bacteria requiring additional antibiotic therapy.
5. Because of the disulfiramlike reaction, patients should avoid *all* products with alcohol. These include many cough syrups, mouthwashes, liquid medications, and foods prepared with alcohol or liqueurs.
6. Although the potential for teratogenic effects exists, metronidazole has been used safely in pregnant women. Paromomycin is a reasonable alternative, because it is poorly absorbed and effective against both trophozoites and cysts. Iodoquinol is contraindicated in pregnancy (Table 17-3).
7. Up to 30 percent of sexually active homosexuals have *E. histolytica* isolated from their stools, but the clinical significance is unclear. Some authorities have shown that a large percentage of the zymodemes in this setting are nonpathogenic *E. histolytica.*
8. For further information regarding drug therapy, contact the Parasitic Disease Division of the Centers for Disease Control, Atlanta, GA 30333; (404) 639-3670.

Suggested Reading

Allason-Jones E, et al. *Entamoeba histolytica* as a commensal intestinal parasite in homosexual men. N Engl J Med 1986; 315:353–356. *The authors found 45 of 225 (20%) stools from homosexual patients to be positive for* E. histolytica. *All of the isolates were found to be nonpathogenic zymodemes by isoenzyme electrophoresis. Stools from 129 heterosexuals were negative for the organism.* Entamoeba histolytica *is a common commensal in the homosexual population.*

Aucott JN, Raydin JI. Amebiasis and "nonpathogenic" intestinal protozoa. Infect Dis Clin North Am 1993; 7:467–485.

A general review of the diagnosis and therapy of amebiasis. Authors favor diloxanide furanoate as the luminal agent of choice. Brief discussion of other pathogenic protozoa of the gastrointestinal tract is included.

Finegold SM, Mathisen GE. Metronidazole in the treatment of anaerobic bacterial infections. Curr Clin Top Infect Dis 1985; 6: 156–183.

An excellent review of the pharmacokinetics, spectrum of activity, and clinical use of metronidazole.

McAuley JB, Juranek DD. Luminal agents in the treatment of amebiasis. Clin Infect Dis 1992; 14:1161–1162.

Correspondence favoring iodoquinol as the luminal agent of choice in the United States.

McAuley JB, Juranek DD. Paromomycin in the treatment of mild-to-moderate intestinal amebiasis. Clin Infect Dis 1992; 15:551–552.

McAuley JB, et al. Diloxanide furanoate for treating asymptomatic *Entamoeba histolytica* cyst passers: 14 years experience in the United States. Clin Infect Dis 1992; 15:464–468.

Positive experience in treating 4371 cyst passers with diloxanide furanoate.

Reed SL. Amebiasis: An update. Clin Infect Dis 1992; 14:385–391.

Excellent review of the diagnosis and management of amebiasis.

Scully BE. Metronidazole. Med Clin North Am 1988; 72:613–621.

Practical applications for the use of metronidazole.

Sullam PM, et al. Paromomycin therapy of endemic amebiasis in homosexual men. Sex Transm Dis 1986; 13:151–155.

Supports the use of paromomycin for mild to moderate (nondysenteric) intestinal amebiasis in the male homosexual population.

Intestinal Nematodes

Thong P. Le and D. Michael Jones

Infection with gastrointestinal nematodes represents a major public health concern both in developed and developing nations throughout the world. It has been estimated that between 1 and 2 billion people are infected with *Ascaris lumbricoides,* hookworm, *Trichuris trichiura, Enterobius vermicularis,* and *Strongyloides stercoralis.* Therefore, it is fortunate that most antihelminthics available today have a broad range of action and can be used as single agents in the patient with multiple parasite infections (Table 18-1). The focus of this chapter is to review the basic elements of intestinal nematode life cycles, the common syndromes associated with their infections, and the methods of diagnosis and treatment (Table 18-2).

Ascaris lumbricoides

Infection with *Ascaris* in humans follows the ingestion of an embryonated egg, usually found in fecally contaminated food or soil. Eggs hatch in the intestine and mature into larvae, which penetrate the intestinal wall and migrate to the capillary beds of the lung. Further migration from the pulmonary parenchyma, up the trachea, and back into the gastrointestinal tract completes the maturation cycle. During this migration to the lung, an intense allergic reaction marked by cough, wheezing, pleuritic chest pain, and transient pulmonary infiltrate may occur.

As with most intestinal worm infections, children harbor heavy worm burdens much more commonly than adults because of their poor hygienic behavior. Clinical disease can be due to damage from heavy worm burden, such as small-bowel obstruction, intussusception, or perforation. However, damage can also be the result of only one worm that has migrated aberrantly into the hepatobiliary tree causing acute cholangitis.

Serial stool examinations are highly sensitive in diagnosing ascariasis, given that each mature female produces enormous numbers of eggs daily (200,000/day). Of note, eggs may be absent in stool during the early pulmonary migration phase.

The treatment of choice is mebendazole, 100 mg twice a day for 3 days. Mebendazole is a broad-spectrum antihelminthic agent of the benzimidazole family that is structurally related to thiabendazole. It is poorly absorbed from the gastrointestinal tract and thus has few systemic side effects except for diarrhea and abdominal pain. The latter symptom may be related to the worm burden and is infrequently observed in mild infections. Mebendazole selectively and irreversibly blocks glucose uptake by the worm and leads to endogenous depletion of glycogen stores. In addition, cytoplasmic microtubular deterioration has been observed by electron microscopy and results in the accumulation of secretory granules, cytoplasmic lysis, and death of the organism.

Alternatives to mebendazole include a single dose of pyrantel pamoate (11 mg/kg with a 1-gm maximum dose) or piperazine citrate (75 mg/kg with a 3.5-gm maximum dose daily for 2 days). Pyrantel

Table 18-1. Dosage (in mg) in treatment of intestinal nematodes

Drug	*Ascaris*	*Strongyloides*	*Trichuris*	*Enterobius*[a]	Hookworms
Mebendazole	100 bid × 3 days	—	100 bid × 3 days	100 × 1 dose	100 bid × 3 days
Pyrantel	11/kg × 1 dose 1-gm max dose	—	—	11/kg × 1 dose 1-gm max dose	11/kg × 1 dose 1-gm max dose
Piperazine	75/kg qd × 2 days 3.5-gm max dose	—	—	—	—
Thiabendazole	—	25/kg bid × 2 days 3-gm max daily dose	—	—	—
Albendazole[b]	400 × 1 dose	? dose	400 × 1 dose	400 × 1 dose	—
Ivermectin[b]	0.2/kg × 1 dose	0.2/kg qd × 1–2 days	0.2/kg × 1 dose	0.2/kg × 1 dose	—

[a]A second dose usually given at 2 weeks for cure.
[b]Not yet approved by the Food and Drug Administration for these indications in the United States.

Table 18-2. Presentation, diagnosis, and treatment of intestinal nematodes

	Ascaris	*Strongyloides*	*Trichuris*	*Enterobius*	Hookworms
Presentation	Asymptomatic Pneumonitis Bowel obstruction Cholangitis	Enteritis Hyperinfection (sepsis)	Asymptomatic Rectal prolapse	Asymptomatic Anal pruritus	Asymptomatic Iron-deficiency anemia
Diagnosis	Eggs in stool	Larva in stool Duodenal aspirate Serum ELISA	Eggs in stool	"Scotch" tape	Eggs in stool Larva in stool
Treatment	Mebendazole Pyrantel Piperazine Albendazole Ivermectin	Thiabendazole Albendazole Ivermectin	Mebendazole Albendazole Ivermectin	Mebendazole Pyrantel Albendazole Ivermectin	Mebendazole Pyrantel

ELISA = Enzyme-linked immunosorbent assay.

is a compound of the amidine group and is minimally absorbed from the intestine. It inhibits neuromuscular transmission and results in spastic paralysis of the worm. This drug is well tolerated and has not been associated with toxic side effects.

Piperazine citrate is one of the oldest antihelminthic drugs still in use. Unlike the other two drugs used in the treatment of ascariasis, piperazine is readily absorbed from the intestines and acts by blocking acetylcholine in the myoneural junctions of the helminths, producing a flaccid paralysis and facilitating the removal of the worm by normal peristalsis. Piperazine is especially useful in cases in which intestinal or biliary obstruction is suspected. Use of mebendazole under these circumstances has been associated with migration of the parasite and onset of bothersome symptoms. Piperazine citrate is well tolerated and has been associated with few side effects. However, with accidental overdose, ataxia, vertigo, confusion, muscular weakness and uncoordination, and myoclonic contractions have been observed. Piperazine may lower the seizure threshold in epileptic patients and should be used with caution in this setting.

Albendazole, the newest member of the benzimidazole family, is also effective in ascariasis with a single 400-mg oral dose. Albendazole is not yet licensed in the United States.

Mebendazole is teratogenic in animals and is contraindicated in pregnancy. Thus, pyrantel is the drug of choice for pregnant women, with piperazine as an alternative (Table 18-3).

Strongyloides stercoralis

The life cycle of *S. stercoralis* is similar to that of the hookworm (see later in text) in all respects but one: The rhabditiform larvae in the intestinal lumen can either be expelled or mature in situ and penetrate the intestinal mucosa or perianal skin, maintaining an "autoinfection" cycle. As a result, infection can persist in the absence of repeated exposure and need not be associated with direct contact with contaminated soil.

Strongyloidiasis occurs predominantly in Southeast Asia and Africa. Host contact with infective feces and warm, moist soil (providing an optimal environment for free-living larvae) represent the two most important factors in the transmission of the disease. Strongyloidiasis occurs in hosts of any age, in a prevalence pattern similar to that of hookworm. Due to the organism's ability to persist in the host, widespread dissemination of the disease to developed nations has occurred. In the United States, former prisoners of war from both Vietnam and World War II have carried the organism, which remained undiagnosed for up to 40 years. In the United States, the overall incidence of infection in the general population is 1 to 2 percent and may reach 5 percent in rural areas.

In otherwise healthy people, *Strongyloides* infection can cause a variety of gastrointestinal symptoms including enteropathy and malabsorption. However, the most significant clinical manifestation is the hyperinfection syndrome in patients who are receiving immunosuppressive agents. The *Strongyloides* filariform larvae may penetrate multiple organs and cause a sepsislike syndrome. In addition, bacterial infections that are polymicrobial (including enteric gram-

Table 18-3. Intestinal nematodes: Pregnancy and breast-feeding

Agent	FDA pregnancy category	Risk vs benefit (by trimester)			Breast-feeding category
		1st	2nd	3rd	
Mebendazole	C1	R >> B	R >> B	R >> B	IV
Piperazine	C2	R >> B	R >> B	R >> B	IV
Pyrantel	C2	R >> B	R >> B	R >> B	IV
Thiabendazole	C1	R >> B	R >> B	R >> B	IV

Food and Drug Administration (FDA) pregnancy categories:
A = Well-controlled studies fail to demonstrate risk to the fetus.
B1 = Animal studies fail to demonstrate risk to the fetus but no human studies are available.
B2 = Animal studies show some risk to the fetus but this is not confirmed in human studies.
C1 = Animal studies show risk to the fetus but no human studies are available.
C2 = Animal and human studies are unavailable.
D = Drugs associated with birth defects but with potential benefits that may outweigh known risks.
X = Drugs associated with birth defects and with potential risk that clearly outweighs potential benefit.
Risk vs benefit: R >> B = Proven or potential risk outweighs potential benefits.
B > R = Potential benefits outweigh potential risks.
R >> B? = Risks may be outweighed by benefits in some circumstances.
? = Risk-to-benefit ratio is unknown.
Breast-feeding categories:
I = Drug does not enter breast milk.
II = Drug enters breast milk but is not known to be harmful in therapeutic doses.
IIIA = Drug may or may not enter breast milk but no adverse effects are expected.
IIIB = Drug may or may not enter breast milk but drug is systemically absorbed.
IV = Drug enters breast milk and poses a potential risk to the neonate.

negative organisms and anaerobes) often supervene as a result of the underlying bowel wall damage.

Diagnosing *Strongyloides* infection requires a high index of suspicion since stool examinations are insensitive in visualizing larvae. Sensitivity can be improved by duodenal sampling with biopsy. Serologic enzyme-linked immunosorbent assay (ELISA) is useful in establishing a diagnosis of infection, although it cannot distinguish acute from chronic disease.

The drug of choice in the treatment of *S. stercoralis* is thiabendazole, a benzimidazole derivative that is rapidly absorbed and excreted in the urine. The mechanism of action is not well understood but may involve inhibition of the parasite-specific enzyme fumarate reductase. Standard treatment with 25 mg/kg twice a day (with a maximum of 3 gm/day) for 2 days is frequently complicated by the onset of side effects, which include dizziness, nausea, vomiting, anorexia, and diarrhea. Bradycardia, hypotension, erythema multiforme, and Stevens-Johnson syndrome have been reported but fortunately occur rarely. Prolonged therapy is usually required in patients with hyperinfestations due to relatively larger parasite burdens. Thiabendazole is teratogenic in animals and the relapse rate is high. Albendazole produces a cure rate of 75 to 80 percent; however, optimal dose and duration of albendazole have not been determined.

Ivermectin, a synthetic derivative of the macrolide mold product avermectin, is safe and active against *Strongyloides*; its mechanism of action is unknown. Its efficacy appears greater than that of either thiabendazole or albendazole with fewer side effects. Ivermectin is safe in pregnancy (see Table 18-3). Ivermectin is not yet approved for the treatment of *Strongyloides* infection.

Trichuris trichiura

Humans are the principal hosts for this infection, which is directly transmitted by the ingestion of eggs. Larval forms hatch in the upper duodenum and attach to the intestinal villi. Following maturation, the worm migrates to the colon without a tissue invasion phase, embeds in the mucosa, and produces eggs.

Despite its highest prevalence in the humid tropics, trichuriasis remains an important public health problem in rural areas of the United States. Soil pollution is the determining factor in the prevalence and intensity of infection in a community and represents an important focus of disease control. As with ascariasis, children between 5 and 15 years of age are affected with the heaviest worm burdens.

Trichuriasis is typically a clinically silent disease. However, it has been associated with anorexia, diarrhea, abdominal pain, and weight loss. Rectal prolapse, frequently a result of particularly heavy infestation, is also associated with this disease and is thought to be a result of prolonged colonic inflammation. Unlike infections with hookworm, blood loss due to *T. trichiura* is usually insignificant since these worms do not actually suck blood. Diagnosis is suggested by barrel-shaped eggs in the stool, which are not as abundant as in *Ascaris* infection.

The preferred treatment of this disease combines the use of mebendazole, 100 mg twice a day for 3 days, and improved community sanitation. In some cases, compliance with this treatment schedule has been poor, and it is currently being replaced with a single 500-mg dose, with reported cure rates ranging from 93 to 100 percent. Side effects associated with single-dose therapy do not differ significantly from those of the traditional regimen. Albendazole is effective with a single 400-mg oral dose.

Enterobius vermicularis

Enterobius infection is prevalent in temperate as well as tropical climates. The adult *Enterobius* lives in the intestinal lumen, does not invade the bowel wall, and, thus, does not invoke eosinophilia or immunoglobulin E (IgE) response. The female migrates out to the perianal area nocturnally and deposits eggs before dying.

Enterobius infection is usually asymptomatic or presents as perianal pruritus, especially in children. Because of constant scratching, *Enterobius* eggs are easily transmissible among individuals by hand-to-hand contact.

Diagnosing *Enterobius* infection is easily accomplished by blotting the perianal area in the early morning with “Scotch tape” and examining the tape under a microscope for the characteristic eggs.

Effective treatment requires one dose of either mebendazole or pyrantel pamoate. Albendazole and ivermectin are also highly effective, but they are not yet approved for this indication. Due to ongoing transmission among family members and on fomites, a second dose of antihelminthics is usually given 2 weeks later for cure.

Hookworm

Hookworm disease is an infection of the small intestine caused by either *Ancylostoma duodenale* or *Necator americanus.* The life cycle of the two organisms is identical and involves penetration of the skin by a filariform larva following prolonged skin-soil contact (5–10 minutes is sufficient). The larvae are carried by the circulation to the lungs and, similar to *Ascaris,* penetrate the alveolar wall, migrate up the trachea, are swallowed, and attach to the intestinal mucosa, where further maturation and egg production occur. Eosinophilic pneumonitis is not as common or as severe as in ascariasis. Hookworms ingest blood and consume up to 0.2 ml of blood per worm per day.

The primary geographic areas of hookworm infection are the tropical and subtropical zones. As a result of relatively effective eradication programs, it is not a major source of concern in the United States even though it persists in the rural Southeast. Unlike other intestinal parasites, hookworm affects adults as well as children. The main epidemiologic factor responsible for the transmission of the disease remains contact with soil contaminated by human feces.

The typical clinical manifestations of hookworm infection are iron-deficiency anemia and hypoproteinemia. This is more commonly seen when a heavy worm burden infects an already malnourished person. Hookworm infection can be diagnosed by visualizing eggs in stool. Hookworm eggs may hatch if the stool specimen is not examined expeditiously, producing larva that must be differentiated from *Strongyloides.*

Treatment with either mebendazole or pyrantel pamoate produces a cure in 76 to 96 percent of cases. As with *Trichuris* infections, single-dose mebendazole (500 mg) has been shown effective in producing high cure rates, although its use may be limited to less heavily parasitized individuals. Dosages for treatment and mechanisms of action of both mebendazole and pyrantel pamoate are the same for hookworm as for the intestinal nematodes described above.

PEARLS AND PITFALLS

1. Hyperinfection with *S. stercoralis* should be considered in any patient, especially one receiving immunosuppressive agents, with polymicrobial sepsis. Ideally, patients from endemic areas should be screened before receiving immunosuppressives with at least an eosinophil count, serial stool examinations, and *Strongyloides* ELISA.
2. Migration of *A. lumbricoides* has been reported following treatment with both mebendazole and thiabendazole but can be avoided by pretreatment with piperazine citrate.
3. It is important to monitor patients receiving theophylline for signs of toxicity while receiving thiabendazole because of altered pharmacodynamics due to competition for metabolism in the liver.
4. Diagnosing *S. stercoralis* infection requires persistence, a high index of suspicion, and more than routine stool examinations.
5. Ivermectin may become the treatment of choice for *Strongyloides* infection in the future.

Suggested Reading

Berk SL, et al. Clinical and epidemiologic features of strongyloidiasis: A prospective study in rural Tennessee. Arch Intern Med 1987; 147:1257–1261.
The incidence of S. stercoralis *was studied in hospitalized and domiciliary patients (N=575). Infected patients, composing 6.1 and 2.9 percent, respectively, were found to have a higher incidence of eosinophilia, heme-positive stools, and complaints of abdominal bloating. A relapse rate of 15 percent was noted in patients treated with standard thiabendazole therapy.*

Botero D. Chemotherapy of human intestinal parasitic diseases. Ann Rev Pharmacol Toxicol 1978; 18:1–15.
The author outlines the nature of the public health problem represented by infection with gastrointestinal parasites, along with the rationale for therapy and the proposed mechanisms of action of each of the drugs.

Evans AC, Hollmann AW, DuPreez L. Mebendazole, 500 milligrams, for single-dose treatment of nematode infestation. South Afr Med J 1987; 72:665–667.
The results of a study using single-dose mebendazole in 217 children with mixed helminth infections are reported. The end points of therapy were reduction of egg production in the stool and total cure. The authors note the fact that the drug was well tolerated and that its use as a public health tool was enhanced by its acceptability.

Genta RM, et al. Strongyloidiasis in U.S. veterans of the Vietnam and other wars. JAMA 1987; 258:49–52.
The prevalence of strongyloidiasis among American veterans was evaluated by an ELISA method and correlated with stool speci-

men examination. The authors stress the importance of screening this population for S. stercoralis *and initiating therapy with thiabendazole if positive results are obtained—before treatment with immunosuppressives.*

Keystone JS, Murdoch JK. Mebendazole: Diagnosis and treatment drugs five years later. Ann Intern Med 1979; 91:582–586.
This excellent review article outlines the history of mebendazole, its mechanism of action, pharmacology, application, and side effects.

Naquira C, et al. Ivermectin for human *Strongyloides* and other intestinal helminths. Am J Trop Med Hyg 1989; 40:304–309.
This large Peruvian study, although not comparative, shows good effectiveness of ivermectin against Strongyloides *and other intestinal nematode infections.*

Xiu LX, Weller PF. *Strongyloides* and other intestinal nematode infections. Infect Dis Clin North Am 1993; 7:655–682.
This is a good, up-to-date, comprehensive review of intestinal nematode infections that are likely to be encountered in the United States.

Chemoprophylaxis of Traveler's Diarrhea

Mark H. Johnston and D. Michael Jones

More than 300 million people travel abroad each year, and diarrhea is the most common medical problem faced by travelers. Depending on the geographic location, up to 50 percent will experience an episode of traveler's diarrhea. Individuals from North America, western Europe, Australia, and South Africa are most susceptible, and they are at highest risk (20–50% attack rate) when traveling to southern Asia, the Middle East, Africa, and Latin America, and at intermediate risk (10–20% attack rate) when traveling to eastern Europe, former Soviet Union countries, Mediterranean countries, China, most of the Caribbean, and probably Israel and Japan.

Traveler's diarrhea has been defined as (1) three loose stools a day, (2) a twofold increase in the number of loose or watery bowel movements, (3) more than two loose stools a day in association with a single gastrointestinal symptom such as cramping, or (4) one loose or watery stool in association with one symptom of an enteric infection. Traveler's diarrhea typically occurs 2 to 3 days after arrival. The symptoms are usually self-limited, and 85 percent of cases resolve untreated in 3 to 4 days. More than half the cases are mild and do not limit the traveler's activities; however, up to 20 percent of the cases may be severe and confine the traveler to bed for 2 to 3 days.

Enterotoxigenic *Escherichia coli* (ETEC) is the most common pathogen and has been isolated in 40 to 70 percent of cases of traveler's diarrhea. The next most frequent organism isolated is *Shigella,* followed by *Salmonella, Campylobacter,* rotaviruses, and *Giardia.* Intestinal parasites, such as *Amoeba, Cryptosporidium,* and *Strongyloides* are isolated from a smaller number of those with traveler's diarrhea. Recently, a new coccidian parasite that invades the small-intestinal epithelial cells has been found in travelers from Asia and provisionally named *Cyclospora cayetanensis.* In total, about 80 percent of traveler's diarrhea is bacterial in origin. Several agents are effective (reducing attack rates by 80–95%) in preventing traveler's diarrhea.

Trimethoprim-Sulfamethoxazole

Several studies are reported on students traveling from the United States to Mexico who were enrolled in double-blind, placebo-controlled trials shortly after arrival. In one trial, subjects were given trimethoprim-sulfamethoxazole (TMP-SMX), 160 mg/800 mg twice a day for 21 days, versus a group given placebo. Diarrhea developed in 16 percent of the TMP-SMX group, compared with 55 percent of the placebo group. The percentage of protection, defined as [(percentage ill with placebo minus percentage ill with active drug) divided by percentage ill with placebo] times 100, was 71 percent in the study group.

In another trial using TMP-SMX, 160 mg/800 mg once a day for 14 days, versus placebo, diarrhea developed in only 2 percent of study patients. Expressed as percent protection, the study group achieved a rate of 95 percent.

MECHANISM OF ACTION AND PHARMACOLOGY

Trimethoprim-sulfamethoxazole works by blocking two steps in the biosynthesis of nucleic acids and proteins essential to many bacteria. Trimethoprim inhibits the enzyme dihydrofolate reductase and blocks the conversion of dihydrofolic acid to tetrahydrofolic acid. Sulfamethoxazole inhibits synthesis of dihydrofolic acid by competing with para-aminobenzoic acid. Most strains of enterotoxigenic *E. coli,* including those that produce both heat-stabile and heat-labile toxins, are susceptible to TMP-SMX. Although resistance to ETEC has occurred, it is rare. TMP-SMX is also active against other enteric pathogens such as *Shigella* and possibly *Salmonella.*

Trimethoprim-sulfamethoxazole is rapidly absorbed following oral administration, with peak blood levels for each component occurring after 1 to 4 hours. The mean serum half-life of each component is approximately 10 hours. Because TMP-SMX is excreted primarily by the kidneys, dosages must be decreased in cases of severe renal insufficiency.

DOSAGE AND ADMINISTRATION

The dosage for adequate chemoprophylaxis of traveler's diarrhea using TMP-SMX is 160 mg/800 mg (one double-strength tablet) daily. The drug must be continued beyond the period of exposure (for 1–2 days) after returning home.

SIDE EFFECTS

Up to 5 percent of people taking TMP-SMX prophylaxis have developed generalized cutaneous eruptions. The gut flora of most people who take TMP-SMX prophylaxis will develop resistance to the drugs during the period of administration. More severe reactions, such as the Stevens-Johnson syndrome and antibiotic-associated colitis, may rarely occur.

Doxycycline

The efficacy of doxycycline in preventing traveler's diarrhea has been extensively studied in regions where most of the ETEC isolated were sensitive to antibiotics, and in regions of the world where antibiotic-resistant ETEC is known to be common. These studies involved US Peace Corps volunteers who had recently arrived in endemic areas. They were treated with doxycycline, 100 mg/day for 21 days. The percent protection achieved in areas where the ETEC was sensitive to antibiotics was approximately 85 percent. The percent protection achieved in areas where antibiotic resistance to ETEC was common was approximately 64 percent.

In all studies the effect of doxycycline lasted only as long as the drug was taken. At the end of the 3-week period of doxycycline prophylaxis, the study patients were as susceptible to traveler's diarrhea as were patients in the placebo groups at the beginning of the studies. Among people taking doxycycline in whom diarrhea developed, episodes were less severe in terms of the number of stools per day and length of illness when compared to people taking placebo.

MECHANISM OF ACTION AND PHARMACOLOGY

Doxycycline is synthetically derived from oxytetracycline. Its antimicrobial effect is believed to result from inhibition of protein synthesis. Most strains of ETEC are susceptible to doxycycline. High levels of doxycycline are secreted into the small bowel, where ETEC colonization occurs. After oral administration doxycycline is virtually completely absorbed and reaches peak serum levels in about 2 hours. The serum half-life of doxycycline is approximately 20 hours. There is no significant difference in serum half-life in people with normal and severely decreased renal function.

DOSAGE AND ADMINISTRATION

The dosage for adequate chemoprophylaxis of traveler's diarrhea using doxycycline is 100 mg/day. The drug must be continued beyond the period of exposure (for 1–2 days) after returning home.

SIDE EFFECTS

The incidence of side effects from doxycycline therapy is less than 1 percent. Side effects include candidial overgrowth, photosensitivity, and gastrointestinal symptoms such as nausea and vomiting. Doxycycline can interfere with tooth development during the last half of pregnancy, infancy, and early childhood; consequently, it is contraindicated in pregnant women and children below the age of 8 (Table 19-1).

Bismuth Subsalicylate

In 1980, DuPont and associates studied the effect of taking a liquid bismuth subsalicylate preparation prophylactically to prevent traveler's diarrhea in a group of US students arriving in Mexico. The study group received 60 ml of a 1.75% bismuth subsalicylate solution orally 4 times a day (4.2 gm active drug per day) for 21 days. Diarrheal illness developed in 23 percent of the study group, compared to 61 percent of the placebo group. The percent protection afforded by bismuth subsalicylate in preventing traveler's diarrhea was 62 percent.

In 1987, DuPont and associates studied the efficacy of bismuth subsalicylate tablets in preventing traveler's diarrhea. They studied a similar subject population of US students arriving in Mexico. One study group received two tablets of bismuth subsalicylate 4 times a day, another group received one tablet of bismuth subsalicylate 4 times a day, and the third group received placebo tablets 4 times a day. Each bismuth subsalicylate tablet contained 262 mg active drug. The study period ran for 3 weeks. In the high-dose bismuth subsalicylate study group (who received 2.1 gm/day active drug), the percent protection afforded against traveler's diarrhea was 65 percent. In the low-dose bismuth subsalicylate group (who received 1.05 gm/day active drug), the percent protection was 40 percent.

MECHANISM OF ACTION AND PHARMACOLOGY

The mechanism of bismuth subsalicylate in preventing traveler's diarrhea is unclear. The drug effectively neutralizes the diarrheagenic effects of crude toxins of *E. coli* and *Vibrio cholerae,* an action probably due to the subsalicylate moiety. Bismuth subsalicylate may

Table 19-1. Chemoprophylaxis of traveler's diarrhea: Pregnancy and breast-feeding

Agent	FDA pregnancy category	Risk vs benefit (by trimester)			Breast-feeding category
		1st	2nd	3rd	
Bismuth	C1	?	?	?	IIIB
Ciprofloxacin	C1	R >> B?	R >> B?	R >> B?	IV
Doxycycline	D	R >> B	R >> B	R >> B	IV
Trimethoprim-sulfamethoxazole	C1	R >> B	R >> B	R >> B	IV

Food and Drug Administration (FDA) pregnancy categories:
A = Well-controlled studies fail to demonstrate risk to the fetus.
B1 = Animal studies fail to demonstrate risk to the fetus but no human studies are available.
B2 = Animal studies show some risk to the fetus but this is not confirmed in human studies.
C1 = Animal studies show risk to the fetus but no human studies are available.
C2 = Animal and human studies are unavailable.
D = Drugs associated with birth defects but with potential benefits that may outweigh known risks.
X = Drugs associated with birth defects and with potential risk that clearly outweighs potential benefit.
Risk vs benefit: R >> B = Proven or potential risk outweighs potential benefits.
B > R = Potential benefits outweigh potential risks.
R >> B? = Risks may be outweighed by benefits in some circumstances.
? = Risk-to-benefit ratio is unknown.

Breast-feeding categories:
I = Drug does not enter breast milk.
II = Drug enters breast milk but is not known to be harmful in therapeutic doses.
IIIA = Drug may or may not enter breast milk but no adverse effects are expected.
IIIB = Drug may or may not enter breast milk but drug is systemically absorbed.
IV = Drug enters breast milk and poses a potential risk to the neonate.

interfere with the colonization factor antigens of ETEC that facilitate adherence to the bowel epithelium.

DOSAGE AND ADMINISTRATION

Bismuth subsalicylate (most commonly marketed as Pepto-Bismol) has been shown to be effective in an oral dosage of 60 mg 4 times a day. The tablet formulation is given in a dosage of two tablets 4 times a day.

SIDE EFFECTS

The most common side effects of bismuth subsalicylate are darkening of the tongue and stool. Mild tinnitus has been reported in study groups taking the medication. In addition, mild nausea and constipation have also been described.

Ciprofloxacin

Ciprofloxacin is a fluoroquinolone. All known gastrointestinal bacterial pathogens have been shown susceptible to ciprofloxacin. The drug is very effective in eliminating the aerobic bacterial flora of the stool, without affecting the anaerobic flora or selecting resistant organisms.

In a placebo-controlled trial involving 181 adults traveling to Mexico, a 5-day treatment with ciprofloxacin at 500 mg twice a day was as efficacious as trimethoprim-sulfamethoxazole in treating enterotoxigenic *E. coli,* invasive enteropathogens, and unknown pathogens. Resistance and adverse reactions are less problematic with ciprofloxacin than with TMP-SMX.

MECHANISM OF ACTION AND PHARMACOLOGY

Ciprofloxacin works by inhibiting bacterial deoxyribonucleic acid (DNA) gyrase. The enzyme is necessary for DNA replication, gene transcription, and aspects of DNA repair and recombination. DNA gyrase is antagonized by nalidixic acid, norfloxacin, and other quinolone agents. Maximum serum concentrations are attained 1 to 2 hours after oral dosing. Urinary excretion of ciprofloxacin is virtually complete within 24 hours after dosing. Approximately 20 to 35 percent of the oral dose is recovered in the feces within 5 days after dosing.

DOSAGE AND ADMINISTRATION

When prophylaxis is indicated, ciprofloxacin (Cipro), 500 mg once a day; ofloxacin (Floxin), 300 mg once a day; or norfloxacin (Noroxin), 400 mg once a day, is recommended. If traveler's diarrhea is moderate to severe, ciprofloxacin, 500 mg twice a day; norfloxacin, 400 mg twice a day; or ofloxacin, 300 mg twice a day, is recommended until symptoms resolve, for up to 3 days.

SIDE EFFECTS

The incidence of side effects from ciprofloxacin is low, and the drug is well tolerated. The most frequent side effect described is nausea, and, less commonly, diarrhea. Most reported studies cite side effects based on dosing at 500 mg twice a day.

Final Recommendations

Most experts do not recommend routine chemoprophylaxis against traveler's diarrhea for every traveler entering an endemic area. The risk of developing traveler's diarrhea when going from low- to high-risk areas (approximately 40%) must be weighed against the known risk of potential side effects when chemoprophylaxis is employed. Groups of travelers who should be considered for chemoprophylaxis when traveling to high-risk areas are (1) people on short, critical business trips; (2) people with underlying health problems (such as achlorhydria or known gastric resection) that may increase their susceptibility to diarrhea; (3) people who have an increased likelihood of complications secondary to dehydration from diarrhea; (4) military personnel; and (5) people who are taking much-needed and hard-earned vacations, honeymoon couples, and others in similar situations.

Chemoprophylaxis against traveler's diarrhea is not recommended when the period of risk will exceed 2 weeks. If chemoprophylaxis is used, it should continue beyond the period of exposure (for 1 or 2 days) after leaving the high-risk area.

PEARLS AND PITFALLS

1. The mainstays of preventive therapy are careful attention to food and beverage selection in high-risk areas. The traveler should avoid uncooked foods, unwashed salads, unpeeled fruits, and unboiled tap water, including ice.
2. Most experts recommend against routine prophylaxis. Instead, when mild symptoms of traveler's diarrhea develop (1–3 loose stools per 24 hours and no associated symptoms), oral rehydration is adequate. For more pronounced symptoms (3–5 loose stools per 24 hours and more notable but not disabling symptoms), the patient can be treated with bismuth subsalicylate, 30 ml every 30 minutes for eight doses, or an opiate drug such as loperamide, 4 mg followed by 2 mg after each unformed passed stool (up to 16 mg/day). For severe traveler's diarrhea, TMP-SMX, one double-strength tablet twice a day for 3 to 5 days, is effective. Alternatives include doxycycline, 100 mg twice a day for 5 days; ciprofloxacin, 500 mg twice a day for 5 days; or furazolidone, 100 mg 4 times a day for adults or 1.25 mg/kg for children. (See the furazolidone section under giardiasis in Chap. 16 for further details.)
3. The opiate derivatives diphenoxylate and loperamide hydrochloride are both effective antiperistaltic agents used in treating mild traveler's diarrhea. Loperamide is the preferred drug because it does not cross the blood-brain barrier and has a lower incidence of side effects.
4. Because many areas of high risk for traveler's diarrhea are also high risk for hepatitis A infection, travelers are advised to receive immune serum globulin before arrival in these endemic areas.
5. Areas of high risk for traveler's diarrhea include Latin America, Africa, the Middle East, and Asia. Low-risk areas include northern Europe, Canada, New Zealand, Puerto Rico, the Bahamas, and the Virgin Islands.

Suggested Reading

Chak Amitabh, Banwell JG. Traveler's diarrhea. Gastroenterol Clin North Am 1993; 22:549–561.
A brief review of traveler's diarrhea.

Consensus Conference. Traveler's diarrhea. JAMA 1985; 253:2700–2704.
A review of the etiologies and therapies of traveler's diarrhea and recommendations for prophylaxis by a panel of experts convened by the National Institutes of Health.

DuPont HL. Nonfluid therapy and selected chemoprophylaxis of acute diarrhea. Am J Med 1985; 79 (suppl 6B):81–90.
A detailed review of the etiologies, treatment, and prophylaxis of traveler's diarrhea.

DuPont HL, Ericsson CD, Johnson PC. Chemotherapy and chemoprophylaxis of traveler's diarrhea. Ann Intern Med 1985; 109:260–261.
A brief review of chemoprophylaxis of traveler's diarrhea.

DuPont HL, et al. Prevention of traveler's diarrhea: Prophylactic administration of subsalicylate bismuth. JAMA 1980; 243:237–241.
A study documenting the efficacy of subsalicylate bismuth solution in preventing traveler's diarrhea.

DuPont HL, et al. Antimicrobial agents in the prevention of traveler's diarrhea. Rev Infect Dis 1986; 8 (suppl):167–171.
A review of four major studies comparing the effects of trimethoprim-sulfamethoxazole, trimethoprim, norfloxacin, and bicozamycin in preventing traveler's diarrhea.

DuPont HL, et al. Prevention of traveler's diarrhea by the tablet formulation of bismuth subsalicylate. JAMA 1987; 257:1347–1350.
A study of chemoprophylaxis of traveler's diarrhea that demonstrated the effectiveness of bismuth subsalicylate tablets.

DuPont HL, et al. Prevention and treatment of traveler's diarrhea. N Engl J Med 1993; 328:1821–1827.
A brief review of traveler's diarrhea.

Ericson CD. Ciprofloxacin or trimethoprim-sulfamethoxazole as initial therapy for traveler's diarrhea. A placebo controlled, randomized trial. Ann Intern Med 1987; 106:216–220.

Farthing MJG. Travelers' diarrhea. Gut 1994; 35:1–4.
A brief review of traveler's diarrhea.

Gorbach SL, et al. Traveler's diarrhea and toxigenic *Escherichia coli.* N Engl J Med 1975; 292:933–936.
The first study demonstrating that a high percentage of cases of traveler's diarrhea are caused by enterotoxigenic E. coli.

Johnson PC, et al. Lack of emergence of resistant fecal flora during successful prophylaxis of traveler's diarrhea with norfloxacin. Antimicrob Agents Chemother 1986; 30:671–674.
A double-blind study demonstrating a percent protection rate of 89 percent using norfloxacin, 400 mg/day for 14 days.

Kean BH. The diarrhea of travelers to Mexico: Summary of five-year study. Ann Intern Med 1963; 59:605–614.
An overview of a 5-year investigation that documented the effectiveness of phthalylsulfathiazole and neomycin in preventing traveler's diarrhea.

Sack RB. Antimicrobial prophylaxis of traveler's diarrhea: A selected summary. Rev Infect Dis 1986; 8 (suppl 2):160–166.
A review of the major studies documenting the efficacy of doxycycline prophylaxis for traveler's diarrhea.

Wolfson JS, Hooper DC. Norfloxacin: A new targeted fluoroquinolone antimicrobial agent. Ann Intern Med 1988; 108:238–251.
A comprehensive review of norfloxacin, including its potential use in preventing traveler's diarrhea.

Ciprofloxacin

John D. Malone

Fluoroquinolones, a class of antibiotics related to nalidixic acid, have been developed through side chain modification of the basic 4-quinolone ring. Ciprofloxacin's cyclopropyl group on position 1 leads to increased tissue penetration and an enlarged bactericidal spectrum compared to norfloxacin, a related fluoroquinolone. Ofloxacin, enoxacin, and lomefloxacin are other fluoroquinolone formulations that have recently been developed.

Due to excellent activity against many common aerobic gram-negative bacteria and high tissue levels in the gastrointestinal tract, ciprofloxacin is a most effective agent against susceptible enteric pathogens.

MECHANISM OF ACTION

Ciprofloxacin's bactericidal action involves inhibition of bacterial deoxyribonucleic acid (DNA) gyrase (topoisomerase). This enzyme reduces the size of bacterial DNA by supercoiling and imposing a second reverse twist on the DNA helix. This compresses the DNA, allowing placement within the bacteria. Bacterial gyrase inhibition results in relaxation of the supercoiled DNA, with rapid cessation of cell division. Rupture and cell lysis are observed in gram-negative bacteria, while staphylococci become enlarged. Other antibacterial mechanisms are also possible.

PHARMACOLOGY

Ciprofloxacin exhibits excellent bactericidal capability against many gram-negative bacteria; in addition, in vivo effectiveness in enteric infections is related to high drug levels achieved in the gastrointestinal tract. Intracellular concentrations, especially in neutrophils, may be 2 to 7 times greater than extracellular levels. This contributes to effectiveness in *Salmonella typhi* infection, because the organism is frequently located in the reticuloendothelial system, especially Peyer's patches. Ciprofloxacin has a bioavailability of 71 percent. One-third is excreted in the urine, and fecal recovery accounts for 15 to 30 percent. Secretion may occur through the intestinal mucosa, since 15 percent of intravenously administered ciprofloxacin may be recovered in the feces. Hepatic degradation to four different metabolites also occurs.

Ciprofloxacin's bile concentration is severalfold higher than serum levels; specifically, common bile duct levels range from 2.5 to 20.0 μg/ml after a single 500-mg dose.

Antimicrobial resistance to ciprofloxacin can develop with *Pseudomonas, Staphylococcus,* and *Enterococcus.* Resistance mechanisms involve a mutation or acquisition of foreign DNA as in chromosome plasmid transference. In fluoroquinolones, such a transference may be minimized due to an actual lethal effect of the drug on plasmid DNA. In the mid-1980s, fewer than 4 of 24,000 strains of gram-negative rods were resistant to ciprofloxacin (excluding *Pseudomonas*).

Clinical failures in streptococcal infections have been reported, especially in pneumococcal pneumonia. Treatment failures have also been reported with *Campylobacter jejuni* infections. Strains of *Neisseria gonorrhoeae* with decreased susceptibilities to ciprofloxacin have been isolated sporadically from patients in the United States. Ciprofloxacin has no anaerobic coverage.

INDICATIONS

Ciprofloxacin is approved by the Food and Drug Administration (FDA) for use in bacterial diarrhea caused by enterotoxigenic *Escherichia coli, C. jejuni, Shigella sonnei,* and *Shigella flexneri.* Other enteric gram-negative rods that cause diarrhea are also very susceptible, including salmonella (especially *S. typhi*), *Yersinia enterocolitica, Pleisomonas shigelloides, Aeromonas* species, and *Vibrio parahemolyticus.* Due to the growing resistance of enteric pathogens to trimethoprim-sulfamethoxazole, ciprofloxacin is an ideal agent for empiric treatment of diarrheal disease, especially in travelers. Chronic carriers of *S. typhi* can be effectively cleared with ciprofloxacin, 750 mg twice a day for one month.

Coverage does not include the intestinal protozoal pathogens such as *Giardia lamblia* and *Entamoeba histolytica.* Viral gastroenteritides (Norwalk agent, calicivirus, enterovirus–Coxsackie, and echovirus) do not respond to ciprofloxacin.

Relapsing diarrhea may occur in human immunodeficiency virus (HIV) infection due to *Salmonella, Shigella,* and *Campylobacter.* Patients with salmonellosis and CD4 lymphocyte cell counts less than 200/μl or septicemia, or both, should be considered for lifelong suppression with ciprofloxacin.

Mycobacterium avium complex (MAC) opportunistic infection can also be treated with ciprofloxacin, 750 mg twice a day, usually in combination with rifampin (600 mg/day) and ethambutol (15 mg/kg/day). Azithromycin (500–1000 mg/day) or clarithromycin (500–1000 mg twice a day) may be substituted for ciprofloxacin and appears to be superior. Lifelong suppression of MAC in patients with acquired immunodeficiency syndrome (AIDS) is often required. Rifabutin, 300 mg/day may be used as prophylaxis. Regimens involving clofazimine and aminoglycosides are alternatives.

Ciprofloxacin or ofloxacin is utilized in combination therapy for multiple drug (isoniazid and rifampin)–resistant *Mycobacterium tuberculosis* infection.

Ciprofloxacin has been used for selective antimicrobial prophylaxis with intensive chemotherapeutic regimens that result in prolonged neutropenia, such as acute leukemia and bone marrow transplants. The drug exhibits excellent activity against enteric gram-negative rods including *Pseudomonas* without suppressing the natural anaerobic bowel and vaginal flora. In addition, ciprofloxacin is well tolerated and does not prolong neutropenia as does trimethoprim-sulfamethoxazole. Failures of ciprofloxacin occur with respiratory, skin, and soft-tissue infections, primarily from streptococci, including fatal pneumococcal pneumonia. The effectiveness of antimicrobial prophylaxis in granulocytopenia is undergoing reappraisal.

Although there are case reports of increased nephrotoxicity with cyclosporine, an extensive review has not supported any adverse interaction.

CONTRAINDICATIONS AND SIDE EFFECTS

According to the manufacturer's guidelines, ciprofloxacin is contraindicated during pregnancy and breast-feeding (Table 20-1), and in children under 18 years of age. Ciprofloxacin is excreted in lactating rats. Arthropathy has developed in immature animals given quinolones. Ciprofloxacin was given to 1500 children and adolescents with cystic fibrosis, typhoid fever, osteomyelitis, and resistant tuberculosis when there were no other treatment options; reversible arthralgia was a rare side effect (2% in most studies).

Other side effects may include central nervous system (CNS) stimulation with insomnia and restlessness, and dizziness or headache, especially when used with caffeine. Crystalluria due to drug precipitation is reported at higher doses (750 mg twice a day); maintaining a well-hydrated state is recommended. Transaminase elevation is reported in 2 percent of patients. Several cases of fulminant hepatic failure related to ciprofloxacin have recently been reported.

Potentially serious drug interactions include elevation of theophylline levels due to competition for hepatic enzymes. Diphenylhydantoin levels may also vary. Increased prothrombin times in individuals receiving warfarin are reported. Ciprofloxacin absorption is impaired by antacids. Compared to other fluoroquinolones, enoxacin has the greatest theophylline interaction, while ofloxacin and lomefloxacin do not exhibit clinically significant interaction.

In cases of renal failure, dosage should be decreased by 50 percent when creatinine clearance is less than 50 ml/minute. Individuals with creatinine clearances less than 30 ml/minute should receive half the dose every 18 hours.

DOSAGE

Recommended dosage for mild, moderate, or severe diarrhea is a 500-mg tablet every 12 hours continued for at least 2 days after signs and symptoms of diarrhea have resolved. Traveler's diarrhea should respond within 24 to 48 hours and should not require more than 5 days of therapy. Loperamide capsules are a beneficial addition, 4 mg initially, then one capsule every 4 hours up to eight capsules per day.

Dosage and duration of treatment for salmonellosis are more controversial, because prolonged excretion of salmonella occurs in antibiotic-treated individuals. Treatment for salmonellosis should be considered in individuals who are likely to have bacteremia, and a longer duration of therapy may be necessary.

PEARLS AND PITFALLS

1. Ciprofloxacin is recommended for use in adults. Use in children should occur only when other medications cannot be used.
2. Ciprofloxacin interferes with theophylline and warfarin metabolism. If a fluoroquinolone is necessary, ofloxacin is least likely to affect theophylline levels.
3. Concomitant antacid administration interferes with ciprofloxacin absorption. Cimetidine slows hepatic metabolism of ciprofloxacin and increases serum levels.
4. Anaerobic and streptococcal coverage is poor; therefore, use in perirectal abscess or intraabdominal infection would require additional coverage with a penicillin or clindamycin. Fatal cases of pneumococcal pneumonia have developed in patients receiving ciprofloxacin.

Table 20-1. Ciprofloxacin: Pregnancy and breast-feeding

Agent	FDA pregnancy category	Risk vs benefit (by trimester)			Breast-feeding category
		1st	2nd	3rd	
Ciprofloxacin	C1	R >> B?	R >> B?	R >> B?	IV

Food and Drug Administration (FDA) pregnancy categories:
A = Well-controlled studies fail to demonstrate risk to the fetus.
B1 = Animal studies fail to demonstrate risk to the fetus but no human studies are available.
B2 = Animal studies show some risk to the fetus but this is not confirmed in human studies.
C1 = Animal studies show risk to the fetus but no human studies are available.
C2 = Animal and human studies are unavailable.
D = Drug associated with birth defects but with potential benefits that may outweigh known risks.
X = Drug associated with birth defects and with potential risk that clearly outweighs potential benefit.
Risk vs benefit: R >> B = Proven or potential risk outweighs potential benefits.
B > R = Potential benefits outweigh potential risks.
R >> B? = Risks may be outweighed by benefits in some circumstances.
? = Risk-to-benefit ratio is unknown.
Breast-feeding categories:
I = Drug does not enter breast milk.
II = Drug enters breast milk but is not known to be harmful in therapeutic doses.
IIIA = Drug may or may not enter breast milk but no adverse effects are expected.
IIIB = Drug may or may not enter breast milk but drug is systemically absorbed.
IV = Drug enters breast milk and poses a potential risk to the neonate.

Suggested Reading

CDC. Decreased susceptibility of *Neisseria gonorrhoeae* to fluoroquinolones—Ohio and Hawaii, 1992–1994. MMWR 1994; 43(no. 18).

Gonococcal organisms with decreased in vitro susceptibilities to ciprofloxacin have decreased susceptibilities to all fluoroquinolones, including ofloxacin, enoxacin, lomefloxacin, and norfloxacin.

Donnelly JP, Maschmeyer G. Selective oral antimicrobial prophylaxis for prevention of infection in acute leukemia. Eur J Cancer 1992; 28A:873.

Ciprofloxacin (1 gm / day) was effective for selective gastrointestinal tract decontamination. Overall effectiveness of therapy is under evaluation.

DuPont HL. Use of quinolones in the treatment of gastrointestinal infections. Eur J Microbiol Infect Dis 1991; 10:325.

Quinolones are optimal therapy for bacterial diarrhea in adults, especially in areas where trimethoprim resistance is high. (46 references)

Eggelston M, Park SY. Review of the Y-quinolones. Infect Control 1987; 8:119.

An excellent review, with table of activity comparing ciprofloxacin against multiple pathogens.

Fuchs S, Simon Z. Fatal hepatic failure associated with ciprofloxacin. Lancet 1994; 343:738.

Ciprofloxacin causes mild reversible transaminase elevation in 2 to 3 percent of patients, supporting a previous case report of fulminant hepatic failure.

Guay DR. The role of fluoroquinolones. Pharmacotherapy 1992; 12:71S.

Ofloxacin and lomefloxacin are clinically insignificant inhibitors of theophylline metabolism. Enoxacin and temafloxacin are less likely to potentiate the anticoagulant effect of warfarin. Extensive and complete review with 262 references.

Hoey LL, Lake KD. Does ciprofloxacin interact with cyclosporine? Ann Pharmacother 1994; 28:93.

Literature review concludes that cyclosporine and ciprofloxacin can be used together safely despite anecdotal case reports of synergistic nephrotoxicity.

Kubin R. Safety and efficacy of ciprofloxacin in paediatric patients—review. Infection 1993; 21:413.

Ciprofloxacin has been given to 1500 children and adolescents with reversible arthralgia as an extremely rare condition. Use in children may include cystic fibrosis, resistant typhoid, osteomyelitis, and multiresistant mycobacterial disease.

Linville D, Emory C. Ciprofloxacin and warfarin interaction. Am J Med 1991; 90:765.

Case report of life-threatening hemorrhage due to the interaction.

McEvoy GK, Litvak K (eds). *American Hospital Formulary Service Drug Information.* Bethesda, MD: American Society of Hospital Pharmacists, 1993. P. 440.

Extensive, complete, thorough ciprofloxacin review. Additional sections on enoxacin, lomefloxacin, ofloxacin, and norfloxacin.

Nelson MR. *Salmonella, campylobacter,* and *shigella* in HIV-seropositive patients. AIDS 1992; 6:1495.

Patients with salmonella who have low CD4 lymphocytes or septice-

mia, or both, should be considered for lifelong prophylaxis with ciprofloxacin.

Peloquin CA. Pharmacology of antimycobacterial drugs. Med Clin North Am 1993; 77:1253.

Ciprofloxacin and ofloxacin are effective in management of multidrug-resistant tuberculosis (MDR-TB) and Mycobacterium avium *complex (MAC). Recommendations from the National Jewish Center for Immunology and Respiratory Medicine are given for these complicated cases.*

Rodvold KA, Piscitelli SC. New oral macrolide and fluoroquinolone antibiotics: An overview of pharmacokinetics, interactions, and safety. CID 1993; 17(suppl 1):S192.

Fluoroquinolones are compared, along with the new oral macrolides, azithromycin and clarithromycin, both of which have fewer adverse gastrointestinal effects than erythromycin.

Wolfson JS, Hooper DC. Overview of fluoroquinolone safety. Am J Med 1991; 91(suppl 6A):153.

Clinically important interactions occur with co-administration of antacids. Ciprofloxacin and enoxacin interact with theophylline.

Acute Diverticulitis

Michael M. Van Ness

Diverticulosis was first described by Cruveilhier in 1849 and has been increasingly recognized since Beer's description in 1904. Several authors, including Rankin, Brown, and Young, estimate the incidence of asymptomatic diverticulosis in Western countries to be 5 percent at age 40, increasing linearly to 50 percent in the ninth decade.

Acute diverticulitis or bacteria-induced perforation and inflammation of colonic diverticuli may be mild and easily treated or serious and life threatening. Acute diverticulitis complicates asymptomatic diverticulosis with increasing frequency as the patient's age increases. Specifically, after 5 years of observation, acute diverticulitis develops in 10 percent of patients. The incidence of acute diverticulitis increases to 35 percent after 20 years of observation.

Although medical therapy is sufficient in the majority of patients, Chappius and Cohn report that 20 percent of all patients with acute diverticulitis develop an abscess, fistula, or recurrent diverticulitis that requires surgical intervention.

PATHOGENESIS AND INCIDENCE

Microperforation of a single diverticulum is believed to be the initial event that causes peridiverticulitis, the initial stage of acute diverticulitis. Because diverticuli are pseudodiverticuli (they do not contain all the layers of the bowel wall but only mucosa and submucosa herniated through the circular muscle layer of the colon), peridiverticulitis may remain confined to the pericolic fat or may develop into a free macroperforation causing frank peritonitis.

Complications of acute diverticulitis include bacteremia and septicemia; abscess formation with extension into the mesentery, adjacent bowel, or bladder; and free perforation with peritonitis. Death is reported by Welch to occur in 5.9 percent of patients with diverticular abscess at the Massachusetts General Hospital. Fistulae may develop with communication into bowel, uterus, vagina, bladder, or skin. Transient colonic obstruction and bleeding may occur but rarely are serious or life threatening.

Incidence figures for complicated diverticular disease are difficult to obtain. In about 8 percent of cases of diverticulitis of the sigmoid colon, small-intestinal complications such as colo-enteric fistulae, small-bowel obstructions, and inflammatory changes of the small bowel from mesenteritis and the associated mass will be seen. Utilizing computed tomographic (CT) scanning of the abdomen in 68 patients with acute diverticulitis, Labs and associates found 13 cases of diverticular abscess and 12 cases of diverticular fistulae.

PRESENTATION AND DIAGNOSIS

The classic presentation for acute diverticulitis includes left-lower-quadrant pain, low-grade fever, leukocytosis, nausea and vomiting, and abdominal distention. Signs of acute diverticulitis reflect the degree of peritoneal inflammation, with variable degrees of abdominal tenderness, rebound, mass, or fullness.

The differential diagnosis includes acute appendicitis, sigmoid carcinoma, ischemic colitis, mesenteric venous thrombosis, pseudomembranous enterocolitis, and idiopathic inflammatory bowel disease.

Although much less prevalent than left-sided diverticulosis, right-sided diverticuli, both acquired and congenital, can perforate, with abscess and fistula formation. In the appropriate clinical setting, the signs and symptoms of right-sided diverticular disease can be easily confused with acute appendicitis as well as less common entities such as Crohn's disease, carcinoid tumor, or ameboma.

Diagnosis of acute diverticulitis depends on the appropriate history, physical findings, and confirmatory studies. Plain abdominal radiographs may show an ileus pattern, mass effect in the left or right lower quadrant, or evidence of small-bowel or colonic obstruction. Rarely, free abdominal air may be present. A water-soluble colonic enema (Hypaque-76, 66% diatriazole meglumine, and 10% diatriazole sodium) is the best study to show "sawtooth" mucosa, fistulae, or perforation. Although difficult for most patients to tolerate during the initial phase of acute diverticulitis, flexible proctosigmoidoscopy may show peridiverticular erythema, edema, and exudate.

COMPLICATIONS

Abscess, perforation, and fistulae are the most common life threatening complications of acute diverticulitis.

The presence of diverticular abscess should be suspected in the patient whose condition fails to improve within 48 hours of initiation of antimicrobial therapy. High spiking temperatures, persistent leukocytosis, and a tender abdominal mass are clues to the diagnosis. Computed tomography is the diagnostic procedure of choice. In the appropriate patient, percutaneous drainage of diverticular abscess will allow stabilization of critically ill patients at high risk for surgical intervention.

Free perforation (stage 3, generalized purulent peritonitis, or stage 4, fecal peritonitis; Table 21-1) of an infected diverticulum is a surgical emergency and requires an aggressive surgical plan carried out in conjunction with intensive medical support. A combination of a primary resection of the involved areas, end colostomy, and Hartmann's closure has the lowest morbidity and mortality and is the surgical procedure of choice.

Unlike abscess and perforation, fistula formation usually occurs between episodes of acute diverticular disease. Relative luminal stenosis and high-pressure segmental pressures contribute to the development of fistulae to adjacent abdominal organs. Recurrent polymicrobial urinary tract infections, pneumaturia (spontaneous passage of gas in the urinary stream), and fecaluria are clues to the presence of a colovesical fistula, usually present in the posterior bladder wall.

Chronic diarrhea, steatorrhea, and small bowel overgrowth suggest the development of colo-enteric fistulae.

Feculent vaginal discharge or gas passage per vagina are supportive of the presence of colo-uterine or colovaginal fistulae.

Elective surgical fistulectomy and resection of the colon involved with diverticular disease are indicated in the presence of fistulae. Under these circumstances, a primary anastomosis should be possible.

Table 21-1. Perforative diverticular disease

Stage 1: Contained pericolic abscess or phlegmonous diverticulitis
Stage 2: Walled-off pelvic abscess secondary to perforation of a pericolic abscess
Stage 3: Generalized purulent peritonitis resulting from rupture of a pericolic or pelvic abscess
Stage 4: Fecal peritonitis

Adapted from EJ Hinchey, PGH Schaal, GK Richards. Treatment of Perforated Diverticular Disease of the Colon. In C Rob (ed), *Advances in Surgery,* vol 12. Chicago: Year Book, 1978. P 85.

Table 21-2. Diverticulitis: Organisms and antibiotics

1. Facultative aerobes
    - Enterobacteriaceae
        - *Escherichia coli*
        - *Klebsiella* species
        - *Proteus* species
        - *Enterobacter*
        - *Citrobacter*
    - Enterococci
2. Obligate anaerobes
    - *Bacteroides fragilis*
    - *Bacteroides melaninogenicus*
    - *Peptococcus*
    - *Peptostreptococcus*
    - *Fusobacterium*
    - *Eubacterium* species
    - *Clostridium* species

Intravenous treatment regimens

1. Chloramphenicol, 50–100 mg/kg/day, and gentamicin, 1.7 mg/kg every 8 hours
2. Clindamycin, 600 mg every 6–8 hours, and gentamicin, 1.7 mg/kg every 8 hours
3. Ceftizoxime (Cefizox), 2 gm every 12 hours (with dosage adjustment for patients with acute or chronic renal failure)
4. Imipenem-cilastatin (Primaxin), 500 mg every 6–8 hours (with dosage adjustment for patients with acute or chronic renal failure)

Elective resection is also indicated for recurrent attacks of diverticulitis, to rule out malignancy, and for the patient under the age of 55 with his or her first attack of diverticulitis. A rare complication of chronic diverticulosis is a giant pseudodiverticulum. These cavities are usually more than 7 cm in diameter, typically arise on the mesenteric border of the sigmoid colon, and are associated with weight loss, intermittent obstructive symptoms, and pain.

MEDICAL THERAPY

As shown in Table 21-2, a multitude of microorganisms are present in acute diverticulitis. Because diverticulitis is a polymicrobial infection, a broad spectrum of antimicrobial activity is required. In a rat model of secondary bacterial peritonitis and abscess formation, Onderdonk found that antibiotics need not be active against every and all organisms to treat diverticulitis and to prevent abscess formation. If the more virulent pathogens are controlled, the synergistic effect of the aerobes and anaerobes on abscess formation can be eliminated. For example, although gentamicin and clindamycin are known to have little or no activity against Enterobacteriaceae and enterococcus, Bartlett and associates have shown this therapy to be effective in an experimental rat model of intraperitoneal infection, suggesting that the enterococcus is not a primary pathogen in secondary peritonitis. Following on this study, both Fass and Levison have treated patients with mixed aerobic and anaerobic infections with gentamicin and clindamycin, with good clinical results.

Acceptable intravenous treatment regimens for patients with uncomplicated diverticulitis are given in Table 21-2.

PEARLS AND PITFALLS

1. The incidence of asymptomatic diverticulosis is estimated to be about 15 percent at age 50 and 35 percent at age 65.
2. The most common site for diverticulosis is the sigmoid colon, where herniation under pressures as high as 90 mm Hg occurs. The locus minoris resistentiae is the penetration site of small arterioles from the circumferential artery present on the antimesenteric side of the colon.
3. The most common fistula in diverticular disease is the colovesical fistula; diverticulosis causes more colovesicular fistulae than any other disease.
4. The second most common fistula associated with diverticular disease is the colocutaneous fistula. Failure to resect all the diseased sigmoid colon is believed to be the proximate cause in over two-thirds of the cases of recurrent colocutaneous fistulae.
5. Percutaneous drainage of diverticular abscesses is a means of preventing urgent surgical intervention in unstable or frail patients. It may have a role in the long-term treatment of patients for whom surgical intervention is contraindicated.
6. Antibiotic therapy of uncomplicated acute diverticulosis should be tailored to cover the large number of pathogens present, keeping in mind the synergism between aerobic and anaerobic bacteria in the development of diverticular abscess.
7. Diverticular abscess and fistulae usually require surgical intervention.
8. Computed tomography is more sensitive and specific than barium enema in the diagnosis of diverticular abscess.
9. Barium enema is more sensitive and specific than computed tomography in the diagnosis of colovesical fistula.

CONCLUSION

The twentieth century has seen many developments, including diverticulosis—now believed to be the result of a Western diet inadequate in terms of dietary fiber. Approximately 20 to 25 percent of all cases of chronic diverticulosis are complicated by acute diverticulitis, with surgical intervention in nearly 20 percent of these cases. Appropriate antibiotic therapy should cover a wide range of potential pathogens. A high index of suspicion is required for early detection of complications of acute diverticulitis, most commonly diverticular abscess and colovesical fistula. Coordination and cooperation between physicians and surgeons optimize patient care.

Suggested Reading

Bartlett JG, et al. Whither the enterococcus? (abstract 297). Washington, DC: Fifteenth Interscience Conference on Antimicrobial Agents and Chemotherapy, September 24–26, 1975.

Evidence to suggest that the enterococcus is not the primary infective agent in a rat model of peritonitis.

Case records of the Massachusetts General Hospital (case 19–1994). N Engl J Med 1994; 330:1376–1381.

A 47-year-old woman admitted with intermittent abdominal pain, vomiting, and weight loss had a giant sigmoid pseudodiverticulum.

Chappuis CW, Cohn I. Acute colonic diverticulitis. Surg Clin North Am 1988; 68:301–313.

A complete and comprehensive review of the incidence (5% in the fifth decade to 50% in the ninth decade), pathogenesis (acquired pulsion-type pseudodiverticula, in that they do not contain all the layers of the bowel wall), diagnosis (left-lower-quadrant pain, fever, leukocytosis), and management of acute diverticulitis.

Crist DW, et al. Acute diverticulitis of the cecum and ascending colon diagnosed by computed tomography. Surg Gynecol Obstet 1988; 166:99–102.

A report of seven patients presenting with right-sided abdominal pain of 2 to 7 days' duration, anorexia, fever, and guarding. Three of the seven had had previous appendectomy. Urgent CT scanning of the abdomen using 10-ml slice thickness after oral administration of 3% sodium diatrizoate showed extraluminal air suggestive of abscess in five of the seven, narrowing of the distal small bowel in three of the seven, and pericolic inflammation in all seven (eccentric in 5, concentric in 2). The authors conclude that CT scanning may be helpful in the evaluation of patients with a clinical history or physical findings atypical of acute appendicitis where right-sided diverticulosis may be present.

Eyer SD, Snover DC, Delaney JP. Diverticulitis in the multiple endocrine neoplasia type II B syndrome. Am J Gastroenterol 1988; 83:183–186.

As evidence that diffuse ganglioneuromatosis involves the entire gastrointestinal tract, the authors report a case of complicated diverticulitis (colovesical fistula) in a 37-year-old woman and review the other three cases described in the medical literature. The authors emphasize that complications of diverticulosis tend to appear in patients with multiple endocrine neoplasia (MEN) IIB earlier than in the general population.

Fass RJ, et al. Clindamycin in the treatment of serious anaerobic infections. Ann Intern Med 1973; 78:853.

Among 19 adults with anaerobic or mixed infections, 18 of the 19 were cured of their infections with clindamycin or clindamycin and gentamicin. Infections included actinomycosis (5), lung abscess (1), soft-tissue abscess (5), osteomyelitis (3), and pneumonia with empyema (5). The only recurrence after therapy was one of the pneumonia with empyema patients.

Fazio VW, et al. Colocutaneous fistula complicating diverticulitis. Dis Colon Rectum 1987; 30:89–94.

The authors emphasize the need to resect the sigmoid colon completely to prevent the development of postoperative colocutaneous fistulae.

Klein S, et al. Extraintestinal manifestations in patients with diverticulitis. Ann Intern Med 1988; 108:700–702.

An extraordinary series of three patients (2 men, 1 woman, aged 54–67 years) who presented with sigmoid diverticulitis complicated by perforation (3 of 3), pericolic abscess (3 of 3), pyoderma gangrenosum (3 of 3), and lower extremity arthritis (3 of 3). All were treated for idiopathic inflammatory bowel disease with systemic corticosteroids, antibiotics, and local steroids without improvement in the extraintestinal manifestations of their disease. All three patients underwent sigmoid colon resection and experienced relief of pyoderma gangrenosum and lower-extremity arthritis. Pathologic examination of the resected specimens showed no evidence of idiopathic inflammatory bowel disease.

Labs JD, et al. Complications of acute diverticulitis of the colon: Improved early diagnosis with computerized tomography. Am J Surg 1988; 155:331–335.

The authors review their experience in the early recognition of complications of diverticulitis in 68 patients hospitalized at the Johns Hopkins Hospital from 1982 to 1984. Uncomplicated diverticular disease occurred in 43 (63%), whereas complications occurred in 25 (13 of the 25 had diverticular abscesses, and 12 of the 25 had colovesical fistulae). Among the 43 with uncomplicated diverticulosis, CT scanning showed segmental and localized thickening of the colonic wall with luminal narrowing, pericolic reaction, and associated distant, scattered diverticula without evidence of abscess or fistulae. Of the 13 patients with diverticular abscess, 10 underwent CT scanning, which confirmed the presence of a mass in all 10 (pericolic fluid collection). Colovesical fistulae were suspected in 12 patients. All 12 underwent CT scanning. Air was present in the bladder, with thickened segments of adjacent sigmoid colon in 11 of the 12. The authors advocate the early use of CT scanning in patients suspected of having complicated diverticulosis.

Levison ME, et al. In vitro activity and clinical efficacy of clindamycin in the treatment of infections due to anaerobic bacteria. J Infect Dis 1977; 135:S79.

The clinical experience at the Medical College of Pennsylvania with clindamycin in anaerobic infections is reviewed.

Ludmerer KM, Kissane JM (eds). Polymicrobial sepsis and jaundice in a 46-year-old man. Am J Med 1986; 81:649–654.

A case description of a 46-year-old white man presenting with polymicrobial bacteremia, bilateral lower-abdominal pain, jaundice, and fever who had acute sigmoid diverticulitis complicated by perforation, peritonitis, and abscess formation. A very clear differential diagnosis is presented as well as speculation on the etiology of diverticulitis including abnormal vascular supply, incomplete diverticular emptying, or local ischemia and perforation. Last, the discussants emphasize that whereas bacteremia occurs regularly when aerobic organisms are inoculated intraperitoneally, abdominal abscess formation requires the presence of both aerobic and anaerobic organisms.

Neff CC, et al. Diverticular abscesses: Percutaneous drainage. Radiology 1987; 163:15–18.
Among 16 patients with known diverticular abscess, the placement of 8 to 12 French gauge catheters percutaneously was used as a temporizing measure in 13 patients operated on 10 days to 6 weeks later and as definitive therapy in 3 high-risk patients. All three were asymptomatic 12 to 29 months later.

Onderdonk AB, Shapiro ME, Finberg RW, et al. Use of a model of intraabdominal sepsis for studies of the pathogenicity of *Bacteroides fragilis.* Rev Infec Dis 1984; 6(Suppl I):591–5.
Abscess formation can be prevented even if prescribed antibiotics are ineffective against some organisms.

Welch CE. Computerized tomography scans for all patients with diverticulitis. Am J Surg 1988; 155:336.
An editorial accompanying the article by Labs and associates. Because of the high mortality associated with diverticular abscess (5.9%), Welch emphasizes that early CT scanning of patients with suspected diverticular abscess may prove beneficial in reducing mortality.

Liver and Pancreatic Disease Drugs

Exciting advances in the pharmacologic therapy of liver, biliary, and pancreatic disease are becoming more frequent. In 1995, we have advanced significantly in our knowledge of the identity and pathogenesis of acute and chronic liver disease compared to a generation ago. We now have increasingly useful agents that were not available in the 1950s. Despite these advances, general supportive measures and a vigilant search for infection and metabolic abnormalities continue to serve as the cornerstone for the treatment of most liver diseases. Careful application of immunosuppressive agents can be beneficial to selected patients. Widespread use of hepatitis B vaccine is strongly recommended and increasingly required of employees. Hepatitis A vaccine should be available soon.

Chronic Autoimmune Liver Disease and Wilson's Disease

Pharmacologic therapy of chronic autoimmune liver disease (CALD, or "lupoid" hepatitis) and Wilson's disease is of unquestioned benefit. Although neither condition is curable, the disease manifestations can be controlled with appropriate therapy.

Prednisone in CALD prolongs life, improves the patient's overall sense of well-being, and reverses abnormal histologic and laboratory findings. Many CALD patients require long-term prednisone therapy. Side effects of chronic, high-dose prednisone therapy can be lessened by dose reduction concurrent with initiation of azathioprine. Azathioprine alone is not effective for inducing a remission in severe, chronic autoimmune liver disease. However, Stellon and associates have shown recently that azathioprine alone may be capable of maintaining a corticosteroid-induced remission.

Penicillamine remains the most effective and best-tolerated copper-chelation and cupric agent. As much as 1000 to 3000 μg copper is excreted per day with initiation of therapy. There is no place in the diagnosis of suspected Wilson's disease for a "penicillamine trial": Liver biopsy is required for diagnosis. Improvement in liver inflammation, dysarthria, intellectual capacity, and tremor may require 6 months of therapy. Penicillamine tolerance is usually very good in patients with Wilson's disease. Only rarely is the lupuslike reaction seen. For severe, refractory penicillamine reactions, prednisone may provide temporary relief and trien (tetraethylene tetramine dihydrochloride) may be substituted for penicillamine. Penicillamine or trien therapy must be continued for life.

Primary Biliary Cirrhosis

Although new and exciting advances have been reported recently, the benefit of pharmacologic therapy for primary biliary cirrhosis (PBC) remains incomplete.

Both Kaplan and Bodenheimer have studied colchicine in patients with PBC. Improvement in liver function and synthesis was apparent. Histology did not improve with therapy. After 4 years of therapy, Kaplan noted a trend toward a decrease in mortality in the colchicine-treated group.

Immunosuppressive therapy of PBC with either penicillamine, prednisone, or azathioprine appears to be of no benefit. On the other hand, Hoofnagle and associates have published results demonstrating benefit from chlorambucil. Biochemical improvement was accompanied by decreases in inflammatory cell infiltrate in treated patients compared with a control group. Whether chlorambucil will decrease mortality and improve survival is unknown.

Ursodeoxycholic acid, a dihydroxyl bile acid that is the stereoisomer of chenodiol, is an expensive, well-tolerated agent that decreases the deleterious effects of cholestasis by increasing bile flow and decreasing aberrant HLA antigen expression. Ursodeoxycholic acid inhibits ileal reabsorption of endogenous bile acids. Best results (improvement in alkaline phosphatase, decreased pruritus, and decreased need for transplantation) were obtained if a dose of 13 to 15 mg/day were given.

Hepatitis B and C

Modification and manipulation of immune mechanisms by prednisone and interferon hold promise for the treatment of viral hepatitis. Perillo and associates treated chronic hepatitis B patients with a steroid withdrawal followed by alpha-2b interferon. Nine of 18 patients cleared all markers of viral replication and remained clear for 9 months. Although longer periods of observation and larger numbers of subjects are needed, Aach believes that this type of immunomodulating therapy is most promising for these patients.

The hepatitis B vaccine (either plasma-derived or recombinant) is now widely available and is recognized to be safe and effective.

Interferon treatment of patients with hepatitis C is imperfect because untreated hepatitis C is likely to progress to cirrhosis in approximately one-third of cases of chronic hepatitis C. The use of interferon is advocated in the following groups: patients with (1) chronic active hepatitis C without histologic cirrhosis, (2) chronic persistent hepatitis C with severe symptoms, and (3) compensated cirrhosis with either chronic active or chronic persistent hepatitis C. With a standard regimen of 3 million units subcutaneously 3 times a week, approximately 40 percent of patients will respond.

Alcoholic Liver Disease

Although there is renewed interest in the use of corticosteroids for acute alcoholic hepatitis, only abstinence, adequate nutrition, and supportive measures (vitamin K, lactulose) are widely accepted therapies.

Disulfiram may be useful in the treatment of chronic alcoholism.

Biliary and Pancreatic Disease

As of this writing, surgical or endoscopic intervention methods are the preferred treatment modalities, with ursodeoxycholic acid,

Table IV-1. Liver and pancreatic disease drugs: Pregnancy and breast-feeding

Agent	FDA pregnancy category	Risk vs benefit (by trimester)			Breast-feeding category
		1st	2nd	3rd	
Colchicine	C1	R >> B	R >> B	R >> B	IV
Corticosteroids	C1	B > R	B > R	B > R	IV
Lactulose	C2	?	?	?	IIIB
Penicillamine	C1	?	?	?	IIIB
Vitamin K	B1	?	B > R	B > R	II

Food and Drug Administration (FDA) pregnancy categories:
A = Well-controlled studies fail to demonstrate risk to the fetus.
B1 = Animal studies fail to demonstrate risk to the fetus but no human studies are available.
B2 = Animal studies show some risk to the fetus but this is not confirmed in human studies.
C1 = Animal studies show risk to the fetus but no human studies are available.
C2 = Animal and human studies are unavailable.
D = Drugs associated with birth defects but with potential benefits that may outweigh known risks.
X = Drugs associated with birth defects and with potential risk that clearly outweighs potential benefit.
Risk vs benefit: R >> B = Proven or potential risk outweighs potential benefits.
B > R = Potential benefits outweigh potential risks.
R >> B? = Risks may be outweighed by benefits in some circumstances.
? = Risk-to-benefit ratio is unknown.
Breast-feeding categories:
I = Drug does not enter breast milk.
II = Drug enters breast milk but is not known to be harmful in therapeutic doses.
IIIA = Drug may or may not enter breast milk but no adverse effects are expected.
IIIB = Drug may or may not enter breast milk but drug is systemically absorbed.
IV = Drug enters breast milk and poses a potential risk to the neonate.

monooctanoin, or methyl tert-butyl ether reserved for patients with severe systemic illnesses that preclude more traditional therapy.

Pancreatic enzyme replacement benefits patients with pancreatic insufficiency and chronic pancreatic pain. Alkalinization of gastric contents preserves lipase, colipase, and trypsin activity as much as possible.

Michael M. Van Ness

Suggested Reading

Aach RD. The treatment of chronic type B viral hepatitis. Ann Intern Med 1988; 109:89–91.
The author reviews the rationale behind the current efforts to induce remission of hepatitis B by manipulation of immune processes.

Bodenheimer H, Schaffner F, Pezzullo F. Evaluation of colchicine therapy in primary biliary cirrhosis. Gastroenterology 1988; 95:124–129.
Biochemical, but not histologic, improvement was noted with colchicine therapy.

Davis GL. Interferon treatment of cirrhotic patients with chronic hepatitis C: A logical intervention. Am J Gastroenterol 1994; 89: 658–660.
An insightful review of a difficult and evolving area.

Hoofnagle JH, et al. Randomized trial of chlorambucil for primary biliary cirrhosis. Gastroenterology 1986; 91:1327–1334.
Chlorambucil improved biochemical and inflammatory parameters, but not the degree of fibrosis or histologic stage of the disease.

Kaplan MM. Primary biliary cirrhosis—a first step in prolonging survival. N Engl J Med 1994; 330:1386–1387.
A thorough review of current therapy for primary biliary cirrhosis.

Kaplan MM, Knox TA. Treatment of primary biliary cirrhosis with low-dose weekly methotrexate. Gastroenterology 1991; 101:1332–1338.
Although methotrexate produces biochemical and clinical improvement similar to that of ursodiol, it cause reversible interstitial pneumonia in 15 to 20 percent of patients.

Kaplan MM, et al. A prospective trial of colchicine for primary biliary cirrhosis. N Engl J Med 1986; 315:1448–1454.
Biochemical improvement in liver function was apparent in the colchicine-treated PBC patients. Side effects were few.

Maddrey WC, et al. Prednisolone therapy in patients with severe alcoholic hepatitis: Results of a multicenter trial. Hepatology 1986; 6:1202.
Prednisolone benefited patients with acute alcoholic hepatitis. Only 2 of 35 prednisolone-treated patients died, compared to 11 of 31 placebo-treated patients.

Perrillo RP, et al. Prednisone withdrawal followed by recombinant alpha interferon in the treatment of chronic type B hepatitis. Ann Intern Med 1988; 109:95–100.
Immunologic priming with prednisone followed by interferon may prove an effective treatment for selected hepatitis B patients.

Poupon RE, et al. Ursodiol for the long-term treatment of primary biliary cirrhosis. N Engl J Med 1994; 330:1342–1347.
Ursodiol use decreases the need for liver transplantation.

Saito T, et al. A randomized controlled trial of human lymphoblastoid interferon in patients with compensated type C hepatitis. Am J Gastroenterol 1994; 89:681–686.
Interferon can benefit patients with compensated cirrhotic hepatitis C.

Stellon AJ, et al. Maintenance of remission in autoimmune chronic active hepatitis with azathioprine after corticosteroid withdrawal. Hepatology 1988; 8:781–784.
Azathioprine, 2 mg/kg, maintained corticosteroid-induced remission in CALD.

Corticosteroids

Michael M. Van Ness

Because many hepatic diseases are believed to occur because of immunologic abnormalities, corticosteroids have been utilized in their treatment. Close analysis of the results of numerous clinical trials of a wide variety of hepatic diseases has shown benefit in only a few, carefully circumscribed situations such as acute attacks of chronic autoimmune liver disease (lupoid hepatitis) and severe alcoholic liver disease. Newer, unproven, but intriguing applications of corticosteroids in conjunction with antiviral therapy have been reported but are not appropriate for routine clinical practice.

MECHANISM OF ACTION

Corticosteroids act by reducing inflammation, inhibiting fibrosis, and minimizing immunologic processes. More specifically, corticosteroids stabilize lyzosomes, reduce the damaging effects of antigen-antibody interactions, increase albumin synthesis, and retard production of type I collagen. In lymphocytes, the corticosteroid–cell membrane receptor complex appears to act by stimulation of transcription of messenger ribonucleic acid (mRNA) coding for an inhibitory protein, resulting in an overall catabolic response.

INDICATIONS

Chronic Autoimmune Liver Disease

Patients with chronic autoimmune liver disease, as defined by Waldenström in the 1950s and modified by Mistilis in 1970, require appropriate, aggressive immunosuppressive therapy. These patients are systemically ill, with fatigue, anorexia, and weight loss. They may exhibit jaundice and splenomegaly as well as spider angiomas, palmar erythema, acne, and right upper-quadrant tenderness. Severely ill patients may present with bleeding, ascites, and encephalopathy. Characteristic laboratory findings include antinuclear antibodies of the immunoglobulin G (IgG) class (50–70% of patients) and antibodies to double-stranded or native deoxyribonucleic acid (DNA; 42% of patients). A marked and broad-banded, polyclonal elevation of gamma globulins is characteristic. Associated organ system involvement includes pulmonary diffusion defects, fibrosing alveolitis, pericarditis, glomerulonephritis, arthritis, urticaria, thyroiditis, and hemolytic anemia.

Results from the Royal Free Hospital, the King's College Hospital, and the Mayo Clinic all clearly show benefit from corticosteroid therapy (Table 22-1). The goal of therapy is to reduce inflammation without causing side effects. Asymptomatic patients with only mild transaminase elevations should not be treated. Stellon and associates have shown that high-dose azathioprine, 2 mg/kg, is as effective as low-dose azathioprine plus corticosteroids in maintenance of remission in chronic autoimmune liver disease. Myelosuppression must be considered with this regimen, as well as pregnancy. Cushingoid features resolve with this type of regimen.

Table 22-1. Corticosteroids in autoimmune liver disease

First week: 10–15 mg prednisolone 3 times a day, or 15–20 mg prednisone 3 times a day

Second week: Clinical and liver test check; if marked improvement is noted, then reduce corticosteroids by $2^{1}/2$-mg increments.

Third week: Clinical and liver test check; if stable, continue dose reduction to maintenance (10–15 mg prednisolone a day, or 20 mg prednisone a day).

Every month: Clinical and liver test check

At 6 months: Liver biopsy

Full remission: Complete corticosteroid withdrawal, slowly (decrease by 2.5 mg/week); restart at full dose if relapse occurs.

No remission: Continue maintenance dose for 6 more months, consider the addition of azathioprine (50–100 mg/day); maximum dose, 20–30 mg prednisolone, or 40–60 mg prednisone with 100 mg azathioprine.

Alcoholic Liver Disease

In mild to moderate alcoholic liver disease, corticosteroids are of no benefit. In the treatment of severe alcoholic hepatitis complicated by encephalopathy, marked icterus, elevated prothrombin time, and ascites, three clinical trials show survival benefit from corticosteroid therapy.

In a study published by Maddrey and associates in 1978, 55 patients were treated in a double-blind manner with either prednisolone (40 mg/day) or placebo. After 32 days of therapy, 6 of the 31 patients receiving placebo died, compared to only 1 of the 24 receiving prednisolone.

To confirm these results, Maddrey conducted a multicenter, double-blind, placebo-controlled trial of methylprednisolone (32 mg/day) therapy. Sixty-six patients who met the criteria for severe alcoholic hepatitis, as defined by the discriminant function formula (DF equal to 32 or more defined severe disease and was calculated as follows: DF = 4.6 × [prothrombin time of the patient − the control + serum bilirubin]) were involved. Eleven of the 31 placebo-treated patients died within the 28-day study period, compared to only 2 of the 35 patients treated with methylprednisolone ($p = 0.006$).

Imperiale and Ramond have both confirmed these results. Hepatic encephalopathy without gastrointestinal bleeding describes the "ideal" patient who benefits from corticosteroid therapy. Ramond and associates' 1992 study confirms this result.

Therefore, in addition to alcohol abstinence, resumption of a nutritious diet, management of alcohol withdrawal phenomena, and treatment of bleeding, infection, and metabolic complications, management of the alcoholic patient with severe disease (DF > 32) might well include corticosteroid therapy.

Viral Hepatitis

Corticosteroids alone have no role in the treatment of acute or chronic hepatitis B or C.

Corticosteroids in conjunction with alpha- and gamma-interferon may be beneficial in the treatment of chronic hepatitis B characterized by active viral replication (positive e antigen). A short course of prednisone (40–60 mg/day for 6 weeks), with an abrupt taper before therapy with alpha and gamma interferon for 4 months, resulted in a greater than 40 percent clearance of the e antigen with concomitant production of e antibody. At this time, this type of therapy, although promising, remains experimental and should only be used in clinical trials under the auspices of experienced researchers.

Corticosteroids are of no benefit when used for the treatment of acute viral hepatitis. Liver necrosis, healing, antibody formation, and recovery are not improved by corticosteroid therapy. The steroid "whitewash," as described by Shaldon and Sherlock (prednisolone, 30, 20, 15, 10, and 5 mg orally, each dose given for 5 days) is inadvisable for even the nonhepatitis B patient with prolonged cholestasis, despite its proven beneficial effect on the morale of both patient and physician. Subsequent studies fail to demonstrate any real benefit from corticosteroids in acute viral hepatitis and suggest interference with the normal immune response, resulting in higher relapse rates and a propensity for development of chronic hepatitis. The use of corticosteroids for uncomplicated viral hepatitis is unjustifiable.

The rationale for use of corticosteroids in fulminant hepatic failure regardless of cause was based on the assumption that the anti-inflammatory action of corticosteroids would reduce hepatocellular necrosis. No benefit is realized by the use of corticosteroids in fulminant hepatic failure; in fact, there is strong evidence of an adverse effect. Corticosteroids should not be used in the treatment of fulminant hepatic failure.

The use of corticosteroids for the chronic, active hepatitis associated with inflammatory bowel disease is controversial. Gray and associates have described the benefits of corticosteroids (decreased symptoms and decreased transaminase values). Corticosteroids alleviated the symptoms of ulcerative colitis and active hepatitis but had no effect on the progression of chronic active hepatitis. Therefore, chronic active hepatitis associated with inflammatory bowel disease is not an indication by itself for corticosteroid therapy.

Primary Biliary Cirrhosis

Although corticosteroids relieve pruritus and might be expected to reduce inflammation in patients with primary biliary cirrhosis, bone thinning precludes their use, except in the very early anicteric phase when patients may experience intense pruritus.

Corticosteroids in combination with immunosuppressive therapy, usually cyclophosphamide, did prove useful in treatment of patients with hepatitis B–associated polyarteritis nodosa. Survival, abdominal pain, neurologic changes, hypertension, arthritis, skin rashes, and renal failure were improved.

ADMINISTRATION

In patients with chronic autoimmune liver disease (lupoid hepatitis), liver biopsy must precede the commencement of corticosteroid therapy—unless severe coagulopathy precludes biopsy, in which case a biopsy must be performed as soon as possible after a remission is obtained. Sherlock recommends 30 mg prednisolone for 1 week, reducing the dose to a maintenance level of 10 to 20 mg as quickly as possible. Higher initial doses are often required, 40 to 60 mg prednisone per day, to induce a remission. Regardless of the initial dose, tapering of the dosage of the corticosteroid used should be based on improvement of the serum transaminase values. Some

Table 22-2. Corticosteroids: Pregnancy and breast-feeding

Agent	FDA pregnancy category	Risk vs benefit (by trimester)			Breast-feeding category
		1st	2nd	3rd	
Azathioprine	D	R >> B	R >> B	R >> B	IV
Corticosteroids	C1	B > R	B > R	B > R	IV

Food and Drug Administration (FDA) pregnancy categories:
A = Well-controlled studies fail to demonstrate risk to the fetus.
B1 = Animal studies fail to demonstrate risk to the fetus but no human studies are available.
B2 = Animal studies show some risk to the fetus but this is not confirmed in human studies.
C1 = Animal studies show risk to the fetus but no human studies are available.
C2 = Animal and human studies are unavailable.
D = Drugs associated with birth defects but with potential benefits that may outweigh known risks.
X = Drugs associated with birth defects and with potential risk that clearly outweighs potential benefit.
Risk vs benefit: R >> B = Proven or potential risk outweighs potential benefits.
B > R = Potential benefits outweigh potential risks.
R >> B? = Risks may be outweighed by benefits in some circumstances.
? = Risk-to-benefit ratio is unknown.

Breast-feeding categories:
I = Drug does not enter breast milk.
II = Drug enters breast milk but is not known to be harmful in therapeutic doses.
IIIA = Drug may or may not enter breast milk but no adverse effects are expected.
IIIB = Drug may or may not enter breast milk but drug is systemically absorbed.
IV = Drug enters breast milk and poses a potential risk to the neonate.

authors prefer prednisolone over prednisone, since the 11-hydroxylation conversion of prednisone to prednisolone must occur in the liver before prednisone can exert its glucocorticoid effect. In practice, there seems to be little advantage of one agent over the other. A suggested regimen for steroid therapy in autoimmune liver disease is presented in Table 22-1.

SIDE EFFECTS

The side effects of chronic corticosteroid therapy are well recognized and include the development of cushingoid or moon facies, diabetes, hypertension, acne, obesity, hirsutism, and striae. Growth retardation in children, diabetes, bone thinning (osteoporosis), and serious infection (fungal infections or reactivation of tuberculosis) are particularly troublesome. In patients with chronic autoimmune liver disease, the addition of azathioprine (50–100 mg/day) may allow reduction in or cessation of corticosteroids.

PEARLS AND PITFALLS

1. The only well-studied and justifiable uses of corticosteroids alone in the treatment of liver disease are in patients with acute or chronic autoimmune liver disease and severe acute alcoholic liver disease.
2. In patients with autoimmune liver disease, azathioprine may allow a reduction in corticosteroid dose so as to ease the complications of long-term corticosteroid use. Azathioprine alone may be useful as a maintenance agent in the treatment of autoimmune liver disease.
3. Long-term use of corticosteroids in patients with primary biliary cirrhosis may lead to serious and severe osteoporosis.
4. Corticosteroids in combination with antiviral cyclosphosphamide or immunomodulating agents (alpha- and gamma-interferon) may prove to be of benefit in the treatment of patients with chronic hepatitis B.
5. Although a more consistent dose-response might be expected from the use of prednisolone instead of prednisone for the treatment of severe liver disease, the advantage of prednisolone over prednisone may be theoretical only.

Suggested Reading

Carithers RL, et al. Methylprednisolone therapy in patients with severe alcoholic hepatitis: A randomized multi-center trial. Ann Intern Med 1989; 110:685.

Selected patients (patients with gastrointestinal bleeding, acute pancreatitis, sepsis, diabetes, or renal failure were not treated) benefit from methylprednisolone.

Czaja AJ, Rakela J, Ludwig J. Features reflective of early prognosis in corticosteroid-treated severe autoimmune chronic active hepatitis. Gastroenterology 1988; 95:448.

Patients who resolved at least one pretreatment laboratory abnormality, improved a pretreatment hyperbilirubinemia, or did not experience biochemical deterioration after 2 weeks of therapy survived at least 6 months in 98 percent of cases.

DeRitis R, et al. Negative results of prednisone therapy in viral hepatitis. Lancet 1964; 1:533.

Sixty-five patients with viral hepatitis received either prednisone, 30 mg/day (N = 34) or placebo (N = 31). No statistically significant differences were observed in the biochemical data, and the disease was not shortened in the treated group of patients.

Dudley FJ, Scheuer PJ, Sherlock S. Natural history of hepatitis-associated antigen-positive chronic liver disease. Lancet 1972; 2:1388.

Corticosteroid treatment in the acute phase of disease appears, in this clinical and pathologic study of 59 patients with hepatitis B, to predispose to relapse and chronicity.

Gray N, et al. Hepatitis, colitis, and lupus manifestations. Am J Dig Dis 1958; 3:481.

A classic description of lupoid hepatitis.

Gregory PB, et al. Steroid therapy in severe viral hepatitis: A double-blind, randomized trial of methyl-prednisolone versus placebo. N Engl J Med 1976; 294:681.

Seven of 15 randomized to methylprednisolone and 2 of 15 randomized to placebo died during the 16-week study period.

Howat AT, et al. The late results of long-term treatment of primary biliary cirrhosis by corticosteroids. Rev Int Hepatol 1966; 16:227.

Corticosteroids had no beneficial effect on the progression of primary biliary cirrhosis, but they did promote the development of osteoporosis in the majority of patients.

Imperiale TF, McCullough AJ. Do corticosteroids reduce mortality from alcoholic hepatitis? Ann Intern Med 1990; 113:299.

Using meta-analysis, the authors concluded that patients with encephalopathy and with gastrointestinal bleeding do benefit from corticosteroid therapy.

Lesesne HR, Bozymicki E, Fallon H. Treatment of alcoholic hepatitis with encephalopathy: Comparison of prednisolone with caloric supplements. Gastroenterology 1978; 79:169.

Women from North Carolina with severe alcoholic liver disease appear to benefit from corticosteroid therapy.

Maddrey W, et al. Corticosteroid therapy of alcoholic hepatitis. Gastroenterology 1978; 75:193.

An early study suggesting the benefit of corticosteroid therapy in patients with severe alcoholic liver disease complicated by encephalopathy.

Maddrey WC, et al. Prednisolone therapy in patients with severe alcoholic hepatitis: Results of a multicenter trial. Hepatology 1986; 6:1202.

Eleven of the 31 placebo recipients died within the 28-day study period, compared with only 2 of 35 methylprednisolone-treated patients.

Madsbad S, et al. Impaired conversion of prednisone to prednisolone in patients with liver cirrhosis. Gut 1980; 21:52.

Mean serum prednisolone concentration was only 53 percent ($p < 0.05$) of that observed in the seven patients with only slightly impaired liver function.

Perrillo RP, et al. Prednisone withdrawal followed by recombinant alpha interferon in the treatment of chronic type B hepatitis: A randomized, controlled trial. Ann Intern Med 1988; 109:95.

A study of 39 patients with chronic hepatitis B in which one group received combination therapy (N = 18) and the other received placebo (N = 21). A statistically significant difference in the rate of clearance of hepatitis B virus (HBV)-DNA and DNA polymerase was seen, in favor of the treatment group.

Ramond M, et al. A randomized trial of prednisolone in patients with severe alcoholic hepatitis. N Engl J Med 1992; 326:507.
Treatment improves survival.

Shaldon S, Sherlock S. Virus hepatitis with features of prolonged cholestasis. Br Med J 1957; II:734.
The steroid "whitewash" should be reserved for the non-hepatitis B and C patient with prolonged cholestasis. This therapy probably has no effect on healing of the liver.

Sherlock S. Chronic hepatitis in Diseases of the Liver and Biliary System, seventh edition, 1985, p. 293, Blackwell Scientific Publications, Oxford.
A comprehensive review with specific recommendations for treatment of chronic autoimmune liver disease.

Stellon AJ, et al. Maintenance of remission in autoimmune chronic active hepatitis with azathioprine after corticosteroid withdrawal. Hepatology 1988; 8:781.
Azathioprine alone may be sufficient at high dose, 2 mg/kg, to maintain remission in chronic autoimmune liver disease.

Azathioprine

Michael M. Van Ness

Azathioprine was once thought to have great potential in the treatment of acute and chronic liver disease. It has been studied in a number of conditions, including primary biliary cirrhosis, acute and chronic autoimmune liver disease, and chronic active hepatitis (C). Despite widespread hopes, the use of azathioprine appears limited to the long-term treatment of patients with chronic autoimmune liver disease and the rare patient with primary biliary cirrhosis who is unable to tolerate colchicine therapy. The side effects of azathioprine are potentially formidable and require a careful follow-up plan.

MECHANISM OF ACTION

Azathioprine is an imidazole derivative of 6-mercaptopurine. It is well established that azathioprine is metabolized first to 6-mercaptopurine in vivo, and then to 6-thioimosinic acid, the putative agent that disrupts deoxyribonucleic acid (DNA) synthesis in lymphocytes. Accordingly, the antimetabolite and immunosuppressive actions result from inhibition of purine-ring biosynthesis.

INDICATIONS

Azathioprine is approved by the Food and Drug Administration for the treatment of severe, active rheumatoid arthritis and acute leukemia, and as an adjunct for the prevention of orthotopic renal transplant rejection. Its use in chronic autoimmune liver disease (CALD) is well established. Efficacy of azathioprine in chronic liver diseases such as primary biliary cirrhosis and chronic hepatitis B is by no means proven.

Primary Biliary Cirrhosis

In 1976, Heathcote and associates published the results of the first prospective, controlled trial of azathioprine in primary biliary cirrhosis (chronic, intrahepatic, nonsuppurative cholangitis). Forty-five patients (stages I, II, or III) were studied from 1968 until 1974. Of the 45, 22 received 2 mg azathioprine per kilogram body weight a day. Although subjective improvement in pruritus and objective improvement in serum aspartate transaminase levels were noted, it was not until the sixth year of the trial that survival benefit could be demonstrated. The statistical power of that survival benefit was low.

Crowe published the preliminary results of a multicenter, double-blind, randomized, placebo-controlled trial of azathioprine in 1980. Azathioprine, 1 mg/kg body weight, up to a maximum of 100 mg/day, was given, with the drug suspended temporarily if leukocyte counts dropped below 2000 cells per microliter or platelet counts dropped below 20,000 cells per microliter. Annual liver biopsies were performed. At the time of the report, 236 patients (all stages of the disease were included) had been entered, with 124 receiving azathioprine and 112 receiving placebo.

Patients at prefibrotic and precirrhotic stages of the disease (stages I and II) were expected to receive the greatest benefit from azathioprine. In an early analysis of the study results, survival, progression to cirrhosis, and symptoms (pruritus, need for cholestyramine treatment, jaundice, edema, and xanthoma formation) were not improved by azathioprine.

The follow-up, final report of this international trial was published in 1985 and concluded that the 1980 preliminary report contained some random imbalance between the two treatment groups that might have obscured benefit of azathioprine therapy in primary biliary cirrhosis. This final report was produced using multivariate Cox regression analysis. Five variables with independent prognostic influence were noted, and a modest benefit of azathioprine was established. The authors conclude that although the benefit of azathioprine on survival is not dramatic, the agent should be considered a valuable medical treatment for primary biliary cirrhosis.

Chronic Autoimmune Liver Disease

Prednisone is the cornerstone of therapy for chronic autoimmune liver disease. Life expectancy, survival, liver function, serologic abnormalities, and hepatic histology improve on immunosuppressive therapy with prednisone alone and prednisone in combination with azathioprine. Toxicity from prednisone alone (osteoporosis, diabetes, cushingoid features) and azathioprine alone (leukopenia, thrombocytopenia) are common (21 and 53%, respectively) but rarely life threatening (less than 10%). The benefits of prednisone alone (prednisone 20 mg) or prednisone in combination with azathioprine (prednisone 10 mg with azathioprine 50 mg) in the treatment of patients with CALD far outweigh the potential complications and side effects.

Stellon and associates published a study documenting maintenance of remission in CALD with azathioprine after corticosteroid withdrawal. Azathioprine, 2 mg/kg, was required. After 1 year of therapy, there was no significant difference with respect to liver function or histology between the "control" group (N = 22) treated with prednisolone and azathioprine (1 mg/kg) and the group of 25 treated with higher doses of azathioprine.

Chronic Hepatitis (non-A, non-B)

Stellon and associates published an intriguing abstract in 1985 comparing the results of azathioprine withdrawal and azathioprine maintenance in a group of 50 patients with prednisone- and azathioprine-induced remission of chronic active hepatitis. Over a median follow-up period of 20 months, reactivation of disease occurred significantly more often in the azathioprine withdrawal group (7 of 27) than in the azathioprine maintenance group (1 of 23). Further studies are needed in this area.

ADMINISTRATION

Azathioprine, 1 mg/kg body weight per day, is given as a single daily oral dose as the initial treatment for chronic autoimmune liver disease and primary biliary cirrhosis. If necessary, the dose can be increased in 1/2-mg/kg/day increments every 4 weeks up to a maximum dose of 2 mg/kg/day.

For treatment of acute flares of chronic autoimmune liver disease, azathioprine should be given in combination with corticosteroids, not as a single agent. For maintenance of remission of chronic autoimmune liver disease, azathioprine in combination with corticosteroids or alone may be efficacious.

Allopurinol interferes with the enzymatic oxidation of azathioprine by xanthine oxidase. Concomitant azathioprine and allopurinol therapy can result in elevated blood levels of azathioprine and increased frequency and severity of side effects. A marked reduction in azathioprine dose (25% of a normal dose) prevents dose-related side effects.

Monitoring of complete blood counts, including platelet counts, during the first months of therapy is required. During the first month of therapy and after incremental dose increases, weekly blood counts should be obtained and will give prompt warning of bone marrow suppression. If either leukocyte, red blood cell, or platelet counts drop significantly, a reduction in dosage or temporary withdrawal of azathioprine is prudent.

SIDE EFFECTS

Azathioprine must be used carefully and the patient followed conscientiously to minimize the side effects that are known to occur with this agent. Hematologic, gastrointestinal, and oncologic complications are well described.

Azathioprine has a dose-related effect on all blood elements. Leukopenia, thrombocytopenia, and anemia are well described and occur in 10 to 20 percent of patients receiving as little as 50 to 100 mg oral azathioprine a day. Weekly monitoring of blood counts starting at initiation of therapy and after incremental increases in dosage is necessary for early detection of bone marrow suppression. Dose reduction or temporary cessation of therapy is required if the white blood cell count drops below 2000 cells per microliter, if the platelet count drops below 20,000 cells per microliter, or if the hematocrit decreases to 30 percent or less.

Azathioprine has been implicated on rare occasions as causing a mixed cholestatic, hepatocellular injury. With the high-dose therapy required in the treatment of renal transplant patients, venoocclusive disease can be seen. Hypersensitivity pancreatitis and vasculitis are well described and are, fortunately, rare (<1% of recipients). After prolonged rise, nodular regenerative hyperplasia has been described. Sterneck and associates suggest that the early and late changes seen with azathioprine represent different stages of drug-induced endotheliitis.

The oncogenicity of azathioprine has long been suspected but never proved. Tage-Jensen and associates reviewed their group's experience with 154 patients with nonalcoholic chronic liver disease, randomized to treatment with either azathioprine or prednisone. Tage-Jensen found that 13 of 39 (33%) azathioprine-treated patients died from malignant neoplasia, compared to only 4 of 32 (13%) prednisone-treated patients, and thus urged caution in the long-term use of azathioprine. In an accompanying editorial, Schaffner refuted this conclusion by noting the lack of statistical evidence implicating azathioprine oncogenicity. Schaffner concludes that "nothing so far reported should prevent us from using a drug that appears to be both potent and remarkably safe."

Aplastic anemia has been noted in a liver-transplant patient receiving azathioprine. Only one of the nine patients reviewed by the Pittsburgh group received azathioprine. The authors conclude that

Table 23-1. Azathioprine: Pregnancy and breast-feeding

Agent	FDA pregnancy category	Risk vs benefit (by trimester)			Breast-feeding category
		1st	2nd	3rd	
Azathioprine	D	R >> B	R >> B	R >> B	IV

Food and Drug Administration (FDA) pregnancy categories:
A = Well-controlled studies fail to demonstrate risk to the fetus.
B1 = Animal studies fail to demonstrate risk to the fetus but no human studies are available.
B2 = Animal studies show some risk to the fetus but this is not confirmed in human studies.
C1 = Animal studies show risk to the fetus but no human studies are available.
C2 = Animal and human studies are unavailable.
D = Drug associated with birth defects but with potential benefits that may outweigh known risks.
X = Drug associated with birth defects and with potential risk that clearly outweighs potential benefit.
Risk vs benefit: R >> B = Proven or potential risk outweighs potential benefits.
B > R = Potential benefits outweigh potential risks.
R >> B? = Risks may be outweighed by benefits in some circumstances.
? = Risk-to-benefit ratio is unknown.
Breast-feeding categories:
I = Drug does not enter breast milk.
II = Drug enters breast milk but is not known to be harmful in therapeutic doses.
IIIA = Drug may or may not enter breast milk but no adverse effects are expected.
IIIB = Drug may or may not enter breast milk but drug is systemically absorbed.
IV = Drug enters breast milk and poses a potential risk to the neonate.

the high incidence of aplastic anemia in the group relates more to the underlying liver disease (non-A, non-B hepatitis) than to any particular drug therapy.

PEARLS AND PITFALLS

1. The clearest indication for azathioprine in the treatment of chronic liver disease is the steroid-sparing effect (and possibly additive efficacy) of azathioprine in patients with chronic autoimmune liver disease.
2. Allopurinol markedly increases the risk of azathioprine toxicity by blocking azathioprine degradation by xanthine oxidase.
3. The utility of azathioprine for the treatment of primary biliary cirrhosis has, by and large, been superseded by colchicine and ursodeoxycholic acid.
4. The use of azathioprine during pregnancy is relatively contraindicated unless the potential benefits far outweigh the potential fetal risks.

Suggested Reading

Alstead EM, et al. Safety of azathioprine in pregnancy—inflammatory bowel disease. Gastroenterology 1990; 99:443–446.
In this retrospective report of 16 patients with inflammatory bowel disease (IBD) receiving azathioprine during pregnancy, no congenital abnormalities were seen.

Bergman SM, et al. Azathioprine and hypersensitivity vasculitis. Ann Intern Med 1988; 109:83–84.
Two patients with end-stage renal disease received azathioprine and developed vasculitis within 8 to 14 days of initiation of drug therapy. Rechallenge precipitated the symptoms of fever, headache, malaise, purpura, and bullae.

Christensen E, et al. Beneficial effect of azathioprine and prediction of prognosis in primary biliary cirrhosis. Gastroenterology 1985; 89:1084–1091.
Using Cox multiple-regression analysis and adjusting for the slight imbalance between the two treatment groups, the long-term therapeutic effect of azathioprine was statistically significant, with azathioprine reducing the risk of dying to 59 percent of that observed during placebo treatment, and improving survival by 20 months in the average patient.

Crowe J, Christensen E, Smith M, et al. Azathioprine in primary biliary cirrhosis: A preliminary report of an international trial. Gastroenterology 1980; 78:1005.
No benefit was seen when the results were analyzed after 18 months of therapy (see Christensen E).

DePinho RA, Goldberg CS, Lefkowitch JH. Azathioprine and the liver: Evidence favoring idiosyncratic, mixed cholestatic-hepatocellular injury in humans. Gastroenterology 1984; 86:162.
Azathioprine has been implicated on rare occasions in causing a mixed cholestatic-hepatocellular injury.

Heathcote J, Ross A, Sherlock S. A prospective controlled trial of azathioprine in primary biliary cirrhosis. Gastroenterology 1976; 70:656–660.
Survival was similar for the first 5 years of the trial, with a significant difference in favor of the treated group in the sixth year.

Lawson DH, et al. Adverse effects of azathioprine. Adv Drug React Ac Pois Rev 1984; 3:161–171.

A thorough review of the pharmacology and side effects of azathioprine. A must before initiation of this type of immunosuppressive therapy.

Schaffner F. The oncogenicity of azathioprine? Hepatology 1988; 8:693.

The author maintains a healthy skepticism over the issue of azathioprine-induced neoplasms.

Stellon AJ, et al. Controlled trial of azathioprine withdrawal in autoimmune chronic active hepatitis. Lancet 1985; 1:668–670.

A beneficial effect of azathioprine (50–100 mg) was demonstrated by the authors. This dose, in combination with corticosteroids, resulted in a relapse rate of only 6 percent in 3 years. Corticosteroid therapy alone resulted in a 33 percent relapse rate.

Stellon AJ, et al. Maintenance of remission in autoimmune chronic active hepatitis with azathioprine after corticosteroid withdrawal. Hepatology 1988; 8:781–784.

The authors show that azathioprine alone is sufficient to maintain a remission of chronic autoimmune liver disease induced by azathioprine and prednisone.

Sterneck M, et al. Azathioprine hepatotoxicity after liver transplantation. Hepatology 1991; 14:806–810.

Drug-induced endotheliitis is the most likely cause of cholestatic jaundice, venoocclusive disease, and nodular regenerative hyperplasia seen with azathioprine.

Tage-Jensen U. Copenhagen Study Group for Liver Diseases. Malignancies following long-term azathioprine treatment in chronic liver disease. Liver 1987; 7:81–83.

Among 154 patients with histologically proven nonalcoholic liver disease, randomized to treatment with either azathioprine or prednisone, the cause of death after a median follow-up period of 91 months was from a malignant neoplasm in 33 percent of the azathioprine group and 13 percent in the prednisone group.

Heavy Metal Antagonists

Michael M. Van Ness

Penicillamine is a useful agent in the treatment of one disease of the gastrointestinal system and may yet prove efficacious in two others. For years it was hoped that the efficacy of penicillamine would be demonstrable in a wide variety of conditions, including all stages of primary biliary cirrhosis. At this time, penicillamine is only indicated for the acute and chronic management of Wilson's disease.

MECHANISM OF ACTION

Penicillamine is an anti-inflammatory agent with antifibrotic actions capable of chelating copper. While the anti-inflammatory and antifibrotic actions remain of unproved benefit, copper chelation has been proved valuable in the treatment of Wilson's disease.

Penicillamine chelation therapy induces urinary copper excretion of 2 to 5 mg/24 hours. With the initiation of therapy and cupriuria, active hepatic inflammation and hemolysis often subside dramatically, although mild elevation of liver-associated enzymes may persist for months. Hepatic fibrosis and portal hypertension are less responsive to penicillamine therapy.

Penicillamine combines with free aldehyde groups in collagen, preventing cross-linking and thereby interfering with collagen formation and collagen tensile strength. It does not prevent collagen synthesis.

Penicillamine has several immune-system effects. Serum immunoglobulin synthesis, polymorphonuclear leukocyte chemotaxis, and C1q binding protein are all reduced by penicillamine. D-Penicillamine also inhibits T-lymphocyte function by suppressing T-cell mitogen response.

INDICATIONS

Wilson's Disease

Penicillamine is the treatment of choice for patients with Wilson's disease. In 1956, Walshe published the first report of penicillamine use in Wilson's disease patients. Most published series of penicillamine therapy for Wilson's disease show good drug efficacy with reversal of psychiatric, neurologic, and hepatic abnormalities.

The drug may be less efficacious in patients who present with liver disease. Scott reported that 9 of 17 adolescent patients presenting with active hepatitis secondary to acute Wilson's disease died despite penicillamine treatment.

Clinical improvement may require 1 to 3 months of therapy. On occasion, a deterioration in neurologic symptoms precedes the gradual long-term amelioration induced by chelation therapy. If such a deterioration is noted, temporary dose reduction or cessation of therapy is *not* suggested, as the risk of a sensitivity reaction is increased with resumption of penicillamine. If therapy must be stopped, an attempt at desensitization with gradually increasing daily doses along with steroid coverage as outlined by Chan and Balan is preferable to the alternative chelating agent triethylene tetramine dihydrochloride (trien). Likewise, avoidance of foods high in copper content (shellfish, organ meats such as liver and kidney, nuts, and mushrooms) and domestically softened water is advisable. Zinc therapy as described by Rossaro and associates is an interesting alternative.

Several other diseases of the liver are characterized by elevated hepatic copper content (greater than 250 mg/dry weight), including primary biliary cirrhosis, extrahepatic biliary obstruction or atresia, intrahepatic cholestasis of childhood, Indian childhood cirrhosis, and toxic hepatitis seen in vineyard workers spraying and inhaling copper salts. Of these conditions, only patients with primary biliary cirrhosis may benefit from penicillamine therapy. Penicillamine would be expected to reduce hepatic copper content and decrease hepatic inflammation. Despite several authors' initial enthusiasm, consistent improvement in liver function and patient survival has not been demonstrated (Table 24-1). In the Mayo Clinic study, Dickson and associates did find a favorable influence on histologic progression of disease with six of seven subjects receiving 1 gm D-penicillamine a day, a low-copper diet, and pyridoxine supplements, showing no progression from stage 1 to stage 2 disease over 12 months, compared to progression seen in 7 of 10 receiving placebo. Side effects may limit the use of penicillamine to patients with a poor prognosis (pruritus, jaundice, rising bilirubin > 7 mg/dl, ascites, and splenomegaly), who are not candidates for liver transplantation. In this group of stage 3 or 4 patients, Epstein and associates have shown improvement in survival, but only after 18 months of therapy. Improvement in liver function, a fall in serum immunoglobulins, and decreased liver copper content were seen.

D-Penicillamine should not be given to patients with asymptomatic primary biliary cirrhosis. In this group, ursodiol or colchicine may prove a more satisfactory alternative.

The use of penicillamine has been studied in noncirrhotic alcoholic liver disease. Although a suggestion of decreased fibrosis was made for patients receiving 1 gm penicillamine a day, neither survival nor rates of recovery from acute alcoholic liver injury were altered by penicillamine therapy. Given its narrow toxic/therapeutic index, penicillamine cannot be recommended for use in patients with noncirrhotic alcoholic liver disease.

Table 24-1. The effect of D-penicillamine on primary biliary cirrhosis

	European (1985)	Mayo Clinic (1985)	Boston (1982)
Number of patients	189	227	52
Dose (gm)	1.2	1.0	1.0
Adverse effects (%)	36	22	31
Histology	NS	ND	ND
Mortality (%; 2-year)	18	12	27
Survival	ND	ND	ND
Length of study (mos)	60	120	28

NS = not stated; ND = no difference in progression between treatment and placebo. Adapted and reprinted with permission of the authors, Cramer GL, et al. Bile Excretory Function, Cholestasis, and Hyperbilirubinemia. In G Gitrick (ed), *Current Hepatology*. Chicago: Year Book, 1987. P 266.

SIDE EFFECTS

Hematologic, gastrointestinal, allergic, and renal abnormalities occur in 5 to 25 percent of patients treated with penicillamine. Thrombocytopenia (4%), leukopenia (2%), and aplastic anemia (< 1%) usually occur early in the treatment course (first 3 months) and necessitate complete blood cell and platelet counts every 2 weeks during this period.

Altered or diminished taste (10%) and epigastric pain, nausea, and diarrhea (15%) are common. Rare (< 1%) gastrointestinal side effects include hepatitis, pancreatitis, and intrahepatic cholestasis.

A systemic lupus erythematosus–like syndrome (< 1%) with rash, fever, anemia, leukopenia, and proteinuria is well described with penicillamine. For patients with Wilson's disease, this syndrome is best treated with a 50 percent dose reduction—*not* cessation, an antihistamine such as diphenhydramine (50 mg orally every 6 hours), and prednisone (20 mg orally every 12 hours). With resolution of the lupuslike syndrome, small incremental increases in the daily penicillamine dosage, with continued steroid coverage, allow restoration of full-dose therapy.

Proteinuria as an early sign of membranous glomerulonephropathy is common enough (6%) to mandate performance of a urinalysis every 2 weeks during the first 6 months of therapy. Proteinuria exceeding 1 gm every 24 hours necessitates progressive dose reduction. If significant proteinuria persists then complete cessation of therapy is required.

Pyridoxine, 25 mg/day, is necessary for patients with Wilson's disease who are receiving penicillamine therapy, to prevent the development of cheilosis, glossitis, seborrhea, neuropathy, and anemia.

Since penicillamine can inhibit iron absorption, menstruating women and children benefit from short courses of iron supplementation (3 months, 325 mg 3 times a day) given 2 hours after penicillamine. Continuous oral iron therapy is inadvisable since iron can inhibit penicillamine absorption.

Successful pregnancies are reported in Wilson's disease patients who received 1 gm penicillamine daily, with no untoward fetal effects (Table 24-2). Discontinuation of the drug has deleterious effects on the mother and should be avoided. Scheinberg and Sternlieb have used penicillamine to preserve hepatic and renal function in over 150 pregnant patients without untoward fetal or maternal side effects. Dose reduction to 250 mg/day for the 6 weeks before a scheduled cesarean section is advisable to restore wound healing to near normal. Breast-feeding by mothers receiving penicillamine should be very strongly discouraged.

ADMINISTRATION

For Wilson's disease, penicillamine, 250 mg 4 times a day 1 hour before meals, is an appropriate starting regimen. If tolerated, then incremental increases of 250 mg/day every 3 to 4 days, to a daily dose of 2 gm/day are suggested. Cupriuresis of more than 2 mg/day is desirable. After 3 months of therapy, the daily dose can be modified to keep the serum copper level lower than 10 μg/dl and the hepatic copper content lower than 55 μg/gm dry liver weight. (Concentrations > 250 μg/gm dry liver weight are usual in patients with homozygous Wilson's disease.)

Table 24-2. Heavy metal antagonists: Pregnancy and breast-feeding

Agent	FDA pregnancy category	Risk vs benefit (by trimester)			Breast-feeding category
		1st	2nd	3rd	
Penicillamine	C1	?	?	?	IIIB
Zinc	C1	?	?	?	IIIB

Food and Drug Administration (FDA) pregnancy categories:
A = Well-controlled studies fail to demonstrate risk to the fetus.
B1 = Animal studies fail to demonstrate risk to the fetus but no human studies are available.
B2 = Animal studies show some risk to the fetus but this is not confirmed in human studies.
C1 = Animal studies show risk to the fetus but no human studies are available.
C2 = Animal and human studies are unavailable.
D = Drugs associated with birth defects but with potential benefits that may outweigh known risks.
X = Drugs associated with birth defects and with potential risk that clearly outweighs potential benefit.
Risk vs benefit: R >> B = Proven or potential risk outweighs potential benefits.
B > R = Potential benefits outweigh potential risks.
R >> B? = Risks may be outweighed by benefits in some circumstances.
? = Risk-to-benefit ratio is unknown.
Breast-feeding categories:
I = Drug does not enter breast milk.
II = Drug enters breast milk but is not known to be harmful in therapeutic doses.
IIIA = Drug may or may not enter breast milk but no adverse effects are expected.
IIIB = Drug may or may not enter breast milk but drug is systemically absorbed.
IV = Drug enters breast milk and poses a potential risk to the neonate.

Maintenance therapy of Wilson's disease usually requires 1500 to 2000 mg penicillamine a day for life.

For treatment of patients with poor-prognosis, primary biliary cirrhosis, the initial daily dose of 125 mg is increased by 125 mg every 2 weeks until the maintenance dose of 500 mg/day is reached. As with patients with Wilson's disease, monitoring of hematologic (complete blood cell and platelet count) and renal function (urinalysis) every week is required during the first weeks of therapy.

PEARLS AND PITFALLS

1. Once penicillamine is initiated for the treatment of Wilson's disease, it should not be stopped unless serious side effects occur, as reinstitution of therapy after a delay of even a few days is associated with potentially severe hypersensitivity side effects.
2. There is no place in the evaluation of a patient suspected of having Wilson's disease for a penicillamine trial.
3. Penicillamine therapy should continue through pregnancy to protect the mother from the hepatic and renal complications of Wilson's disease.
4. Liver transplantation is a real therapeutic option for the younger patient with severe hepatic disease unresponsive to penicillamine therapy.
5. Penicillamine may benefit patients with stage 3 or 4 primary biliary cirrhosis who are not candidates for hepatic transplantation.
6. Indications for D-penicillamine therapy in nongastrointestinal diseases include cystinuria and severe active rheumatoid arthritis that is unresponsive to conventional therapy.
7. Penicillamine should be given at least 1 hour before or 2 hours after meals and at least 1 hour apart from snacks or other drugs.

Suggested Reading

Balan V, et al. Survival in Wilson's disease is less than expected: An analysis of 127 patients followed long term. Gastroenterology 1994; 106:A863.

Compared to an expected 15-year survival of 99 percent, patients with Wilson's disease who were treated with penicillamine had a 15-year survival of 74 percent.

Berry WR, et al. Effects of penicillamine therapy and low copper diet on dysarthria in Wilson's disease (hepatolenticular degeneration). Mayo Clin Proc 1974; 49:405–408.

Improvement in general neurologic status by penicillamine, 750 to 1500 mg/day, was graded by voice recordings, intention tremor, and rigidity.

Brewer GJ, et al. Oral zinc therapy for Wilson's disease. Ann Intern Med 1983; 99:314–320.

Although not approved for maintenance therapy for Wilson's disease, oral zinc (150 mg/day in divided doses) is shown in this article to maintain a neutral or negative copper balance in five of five patients.

Chan C-Y, Balan AL. Penicillamine hypersensitivity: Successful desensitization of a patient with severe hepatic Wilson's disease. Am J Gastroenterol 1994; 89:442–444.

Concurrent prednisone therapy, 30 mg/day, with stepwise increases in penicillamine, 125 mg every 3 days, resulted in success-

ful desensitization to penicillamine and avoidance of liver transplantation.

Cossack ZT. The efficacy of oral zinc therapy as an alternative to penicillamine for Wilson's disease. N Engl J Med 1988; 318:322.
In a letter, the author proposes zinc as an effective alternative therapy for patients with Wilson's disease who (1) develop renal failure, (2) are pregnant, (3) need adjunctive therapy to prevent zinc deficiency, (4) require penicillamine dose reduction, and (5) face intolerable toxicities. A response refuting these suggestions is given by Scheinberg and Sternlieb.

Dickson ER, Fleming CR, Ludwig J. Primary Biliary Cirrhosis. In H Popper, F Schaffner (eds), *Progress in Liver Disease,* vol 6. New York: Grune & Stratton, 1978. p 487.
The initial report of the efficacy of penicillamine benefiting early-stage primary biliary cirrhosis (PBC) has not stood the test of time.

Epstein O, et al. Reduction of immune complexes and immunoglobulins induced by D-penicillamine in primary biliary cirrhosis. N Engl J Med 1979; 300:274–278.
Twenty-eight patients randomly allocated to receive either penicillamine, 600 to 900 mg/day, or placebo for 24 months demonstrated significant reductions in immunoglobulins (Ig) A, M, and G concentrations; bilirubin values; and serum aspartate transaminase levels. The authors conclude that penicillamine may favorably change the course of primary biliary cirrhosis by these immunologic manipulations, in addition to the drug's copper-chelating action.

Resnick R, et al. Preliminary observations of D-penicillamine therapy in acute alcoholic liver disease. Digestion 1974; 11:257.
Despite a modest improvement in liver histology ascribable to penicillamine therapy, the drug cannot be recommended in this patient population.

Rossaro L, et al. Zinc therapy in Wilson's disease: Observations in five patients. Am J Gastroenterol 1990; 85:665–668.
Oral zinc therapy, 220 mg orally 3 times a day, was well tolerated, reduced symptoms, and promoted copper excretion.

Scheinberg IH, Sternlieb I. Letter. N Engl J Med 1988; 318:323.
A response to the letter of Cossack cited previously, emphasizing that (1) in more than 400 patients with Wilson's disease, only one has suffered renal failure (secondary to nephrocalcinosis); (2) penicillamine-induced proteinuria occurs in only about 4 percent of patients; (3) penicillamine has been given to more than 150 pregnant women without untoward effect; (4) no zinc deficiency has ever been observed during penicillamine therapy; and (5) trientine is the only other drug approved by the United States Food and Drug Administration for treatment of Wilson's disease.

Scott J. Wilson's disease presenting as chronic active hepatitis. Gastroenterology 1978; 74:645–651.
A series of 17 teenage patients presenting with chronic hepatitis, emphasizing the serious nature of this form of the disease. Nine of the 17 died of liver failure within weeks of the initiation of treatment with penicillamine.

Stremmel W, et al. Wilson's disease: Clinical presentation, treatment, and survival. Ann Intern Med 1991; 115:720–726.
Long-term survival of Wilson's disease patients treated with penicillamine is equal to that of a matched control group at 30 years.

Colchicine

Michael M. Van Ness

Therapeutic options for patients with primary biliary cirrhosis (PBC) and non-PBC cirrhosis have been limited by the effectiveness of the available agents and the toxicities of potential therapeutic candidates. Recently, the anti-inflammatory and antifibrotic agent colchicine has shown promise in decreasing the morbidity and mortality associated with both primary and non-PBC cirrhosis. These preliminary studies found little toxicity with colchicine and offer hope that a more effective and well-tolerated therapy may be available. Combination therapy with colchicine and ursodiol is an exciting prospect.

MECHANISM OF ACTION

Although many of the actions of colchicine are well characterized, its mechanism of action in liver disease is unknown. Colchicine is derived from the autumn crocus and was first isolated in 1820. Among its many actions, it binds to tubulin, blocks mitosis, and inhibits polymorphonuclear leukocyte function. Colchicine accumulates intracellularly in human lymphocytes (16 times the serum concentration).

With respect to primary biliary cirrhosis, colchicine corrects the deficiency of concanavalin A–induced suppressor cell function characteristic of these patients. It decreases elevated levels of interleukin-1 in monocytes. For example, colchicine decreases interleukin-1 levels in monocytes from patients with primary biliary cirrhosis by 50 percent.

In patients with cirrhosis, colchicine increases the level of cathepsin B and D and hydroxyproline in hepatic tissue. Colchicine also increases liver blood flow as measured by an indirect, noninvasive method. It interferes with transcellular movement of collagen, reduces the activity of hepatic collagen-processing enzymes in rats, and stimulates collagenase production in vitro.

PHARMACODYNAMICS

Colchicine is well absorbed after oral ingestion and is excreted in bile, stool, and urine. The drug half-life is 24 to 36 hours. Intracellular drug concentrations are significantly higher than serum concentrations and are maintained for several days after cessation of drug therapy.

INDICATIONS

Primary Biliary Cirrhosis

Colchicine may have a useful role in the treatment of primary biliary cirrhosis (Table 25-1). The first uncontrolled clinical trial of colchicine was reported in 1980 by Koldinger. He found significant decreases in hepatic enzymes in five patients with primary biliary cirrhosis treated with 0.6 mg twice a day for up to 40 months. After 12 months of therapy, the serum alkaline phosphatase levels decreased an average of 2.7 times the upper limit of normal (from a mean of 8.6 times the upper limit of normal, to 4.9 times the upper limit of normal).

Table 25-1. Controlled trials of colchicine in cirrhosis

Author	Number	Follow-up (mos)	Dose (mg)	Improved?
Primary biliary cirrhosis				
Koldinger (1980)	5	40	0.6 bid	Biochemically
Warnes et al. (1987)	64	23	1 mg/day 5 days a wk	Biochemically; pathologically? survival?
Kaplan et al. (1986)	60	24	0.6 bid	Biochemically; not survival
Bodenheimer et al. (1988)	57	33	0.6 bid	Biochemically; not pathologically
Nonprimary biliary cirrhosis				
Kirshenobich et al. (1988)	100	14	1 mg/day 5 days a wk	Biochemically; pathologically; survival
Kirshenobich et al. (1979)	43	—	1 mg/day 5 days a wk	Biochemically; pathologically; survival
Bahgat et al. (1985)	96	—	—	No benefit

This encouraging preliminary report was followed by Warnes' report. In a group of 64 patients, half treated with colchicine (1 mg/day) and half treated with placebo, significant improvement in serum albumin, immunoglobulin, and bilirubin levels were accompanied by a decreasing trend in mortality in the colchicine-treated group. Diarrhea developed in one-fourth of the colchicine-treated patients.

Kaplan's group reported the results of their double-blind, randomized, placebo-controlled trial of colchicine (0.6 mg twice a day) in 1986. They found improvement in serum enzymes (alkaline phosphatase and serum alanine aminotransferase) and liver function (bilirubin, cholesterol, and albumin), as well as a statistically significant improvement in mortality. Interestingly, there was no accompanying improvement in liver histology (inflammation or fibrosis) in those colchicine-treated patients who underwent serial liver biopsy.

A second placebo-controlled trial of colchicine confirmed Kaplan's findings. Bodenheimer and associates gave 57 patients either placebo or colchicine, 0.6 mg twice a day, for 4 years. Patients were evaluated every 3 months and underwent liver biopsy annually. Apparent were decreases in both alkaline phosphatase (mean alkaline phosphatase pretreatment was 281 IU/liter and, post-treatment, 112 IU/liter) and serum alanine aminotransferase (last–first ratio in the colchicine cohort was 0.68, compared to 0.94 in the placebo cohort; $p < 0.0001$). The mean rise in serum bilirubin levels was slowed (0.54 mg/dl/year in the colchicine group, versus 1.77 mg/dl/year in the placebo group). Like Kaplan, Bodenheimer noted no improvement in the histologic progression of the disease. Few side effects were encountered except diarrhea, which responded to colchicine dose reduction.

In a recent review of the subject of colchicine therapy for primary biliary cirrhosis, Wiesner and associates conclude that treatment with colchicine appears to be associated with hepatic biochemical and functional improvement and a trend toward increased survival. The failure of colchicine to ameliorate clinical symptoms or to halt histologic progression of the disease precludes an enthusiastic endorsement of colchicine therapy for primary biliary cirrhosis.

Cirrhosis (Nonprimary Biliary Cirrhosis)

In 1979, Kirshenobich published the preliminary results of a double-blind, randomized, placebo-controlled study of colchicine, 1 mg orally 5 days a week, in the treatment of cirrhosis. Improvement in hepatic biochemical function (albumin), histology, and survival created considerable interest in the utility of colchicine as an antifibrotic and anti-inflammatory drug for cirrhosis.

A follow-up study by Bahgat in Egypt was less enthusiastic. Despite Kirshenobich's initial results, Bahgat noted no improvement clinically, biochemically, or histopathologically in 96 patients with biopsy-proved, chronic, active hepatitis treated with either corticosteroids, azathioprine, corticosteroids and azathioprine, chlorambucil, 5-fluorouracil, isoprinosine, or colchicine, compared to placebo. Given the number of treatment options in this study and the small number of patients enrolled in each arm, the possibility of a type II error encourages further work in the area.

In 1988, Kirshenobich reported the final results of 100 Mexican patients (45 with alcoholic cirrhosis, 41 with posthepatic cirrhosis, and 14 with cirrhosis of various etiologies) treated with either pla-

Table 25-2. Colchicine: Pregnancy and breast-feeding

Agent	FDA pregnancy category	Risk vs benefit (by trimester)			Breast-feeding category
		1st	2nd	3rd	
Colchicine	C1	R >> B	R >> B	R >> B	IV

Food and Drug Administration (FDA) pregnancy categories:
A = Well-controlled studies fail to demonstrate risk to the fetus.
B1 = Animal studies fail to demonstrate risk to the fetus but no human studies are available.
B2 = Animal studies show some risk to the fetus but this is not confirmed in human studies.
C1 = Animal studies show risk to the fetus but no human studies are available.
C2 = Animal and human studies are unavailable.
D = Drug associated with birth defects but with potential benefits that may outweigh known risks.
X = Drug associated with birth defects and with potential risk that clearly outweighs potential benefit.
Risk vs benefit: R >> B = Proven or potential risk outweighs potential benefits.
B > R = Potential benefits outweigh potential risks.
R >> B? = Risks may be outweighed by benefits in some circumstances.
? = Risk-to-benefit ratio is unknown.
Breast-feeding categories:
I = Drug does not enter breast milk.
II = Drug enters breast milk but is not known to be harmful in therapeutic doses.
IIIA = Drug may or may not enter breast milk but no adverse effects are expected.
IIIB = Drug may or may not enter breast milk but drug is systemically absorbed.
IV = Drug enters breast milk and poses a potential risk to the neonate.

cebo or colchicine, 1 mg/day 5 days a week. The cumulative 5-year survival rate for the colchicine group was 75 percent, compared to a 34 percent survival rate in the placebo group. Improvement in the hepatic histology was apparent in 60 percent of the 30 colchicine-treated patients undergoing repeat biopsy. No improvement in liver histology was apparent in the 14 placebo-treated patients who underwent repeat biopsy.

Enthusiasm generated by Kirshenobich's article must be tempered by Boyer and Ransohoff's accompanying editorial. They note a higher mean serum albumin level in the colchicine group at the start of the study, a high rate of patients lost to follow-up—20 percent in both treatment groups, and a lack of nutritional or compliance data. Because of these study deficiencies, Boyer and Ransohoff do not yet endorse colchicine as a treatment for nonprimary biliary cirrhosis liver disease.

SIDE EFFECTS AND CONTRAINDICATIONS

From the experience of using colchicine in the treatment of acute gout, it is well known that diarrhea, nausea, and abdominal pain occur frequently with doses of 4 to 6 mg in a 24-hour period. With the dosages used for chronic liver disease, 0.6 mg twice a day or 1 mg once a day, as many as one-third of patients experience an increase in bowel frequency and liquidity. Dose reduction to 0.6 mg once a day is appropriate in this situation. If diarrhea persists, then cessation of therapy may be necessary.

Rarely reported side effects include alopecia, aplastic anemia, myopathy, angioneurotic edema, epistaxis, and azoospermia. A recent case report by Finklestein and associates of profound granulocytopenia in a 76-year-old woman with primary biliary cirrhosis receiving colchicine, 0.6 mg twice a day for 2 months, emphasizes the potential for agranulocytosis with this agent. Bone marrow examination revealed moderate hypocellularity of all cell lines. With cessation of colchicine therapy, the patient recovered.

PEARLS AND PITFALLS

1. Although not approved by the Food and Drug Administration for the treatment of primary biliary cirrhosis, colchicine, 0.6 mg twice a day, may have benefit in terms of mortality and liver function in these patients.
2. Overdoses of colchicine (as little as 7 mg orally) have been associated with death.
3. Diarrhea from colchicine usually responds to a 50 percent dose reduction.

Suggested Reading

Akriuiadis EA, et al. Failure of colchicine to improve short-term survival in patients with alcoholic hepatitis. Gastroenterology 1990; 99:811–818.

Colchicine did not decrease 30-day mortality in moderately to severely ill patients with acute alcoholic hepatitis.

Bahgat MH, et al. Comparative study of different types of treatments in chronic active hepatitis. Chemioterapia 1985; 4:227–235.

A study of 96 patients with biopsy-proven chronic active hepatitis treated with either steroids, azathioprine, chlorambucil, 5-FU, colchicine or isoprinosine. No benefit was demonstrated (beta error?).

Bodenheimer H, Schaffner F, Pezzullo J. Evaluation of colchicine therapy in primary biliary cirrhosis. Gastroenterology 1988; 95: 124–129.

A double-blind, placebo-controlled trial of colchicine, 0.6 mg orally twice a day, in 57 patients with various stages of primary biliary cirrhosis, demonstrating significant improvement in serum alkaline phosphatase (AP) levels (mean AP pretreatment, 281 IU/liter; post-treatment, 112 IU/liter), mean annual rise in bilirubin levels (0.54 mg/dl/year in the colchicine group, versus 1.77 mg/dl/year in the placebo group), and serum alanine aminotransferase values (last–first ratio in the colchicine cohort, 0.68, compared to 0.94 in the placebo cohort; $p < 0.0001$). No difference in histologic progression was demonstrable. In contrast to penicillamine (an antifibrotic, immunosuppressive drug with the potential for severe and frequent side effects), no serious side effects were experienced in this trial. Diarrhea responded to colchicine dose reduction.

Boyer JL, Ransohoff DF. Is colchicine effective therapy for cirrhosis? N Engl J Med 1988; 318:1751–1752.

An editorial critical of the Kirshenobich article pointing out that chance, bias, and biologic factors may have unintentionally improved survival in the colchicine treatment group. The authors note that a higher mean serum albumin level in the colchicine group (567 versus 510 μ/liter), a high rate of patients lost to follow-up (20% in both groups), and a lack of nutritional or compliance data weaken the endorsement of colchicine as treatment for cirrhosis.

Finklestein M, et al. Granulocytopenia complicating colchicine therapy for primary biliary cirrhosis. Gastroenterology 1987; 93:1231–1235.

Granulocytopenia developed in a 76-year-old woman with primary biliary cirrhosis and adult polycystic liver disease 2 months after she started colchicine therapy (0.6 mg bid po). Granulocytopenia reversed 4 days after the drug was stopped. Bone marrow examination revealed moderate hypocellularity of all cell lines and striking dysplastic changes in the late myeloid and erythroid series. There was no apparent toxicity of other organ systems, and the patient recovered fully.

Hoofnagle JH, Davis GL, Schafer DF, et al. Randomized trial of chlorambucil for primary biliary cirrhosis. Gastroenterology 1986; 91:1327–1334.

A prospective randomized trial of 24 patients treated with either placebo or chlorambucil, 10 mg/day for 10 days, then 2 mg/day and followed for 2 years. Decreased hepatic inflammation and improved liver function were seen in the chlorambucil group.

Kaplan MM. Another treatment for primary biliary cirrhosis. Gastroenterology 1987; 92:255–257.

An editorial accompanying the Hoofnagle chlorambucil article reviewing the role of immunosuppressive therapy in the treatment of PBC, which helps to put in perspective the potential utility of colchicine in the treatment of PBC.

Kaplan MM, et al. A prospective trial of colchicine for primary biliary cirrhosis. N Engl J Med 1986; 315:1448–1454.

Sixty patients with primary biliary cirrhosis were entered in a double-blind, randomized, controlled trial. Thirty patients had early disease (stages 1 and 2) and 30 had advanced disease (stages 3 and 4). Fifteen patients with early disease and 15 with advanced disease received colchicine (0.6 mg bid) and the remainder received placebo. Patients were studied every 2 months, and at 2 years underwent repeat liver biopsy. During the 2-year study period the colchicine-treated patients had improvement in levels of serum albumin, serum bilirubin, alkaline phosphatase cholesterol, and aminotransferase. However, there was no such improvement in the severity of symptoms or physical findings; moreover, there was no significant difference in the histologic changes noted at liver biopsy in the two treatment groups. At 4 years after entry, the cumulative mortality from liver disease was 21 percent in patients given colchicine and 47 percent in those given placebo.

Kirshenobich P, Uribe M, Suarez GI, et al. Treatment of cirrhosis with colchicine: Double-blind, randomized trial. Gastroenterology 1979; 77:532.

Early report of benefit of colchicine therapy for alcoholic and cryptogenic cirrhosis.

Kirshenobich D, et al. Colchicine in the treatment of cirrhosis of the liver. N Engl J Med 1988; 318:1709–1713.

A randomized, double-blind, placebo-controlled trial of 100 Mexican patients, 45 with alcoholic cirrhosis, 41 with posthepatitic cirrhosis, and 14 with cirrhosis of various etiologies, treated with either placebo or colchicine, 1 mg/day 5 days a week. All patients but one were Childs' class A or B. Analysis of mortality utilizing the intent-to-treat rule showed marked improvement in the colchicine group, with cumulative 5-year survival rates of 75 percent, compared to a 34 percent survival rate in the placebo group. On repeat liver biopsy of 30 colchicine-treated patients, improvement in histology was apparent in 9 (30%), was normal in 2 (7%), and showed only minimal portal fibrosis in 7 (23%). No improvement in liver histology was apparent in 14 placebo-treated patients who underwent repeat liver biopsy.

Klion FM, et al. Prediction of survival of patients with primary biliary cirrhosis. Examination of the Mayo Clinic model on a group of patients with known end point. Gastroenterology 1992; 102:310–313.

The authors' data confirm the accuracy of the Mayo Clinic model when measured more than 2 years before death.

Koldinger RE. Treatment of primary biliary cirrhosis with colchicine. Gastroenterology 1980; 78:1309A.

Preliminary study suggesting benefit of colchicine in PBC patients.

Tapalaga D, et al. Colchicine treatment effects on liver cirrhosis assessed by liver blood flow measurements. Med Interne 1986; 24:69–73.

In a group of 22 patients with liver cirrhosis, the hemodynamic changes associated with cirrhosis were studied before and after 24 months of antifibrotic treatment with colchicine (1 mg/day, 5 days a week). The liver blood flow was estimated every year by a noninvasive radioisotopic method. A significant improvement of the liver blood supply was noted. The simultaneous and favorable changes of liver chemistries and hemodynamic parameters suggest that the perfusion improvement might explain the tendency of the biochemical data to improve.

Warnes TW, et al. A controlled trial of colchicine in primary biliary cirrhosis. J Hepatol 1987; 5:1–7.

Colchicine (1 mg/day) was given to 64 patients with PBC in a double-blind, placebo-controlled trial. In comparison with placebo, colchicine produced a beneficial effect on serum albumin and bilirubin levels at 3 months in patients who had abnormal liver function (bilirubin >20 μmole/liter) at entry. In patients with normal liver function at entry, beneficial effects were noted on total globulin levels at 3 months and on immunoglobulin G levels at 3 and 6 months. At 18 months, survival estimates in the colchicine and placebo groups were 84 and 69 percent, respectively.

Wiesner RH, et al. Clinical and statistical analyses of new and evolving therapies for primary biliary cirrhosis. Hepatology 1988; 8:668–676.

A rigorous analysis and critique of the therapeutic trials in PBC, with special attention to colchicine. In light of the intent-to-treat rule, the authors conclude that there currently is no effective therapy for PBC.

Vitamin K

Margaret Andrea Wise and Michael M. Van Ness

Vitamin K is one of four fat-soluble vitamins required by the liver for synthesis of clotting factors. It was first recovered from hog liver fat and alfalfa. Two forms of vitamin K are known. Vitamin K_1 (phytonadione), 2-methyl-3-phytyl-1,4-naphthoquinone, is found in vegetable products such as broccoli, cabbage, lettuce, spinach, and kale. Vitamin K_2 (menaquinone) is synthesized by intestinal gram-positive bacteria, has as its side chain 2 to 13 phenyl units, and is about 60 percent as potent as vitamin K. *Koagulation vitamin* is the name Dam gave vitamin K in 1929 while studying bleeding tendencies in chickens fed fat-free diets. Subsequent studies in animals and humans showed a correlation between hemorrhage and decreased prothrombin level. Thirty years passed before it was determined that vitamin K is required for production of the prothrombin precursor of active prothrombin.

MECHANISM OF ACTION

Vitamin K is essential for the production of prothrombin. It acts to convert glutamic acid residues on the precursor protein of prothrombin to gamma-carboxyglutamic acid residues, a conversion required for the activation of prothrombin. This conversion allows the peptide to build calcium, a step essential for phospholipid surface building and initiation of the clotting cascade.

Bile salts are necessary for the absorption of vitamin K. From the small intestine, it is carried by lipoproteins in the lymph and stored in the liver.

In the absence of vitamin K, the vitamin K–dependent blood clotting factors—prothrombin (II), proconvertin (VII), plasma thromboplastin (Christmas factor, IX), and the Stuart factor (X)—are biologically inactive.

Anticoagulant drugs such as warfarin sodium act as antagonists to vitamin K by disrupting hepatic production of prothrombin and the other vitamin K–dependent clotting factors, by inhibiting conversion of glutamic acid residues on the precursor protein to gamma-carboxyglutamic acid residues. Acarboxyprothrombin, an inactive prothrombin precursor, accumulates in the blood during warfarin (Coumadin) therapy and lacks the calcium-binding capacity necessary to bind to phospholipid surfaces and initiate the clotting cascade.

INDICATIONS

Vitamin K is indicated for treatment of hypoprothrombinemia as a result of inadequate vitamin K intake, absorption, or utilization.

Infants may have a low prothrombin level immediately after birth as a result of a sterile gut. Because dietary deficiency is rare and hepatic stores are quickly filled, vitamin K supplementation after the perinatal period is rarely necessary.

Impaired bile salt production may occur in serious liver disease. Cirrhosis and hepatitis may be accompanied by decreased production of vitamin K–dependent clotting factors despite adequate dietary levels of vitamin K. Since bile is needed for the absorption of vitamin

K_1, hepatic or biliary obstruction may limit its uptake. With cholestatic liver disease, the major defect is malabsorption of vitamin K, and parenteral supplementation is useful. With severe hepatocellular disease, the major defect is inadequate carboxylation of glutamyl precursors of precoagulant factors, and parenteral supplementation is ineffective.

Vitamin K is useful to antagonize the effects of anticoagulant therapy with Coumadin.

DOSAGE AND ADMINISTRATION

Vitamin K_1 (phytonadione) is available as Mephyton in 5-mg tablets for oral administration; as ampules of Konakion, either 2 or 10 mg/ml, for intramuscular administration; or as AquaMEPHYTON, 2 or 10 mg/ml, for intravenous therapy.

A single intramuscular dose of 0.5 to 1.0 mg is recommended for the normal newborn infant.

Generally, vitamin K, 10 mg/day orally or intravenously, is recommended in patients with biliary tract obstructive disease from either congenital defects (extrahepatic biliary atresia), tumors (Klatskin tumor, cholangiocarcinoma, or pancreatic carcinoma), or stone (choledocholithiasis).

In children with hypoprothrombinemia from intestinal malabsorption or drug therapy, dosages range from 2 mg for infants to 5 to 10 mg for older children, either orally or parenterally. If the deficiency is due to prolonged hyperalimentation, the proper child's dose is 2 to 5 mg intramuscularly on a weekly basis.

Vitamin K may be useful in overcoagulated patients. Depending on the clinical manifestations, overdose may be treated by complete withdrawal of the anticoagulant agent, by a decrease in anticoagulant dosage, or by a single (1–5 mg) dose of vitamin K. With massive bleeding, 20 to 40 mg vitamin K is indicated, with repeated dosing every 4 hours until hypoprothrombinemia is reversed.

There is no recommended daily allowance for vitamin K. Although the total amount needed appears to be small, what is obtained from the diet is supplemented by vitamin K_2 manufactured by the intestinal flora. Little vitamin K is stored in the liver or elsewhere in the body. If a patient is receiving oral vitamin K replacement due to obstruction of bile flow, the bile salts (ox bile, 250–500 mg 3 times a day; Bilezyme, one to two tablets 3 times a day) must be given concurrently.

SIDE EFFECTS

Phytonadione (vitamin K_1) and menaquinone (vitamin K_2) are nontoxic even in large doses. Parenteral administration should be slow (5–10 minutes) to avoid flushing, dyspnea, chest pain, and cardiovascular collapse (rarely seen).

PEARLS AND PITFALLS

1. Vitamin K is essential for the activation of precursors of the vitamin K–dependent factors II, VII, IX, and X.
2. Vitamin K promotes the conversion of protein glutamic acid side chain moieties to the carboxyglutamic acid required for calcium building, surface phospholipid binding, and initiation of the clotting cascade.
3. Rapid infusion of vitamin K can cause flushing, chest pain, dyspnea, and, rarely, death.

Table 26-1. Vitamin K: Pregnancy and breast-feeding

Agent	FDA pregnancy category	Risk vs benefit (by trimester)			Breast-feeding category
		1st	2nd	3rd	
Vitamin K	B1	?	B > R	B > R	II

Food and Drug Administration (FDA) pregnancy categories:
A = Well-controlled studies fail to demonstrate risk to the fetus.
B1 = Animal studies fail to demonstrate risk to the fetus but no human studies are available.
B2 = Animal studies show some risk to the fetus but this is not confirmed in human studies.
C1 = Animal studies show risk to the fetus but no human studies are available.
C2 = Animal and human studies are unavailable.
D = Drug associated with birth defects but with potential benefits that may outweigh known risks.
X = Drug associated with birth defects and with potential risk that clearly outweighs potential benefit.
Risk vs benefit: R >> B = Proven or potential risk outweighs potential benefits.
B > R = Potential benefits outweigh potential risks.
R >> B? = Risks may be outweighed by benefits in some circumstances.
? = Risk-to-benefit ratio is unknown.
Breast-feeding categories:
I = Drug does not enter breast milk.
II = Drug enters breast milk but is not known to be harmful in therapeutic doses.
IIIA = Drug may or may not enter breast milk but no adverse effects are expected.
IIIB = Drug may or may not enter breast milk but drug is systemically absorbed.
IV = Drug enters breast milk and poses a potential risk to the neonate.

4. There is no recommended daily allowance for vitamin K.
5. Hypoprothrombinemia can occur in patients receiving antibiotics, by inhibiting production of vitamin K_2 by intestinal flora.
6. Oral vitamin K should be supplemented by bile salts in patients with a completely obstructed extrahepatic biliary tree. Either drinking bile collected from percutaneous drainage or exogenous bile salt replacement is a satisfactory option.
7. Parenteral vitamin K is ineffective in severe parenchymal liver disease.

Suggested Reading

Friedman P. Vitamin K. In MI Arias et al. (eds), *The Liver Biology and Pathobiology*. New York: Raven, 1982. Pp 359–365.
A commentary on the history and pharmacology of vitamin K in humans, in health and disease.

Hardman RH. Metabolism of Vitamins by the Liver in Normal and Pathologic Conditions. In D Zakim, TD Boyer (eds), *Hepatology: A Textbook of Liver Disease*. Philadelphia: Saunders, 1982. Pp 185–189.
A discussion of the pharmacokinetics of vitamin K.

Hull RD, Raskah GE, Hirsh J. Thrombosis and Anticoagulation. In JH Stein (ed), *Internal Medicine* (2nd ed). Boston: Little, Brown, 1987. Pp 1026–1027.
A discussion of vitamin K in anticoagulant therapy.

Mandel HG, Cohn VH. Fat-Soluble Vitamins—Vitamins A, K, E. In A Goodman et al. (eds), *Goodman and Gilman's The Pharmacological Basis of Therapeutics* (6th ed). New York: Macmillan, 1980. Pp 1592–1596.
A complete description of the pharmacology and mechanism of action of vitamin K.

McEvoy GK, Pharm D (eds). *American Hospital Formulary Service Drug Information*. Bethesda, MD: American Society of Hospital Pharmacists, 1988. P 2122.
A discussion of the uses and dosages of vitamin K.

Shiau YF. Lipid Digestion and Absorption. In LR Johnson (ed), *Physiology of the Gastrointestinal Tract,* vol 2 (2nd ed). New York: Raven, 1987. Pp 1546–1547.
A synopsis of the absorption of fat-soluble vitamins.

White GC II, Levin J. Disorders of Blood Coagulations. In JH Stein (ed), *Internal Medicine* (2nd ed). Boston: Little, Brown, 1987. Pp 1018–1023.
A discussion of vitamin K in blood dyscrasias.

Vaccination Agents

James A. Butler and D. Michael Jones

Hepatitis A

Hepatitis A (HAV) is endemic in all parts of the world, but it is most common in developing countries. Transmission is primarily through the fecal-oral route. Although 23,000 cases were reported in the United States in 1992, the total incidence of hepatitis A infection is much higher since many infections are subclinical. Of children infected under the age of 5, 90 percent remain completely or nearly asymptomatic. However, icteric hepatitis develops in 70 to 80 percent of adults, resulting in significant morbidity and economic losses. Death from fulminant hepatitis occurs in 0.01 to 0.1 percent of infections.

IMMUNOGLOBULIN

Immunoglobulin (Ig) is obtained by cold ethanol fractionation of human plasma. It does not transmit human immunodeficiency virus (HIV), hepatitis B, or other infectious diseases. At present (pending approval of an HAV vaccine), it is indicated for pre- or postexposure prophylaxis of hepatitis A. Immunoglobulin can prevent hepatitis A if given before exposure or within 2 weeks of exposure.

Persons traveling to countries where HAV is prevalent should receive Ig before departure. For trips of less than 3 months, the recommended dose is a single intramuscular injection of 0.02 ml/kg. For prolonged trips the dose is 0.06 mg/kg every 5 months.

Postexposure prophylaxis is used for household and sexual contacts of infected patients, co-workers of infected food handlers, and individuals exposed during a common source outbreak. It is also indicated for workers and attendees at day care centers (attended by children in diapers) and institutions for custodial care where a case has been recognized. Immunoglobulin is not indicated for school, office, or factory contacts, and is not recommended for hospital staff unless an infected patient is fecally incontinent. The dose of Ig is 0.02 mg/kg intramuscularly. Because only one-half the cases of acute hepatitis reported are due to hepatitis A, an attempt should be made by serologic testing to document that the index case indeed has hepatitis A before prophylaxing contacts.

HEPATITIS A VACCINE

At least two vaccines are nearing approval for distribution in the United States, and one of these (manufactured by SmithKline Beecham) has already been released in Europe. Both these vaccines are made from cell culture–derived HAV that has been formalin deactivated, purified, and conjugated with alum. The recommended primary course consists of two doses given 2 to 4 weeks apart. A booster dose given 6 to 12 months later is thought to provide long-term protection. Multiple trials have documented the high immunogenicity of these vaccines and have found few side effects. Two doses of vaccine have produced antibody titers 50 to 100 times greater than occur with a single dose of Ig, and measurable titers have been documented 4 years after immunization.

INDICATIONS

It is unclear for what indications the HAV vaccine will be approved, but it is obvious that it will take the place of Ig in many situations. Possible indications may include travelers to developing countries, military personnel, medical personnel, staff at day care centers, staff and patients at custodial institutions, kitchen personnel, sewage workers, and intravenous drug users.

Hepatitis B

Although the incidence of hepatitis B virus (HBV) infection in the United States has declined since the peak of 26,611 reported cases in 1985, the consequences of acute and chronic infection with this virus are still a major problem in this country. As most cases are subclinical and many are unreported, the true incidence of infection is estimated to be over 200,000 cases per year. Of those infected, 25 percent become clinically ill. More than 10,000 require hospitalization, and approximately 250 die of fulminant disease each year.

Overall, between 6 and 10 percent of persons infected with HBV become chronic carriers, but among children this percentage is much higher. Of infants infected with hepatitis B, 90 percent will become chronically infected. Currently there is an estimated pool of 750,000 to 1 million carriers in the United States. Chronic active hepatitis occurs in over 25 percent of these carriers. It is estimated that 4000 persons die from hepatitis B–related cirrhosis each year in this country, and more than 800 die from hepatitis B–related liver cancer.

HEPATITIS B IMMUNE GLOBULIN

Hepatitis B immune globulin (HBIG) is a sterile solution of antibodies from human plasma that contains high titers of hepatitis B surface antibody (usually in excess of 1:100,000). It provides temporary passive protection and is indicated only after acute intense exposure to hepatitis B virus such as (1) needle-sticks, mucous membrane contact, or swallowing hepatitis surface antigen–positive blood or secretions; (2) sexual contact with people who have active hepatitis B replication; or (3) contact of infants of mothers with acute or chronic hepatitis B. The dose is 0.06 ml/kg intramuscularly. The perinatal dose is 0.5 ml intramuscularly. All these situations require the simultaneous administration of hepatitis B vaccine. There is no evidence that acquired immunodeficiency syndrome has been transmitted by hepatitis B immune globulin, and it is not contraindicated in pregnancy.

HEPATITIS B VACCINES

Two types of hepatitis B vaccine have been licensed in the United States, but plasma-derived hepatitis B vaccine, Heptavax (Merck Sharpe & Dohme), is no longer produced. A genetically engineered hepatitis B vaccine is now available as Recombivax HB (Merck Sharpe & Dohme) and Engerix-B (SmithKline Beecham). The yeast *Saccharomyces cerevisias* (common baker's yeast) was genetically altered by the addition to its genome of a plasmid containing the deoxyribonucleic acid (DNA) coding for the hepatitis B surface antigen. Hepatitis B surface antigen is then prepared by lysing yeast cells, separating the yeast component from antigen by hydrophobic interaction, purifying the hepatitis B surface antigen by sterile filtration, and sterilizing with formalin. Depending on the formulation, the vaccine contains 10 to 40 μg hepatitis B surface antigen per milliliter.

INDICATIONS

The vaccine is recommended for (1) health care workers who have a significant risk of exposure to blood or needle-sticks; (2) residents and staff of institutions for the developmentally disabled; (3) hemodialysis patients; (4) recipients of multiple units of blood products or component products, such as hemophiliac patients; (5) homosexual men; (6) intravenous drug users; (7) household members and sexual contacts of hepatitis B virus carriers; (8) infants born to hepatitis B virus–positive mothers; and (9) all nonimmunized people after exposure to hepatitis B virus from needle-sticks. It is also important to consider the vaccine for (1) prison inmates, (2) heterosexuals with multiple partners, and (3) international travelers to areas where hepatitis B virus is endemic. In November 1991, the Centers for Disease Control recommended that all newborns, regardless of the hepatitis B status of their mothers, receive immunization against hepatitis B.

The vaccine is usually administered as a three-dose series. The second and third doses are given 1 and 6 months after the first. The dose of each injection in adults is 10μg (1 ml) Recombivax HB or 20 μg (1 ml) Engerix-B. Infants should be given the first dose at birth, the second dose at 1 to 2 months, and the third dose at 6 to 18 months. Dosages for infants and children vary considerably with each manufacturer. Newborns of mothers positive for hepatitis B surface antigen should receive the three-dose series on the same schedule; however, the first dose should be given as soon as possible after birth (usually within the first 12 hours of life), with a single dose of hepatitis B immune globulin (0.5 ml) given intramuscularly at a second site. The vaccine and immune globulin should not be given in the same muscle group. For hemodialysis and immunosuppressed patients, a 40-μg dose should be used for each of the three injections.

CLINICAL TRIALS

Clinical trials have shown that 80 to 95 percent of healthy adult vaccine recipients will have a positive antibody response and that a positive antibody response predicts complete protection against hepatitis B infection. Long-term studies performed with the plasma-derived vaccine have shown that this protection persists for at least 9 years, even though anti-HBs titers have often gradually declined to below measurable levels.

The response rates of immunocompromised patients are lower (50–60%), even with the 40-μg vaccine dose studied in patients undergoing hemodialysis. Furthermore, these patients may lose their protection if antibody titers fall below 10millionIU/ml. People who do not complete the full complement of vaccine doses or who are already incubating hepatitis B at the time of vaccination are also less likely to have a satisfactory response to the vaccine.

Table 27-1. Vaccination agents: Pregnancy and breast-feeding

Agent	FDA pregnancy category	Risk vs benefit (by trimester)			Breast-feeding category
		1st	2nd	3rd	
Hepatitis B vaccine	C2	B > R	B > R	B > R	I

Food and Drug Administration (FDA) pregnancy categories:
A = Well-controlled studies fail to demonstrate risk to the fetus.
B1 = Animal studies fail to demonstrate risk to the fetus but no human studies are available.
B2 = Animal studies show some risk to the fetus but this is not confirmed in human studies.
C1 = Animal studies show risk to the fetus but no human studies are available.
C2 = Animal and human studies are unavailable.
D = Drug associated with birth defects but with potential benefits that may outweigh known risks.
X = Drug associated with birth defects and with potential risk that clearly outweighs potential benefit.
Risk vs benefit: R >> B = Proven or potential risk outweighs potential benefits.
B > R = Potential benefits outweigh potential risks.
R >> B? = Risks may be outweighed by benefits in some circumstances.
? = Risk-to-benefit ratio is unknown.
Breast-feeding categories:
I = Drug does not enter breast milk.
II = Drug enters breast milk but is not known to be harmful in therapeutic doses.
IIIA = Drug may or may not enter breast milk but no adverse effects are expected.
IIIB = Drug may or may not enter breast milk but drug is systemically absorbed.
IV = Drug enters breast milk and poses a potential risk to the neonate.

Neither 5-year booster doses of vaccine in the patient with normal immune status nor serologic testing to assess antibody levels are routinely recommended. Testing for immunity following vaccination is recommended only for persons in whom suboptimal response to the vaccine is anticipated. Semiannual antibody testing should be employed in hemodialysis patients, with a booster dose given when antibody levels decline below 10 million IU/ml.

In the vaccinated person who experiences percutaneous or needle exposure to hepatitis surface antigen–positive blood, serologic testing to assess immune status is recommended unless testing within the previous 12 months has indicated adequate levels of antibody. If the exposed person is tested and found to have an inadequate antibody level (< 10 million IU/ml), treatment with hepatitis B immune globulin and a booster dose of vaccine is indicated.

SIDE EFFECTS AND CONTRAINDICATIONS

Hepatitis B vaccines are safe; minor side effects occur with equal frequency after vaccine and placebo injections. Soreness at the injection site occurs in 25 percent of patients. Mild systemic reactions (fever, headache, fatigue, or nausea) are seen in 15 percent. These side effects occur with equal frequency after plasma-derived and recombinant vaccines and placebo injections. There may be an association between Guillain-Barré syndrome and receipt of the first dose of plasma-derived vaccine, but this has not been seen with the recombinant vaccines. Since these vaccines contain only noninfectious hepatitis B surface antigen particles, vaccination of pregnant women entails no additional risk to either the mother or the fetus (Table 27-1).

PEARLS AND PITFALLS

1. Neither Ig, HBIG, nor HBV vaccine has ever been shown to transmit viral hepatitis or HIV.
2. Intramuscular injection of HBV vaccine is preferable to injection into subcutaneous fat, because a measurable increase in seroconversion rates and serum titers is seen with intramuscular injections. Therefore, deltoid muscle injection is strongly preferred over buttock injection.
3. Inadvertent immunization of hepatitis B carriers produces neither therapeutic nor adverse effects.
4. The only population in whom prevaccination serologic screening for hepatitis B is cost-effective are those groups at high risk, such as homosexual men and intravenous drug users.

Suggested Reading

Alter H. The evolution, implication, and applications of the hepatitis B vaccine. JAMA 1982; 247:2272–2275.

An in-depth account of the evolution of and indications for hepatitis B vaccine.

Centers for Disease Control. Protection against viral hepatitis: Recommendations of the Immunization Practices Advisory Committee (ACIP). MMWR 1990; 39 (no. RR-2):1–26. Ann Intern Med 1985; 103:391–402.

Detailed, specific indications for the use of immune globulins, hepatitis B vaccine, and screening.

Centers for Disease Control. Hepatitis B virus: A comprehensive strategy for eliminating transmission in the United States through universal childhood vaccination: Recommendations of the Immunization Practices Advisory Committee. MMWR 1991; 40 (no. RR-13):1–25.

A discussion of the immunogenicity, safety, efficacy, and precautions in the recombinant vaccine and the rationale for universal childhood vaccination.

Dienstag J, et al. Hepatitis B vaccine in health care personnel: Safety, immunogenicity, and indicators of efficacy. Ann Intern Med 1984; 101:34–40.

A double-blind trial of 1330 high-risk health care personnel, which confirmed the plasma vaccine's safety and efficacy.

Margolis HS, Alter MJ, Hadler SC. Hepatitis B: Evolving epidemiology and implications for control. Semin Liver Dis 1991; 11:84–92.

An excellent, detailed summary of hepatitis B epidemiology and prevention.

Sjogren M. The success of hepatitis A vaccine. Gastroenterology 1993; 104:1214–1216.

A concise overview of the development and effectiveness of the hepatitis A vaccine.

Werzberger A, et al. A controlled trial of a formalin-inactivated hepatitis A vaccine in healthy children. N Engl J Med 1992; 327: 453–457.

A placebo-controlled, double-blind study of over 1000 children showing the efficacy and safety of a hepatitis A vaccine.

Disulfiram

Michael M. Van Ness

Disulfiram (Antabuse) is used as an adjunctive therapy in the treatment of chronic alcoholism. Some clinical trials support the short-term effectiveness of disulfiram when employed with behavioral and psychological counseling; however, there is no evidence that the drug is effective in sustaining continuous abstinence or delaying the resumption of drinking. Nevertheless, disulfiram is utilized by many alcohol rehabilitation programs in the United States and abroad.

Originally used as a rubber antioxidant during the late-1800s, disulfiram was first used clinically as a scabicide in the 1930s. Forty-five years ago, two Danish physicians, Wald and Jacobsen, accidentally and subjectively experienced the "Antabuse-alcohol" reaction while attending a cocktail party. At the time, they were investigating the potential use of disulfiram as an antihelminthic. Subsequent investigations suggested promise for the use of disulfiram in the treatment of alcoholism.

MECHANISM OF ACTION

Disulfiram blocks the oxidation of alcohol by interfering with the conversion of acetaldehyde to acetic acid by aldehyde dehydrogenase. This blockade results in an increase of blood acetaldehyde levels that is 5 to 10 times higher than that of control subjects who ingest no alcohol. The increased acetaldehyde level is responsible for what is called *acetaldehyde syndrome* or the *Antabuse-ethanol reaction.*

The onset of symptoms usually occurs within 5 to 10 minutes and the duration of the reaction ranges from 30 minutes to several hours. The severity of the reaction is individually specific and dependent on the amount of ethanol and disulfiram ingested.

SIDE EFFECTS

Adverse reactions in the absence of alcohol include allergic reactions, acneform eruptions, dermatitis, urticaria, optic neuritis, peripheral neuritis, polyneuritis, fatigue, tremor, restlessness, decreased sexual potency, garliclike or metallic taste, psychotic reactions, and mild gastrointestinal disturbances. Cases of reversible hypertension have been reported, as well as cholestatic and fulminant hepatitis. The risk of disulfiram toxicity may be increased by concurrent omeprazole therapy.

INDICATIONS AND ADMINISTRATION

Disulfiram is indicated for use in selected patients in the treatment of chronic alcoholism. Individuals who are highly motivated to abstain from ethanol may benefit from the ethanol-sensitizing effects of disulfiram. Such an individual should abstain from ethanol for at least 12 hours before receiving an initial dose of 500 mg/day, given in a single dose for 1 to 2 weeks. A maintenance regimen follows, with an average amount of 250 mg/day (range 125–500 mg) and should not exceed 500 mg. The preferred mode of delivery is crushed tablets, well mixed with liquid.

PEARLS AND PITFALLS

1. Disulfiram inhibits the drug-metabolizing enzymes of the microsomal system, which can result in toxic levels of a second drug taken in usual doses concurrently (Table 28-1).
2. There are certain drugs that are known to exhibit a disulfiramlike reaction in the presence of ethanol.
3. Marijuana has been reported to interact adversely with disulfiram.
4. Because of the disulfiram-ethanol reaction, extreme caution is necessary for patients with such disorders as diabetes mellitus, epilepsy, hypothyroidism, cerebral damage, nephritis, and liver disease.
5. Patients who are allergic to rubber should be evaluated for hypersensitivity to disulfiram, which is a rubber antioxidant. Also, there is a reported case of disulfiram intoxication in a child, characterized by lethargy or somnolence, weakness, hypotonia, and vomiting, which began 12 hours after ingestion and progressed to stupor and coma.
6. The former practice of inducing the first disulfiram-ethanol reaction in a patient being started on disulfiram no longer holds the popularity of previous years. Disulfiram should never be used as the sole therapy for alcoholism without supportive counseling or psychotherapy, for success is unlikely. Never administer disulfiram to an intoxicated patient.
7. Finally, the patient must be fully informed of the objectives, potential adverse effects, and rationale of treatment.

Table 28-1. Drugs with biotransformation inhibited by disulfiram

Chlordiazepoxide (Librium)
Clorazepate dipotassium (Tranxene)
Diazepam (Valium)
Flurazepam (Dalmane)
Halazepam (Paxipam)
Isoniazid (INH, Nydrazid)
Phenytoin (Dilantin)
Prazepam (Centrax)
Rifampin (Rifadin, Rimactane)
Terfenadine (Seldane)
Thiopental (Pentathal)
Tranylcypromine (Parnate)
Warfarin (Athrombin-K, Coumadin, Panwarfin)

From WF von Oettingen, *The Diphasic Alcohols: Their Toxicity and Potential Dangers in Relation to Their Chemical Constitution and Their Fate in Metabolism.* Public Health Bulletin No. 281. Washington, DC: US Government Printing Office, 1943. P 185.

Table 28-2. Disulfiram: Pregnancy and breast-feeding

Agent	FDA pregnancy category	Risk vs benefit (by trimester)			Breast-feeding category
		1st	2nd	3rd	
Disulfiram	B1	?	?	?	IIIB

Food and Drug Administration (FDA) pregnancy categories:
A = Well-controlled studies fail to demonstrate risk to the fetus.
B1 = Animal studies fail to demonstrate risk to the fetus but no human studies are available.
B2 = Animal studies show some risk to the fetus but this is not confirmed in human studies.
C1 = Animal studies show risk to the fetus but no human studies are available.
C2 = Animal and human studies are unavailable.
D = Drug associated with birth defects but with potential benefits that may outweigh known risks.
X = Drug associated with birth defects and with potential risk that clearly outweighs potential benefit.
Risk vs benefit: R >> B = Proven or potential risk outweighs potential benefits.
B > R = Potential benefits outweigh potential risks.
R >> B? = Risks may be outweighed by benefits in some circumstances.
? = Risk-to-benefit ratio is unknown.

Breast-feeding categories:
I = Drug does not enter breast milk.
II = Drug enters breast milk but is not known to be harmful in therapeutic doses.
IIIA = Drug may or may not enter breast milk but no adverse effects are expected.
IIIB = Drug may or may not enter breast milk but drug is systemically absorbed.
IV = Drug enters breast milk and poses a potential risk to the neonate.

Suggested Reading

Benitz WE, et al. Disulfiram intoxication in a child. I. Pediatrics 1984; 3:487–488.
A case study of the unique features associated with disulfiram intoxication in a child.

Brown CG, et al. Delirium with phenytoin and disulfiram administration. Ann Emerg Med 1983; 12:25.
A case study of delirium secondary to drug toxicity in a patient taking maintenance doses of both phenytoin (Dilantin) and disulfiram (Antabuse).

Eneanya OI, et al. The actions and metabolic fate of disulfiram. Ann Rev Pharmacol 1981; 21:525–596.
An extensive review of many pharmacologic aspects of disulfiram.

Ferko AP. Present status of disulfiram. Am Fam Physician 1983; 6:183–185.
A pharmacologic review and the clinical use of disulfiram.

Fuller RK. Disulfiram treatment of alcoholism. JAMA 1986; 11: 1449–1455.
A Veterans Administration cooperative study.

Hajila R. Disulfiram reaction precipitated by omeprazole. Can Med Assoc J 1990; 143:1207.
The addition of omeprazole appeared to precipitate an Antabuse-like reaction.

Kannangara DW, et al. Disulfiramlike reactions with newer cephalosporins: Cefmenoxime. Am J Med Sci 1948; 2:45–47.
A case report of a disulfiramlike reaction with cefmenoxime.

Kitson TM. The disulfiram-ethanol reaction. J Stud Alcohol 1977; 1:96–113.
A detailed review of the disulfiram-ethanol reaction.

Lacoursiere RB, Swatek R. Adverse interaction between disulfiram and marijuana. Am J Psychiatry 1983; 140:2.
A case report of a hypomaniclike reaction in a patient taking disulfiram and marijuana simultaneously.

Rothrock JF, et al. Fulminant polyneuritis after overdose of disulfiram and ethanol. Neurology 1984; 34:357–359.
A case report of severe sensorimotor polyneuritis after simultaneous ingestion of ethanol and disulfiram in high doses.

Schade RR, et al. Fulminant hepatitis associated with disulfiram. Arch Intern Med 1983; 6:1271–1273.
A case study of disulfiram's causing hepatitis in a man with previously normal hepatocellular function.

Volicer L, Nelson KL. Development of reversible hypertension during disulfiram therapy. Arch Intern Med 1984; 6:1294–1296.
A case study of an alcoholic patient who had a gradual increase in blood pressure while he was being treated with disulfiram.

Wald J, Jacobsen E. A drug sensitizing the organism to ethyl alcohol. Lancet 1948; 2:1001–1004.
The original article revealing the potential use of disulfiram in the treatment of alcoholism.

Lactulose

Frank A. Hamilton

Lactulose is a synthetic disaccharide analogue of lactase, which acts as a laxative by stimulating colonic peristalsis. Unlike the other laxatives described in this book, lactulose has the unique property of detoxifying ammonia and is therefore an ideal agent for therapy in portal-systemic encephalopathy. The clinical diagnosis of hepatic encephalopathy or portal-systemic encephalopathy is suggested by the insidious development of mental changes, asterixis, elevated blood ammonia levels, and fetor hepaticus in patients with cirrhosis of the liver. In contrast, portal-systemic encephalopathy can occur abruptly in patients with previously normal livers that have sustained an acute injury, such as fulminant viral hepatitis or a toxin-induced liver injury.

One factor that contributes to the induction of hepatic coma is ammonia, an intermediate in the metabolism of nitrogen. Ammonia production in the gut is attributed to the action of bacterial ureases on ingested protein and blood entering into the gastrointestinal tract. Normally, ammonia is brought to the liver via the portal vein and converted to urea; however, when the liver is significantly impaired, absorbed ammonia circulates to the brain, bypassing detoxification in the liver, with resultant neurophysiologic changes.

Perhaps the most important measures in the management of hepatic encephalopathy are eliminating exogenous sources of ammonia by restricting dietary protein, controlling gastrointestinal bleeding, and reducing the number of ammonia-producing enteric bacteria. For many years, the antibiotic neomycin was used to suppress ammonia-producing colonic bacteria. This form of treatment is effective in reducing ammonia levels and improving the neurologic status of the patient, although neomycin may cause otoxicity (which is usually irreversible) and nephrotoxicity. Over the last 25 years, clinical studies have clearly demonstrated the effectiveness of lactulose in reducing ammonia levels in most patients with portal-systemic encephalopathy. The safety profile of lactulose is superior to that of neomycin.

MECHANISM OF ACTION

The exact mechanism of action of lactulose is not clear. When lactulose is administered orally, it is not hydrolyzed to its constituent monosaccharides in the small intestine, but passes unabsorbed and unchanged into the colon. There it is hydrolyzed by the action of enteric bacteria to galactose and fructose. These monosaccharides undergo further breakdown to produce hydrogen, lactate, and short-chain free acids (SCFA). These acids stimulate colonic motility, with resultant catharsis, and thereby inhibit coliform growth and ammonia production. Vince and associates showed that lactulose exerts its beneficial effect by lowering the colonic pH, thereby creating a pH gradient favoring nonionic diffusion of ammonia and reducing its absorption. Also, Mortensen has recently shown that with lactulose, there is enhanced colonic acidification and subsequently increased f‑cal ammonia secretion.

DOSAGE AND ADMINISTRATION

In the adult, therapy with lactulose is initiated with an oral dose of 30 to 45 ml 3 times a day. After 2 days this dosage may be adjusted so that the patient produces two or three soft stools per day. In a double-blind trial, Atterbury and associates demonstrated that the hourly administration of 30 to 45 ml lactulose syrup is as effective and rapid in action as neomycin in the acute setting of portal-systemic encephalopathy. In infants and children the dosage and efficacy have not been established.

An alternate route for lactulose administration is as a retention enema. This route is indicated when the danger of aspiration exists during impending coma or advanced stages of portal-systemic encephalopathy. It is given as a mixture of 300 ml lactulose with 700 ml water or normal saline. Studies by Kersh and Rifkin demonstrated the effectiveness of the rectal route in patients with portal-systemic encephalopathy, with improvement in mental status within 2 hours.

Since lactulose contains galactose (< 2.2 gm/15 ml) and lactose (< 1.2 gm/15 ml), its administration should be cautious in the diabetic patient. In addition, when lactulose therapy is instituted, other laxatives should be avoided because the appearance of loose stools may give the clinician a false sense that a therapeutic effect of lactulose has been achieved.

In a minority of patients, lactulose alone may not be effective in portal-systemic encephalopathy. Supporting studies from several investigators demonstrate that the concomitant use of neomycin and lactulose is additive in reducing ammonia levels, with subsequent improvement in mental status. In an earlier study, Weber and associates demonstrated that the combined use of neomycin and lactulose reduced urea production in cirrhotic patients. When lactulose is used for long-term management of chronic portal-systemic encephalopathy, the prudent clinician will follow serum electrolytes in elderly patients to monitor for potential complications such as hypokalemia and hypernatremia.

SIDE EFFECTS

The commonly encountered side effects are gaseousness, abdominal distention, flatulence, belching, and abdominal cramping. Nausea and vomiting occur occasionally. See Table 29-1 for effects in pregnancy and breast-feeding.

PEARLS AND PITFALLS

1. Lactulose, a synthetic disaccharide analogue of lactose, is metabolized by colonic bacteria and traps ammonia in the gastrointestinal lumen in an ionized form.
2. In addition to lactulose, adjunctive measures in the management of hepatic encephalopathy include dietary protein restriction, cessation of gastrointestinal bleeding, and reduction of ammonia producing colonic bacteria.
3. Lactulose works not only by trapping ammonia in the colonic lumen by converting it to an ionized form; it also decreases colonic bacteria by stimulating colonic motility and by stimulating catharsis.
4. In addition to oral therapy sufficient to produce two to four soft, liquid bowel movements a day, lactulose can be given as a retention enema for patients at risk for aspiration from central nervous

Table 29-1. Lactulose: Pregnancy and breast-feeding

Agent	FDA pregnancy category	Risk vs benefit (by trimester)			Breast-feeding category
		1st	2nd	3rd	
Lactulose	C2	?	?	?	IIIB
Neomycin	C1	?	?	?	IIIA

Food and Drug Administration (FDA) pregnancy categories:
A = Well-controlled studies fail to demonstrate risk to the fetus.
B1 = Animal studies fail to demonstrate risk to the fetus but no human studies are available.
B2 = Animal studies show some risk to the fetus but this is not confirmed in human studies.
C1 = Animal studies show risk to the fetus but no human studies are available.
C2 = Animal and human studies are unavailable.
D = Drug associated with birth defects but with potential benefits that may outweigh known risks.
X = Drug associated with birth defects and with potential risk that clearly outweighs potential benefit.
Risk vs benefit: R >> B = Proven or potential risk outweighs potential benefits.
B > R = Potential benefits outweigh potential risks.
R >> B? = Risks may be outweighed by benefits in some circumstances.
? = Risk-to-benefit ratio is unknown.

Breast-feeding categories:
I = Drug does not enter breast milk.
II = Drug enters breast milk but is not known to be harmful in therapeutic doses.
IIIA = Drug may or may not enter breast milk but no adverse effects are expected.
IIIB = Drug may or may not enter breast milk but drug is systemically absorbed.
IV = Drug enters breast milk and poses a potential risk to the neonate.

system (CNS) abnormalities. A mixture of 300 ml lactulose and 700 ml water should be given per rectum and held for at least 20 minutes.
5. The addition of neomycin to lactulose may benefit patients who continue to manifest CNS changes.
6. Chronic use of lactulose is associated with hypokalemia and hypernatremia. Serial electrolyte determinations are required with chronic use of lactulose.

Suggested Reading

Atterbury CE, Maddrey WC, Conn HO. Neomycin-sorbitol and lactulose in the treatment of acute portal-systemic encephalopathy: A controlled, double-blind clinical trial. Am J Dig Dis 1978; 28: 398–406.

Neomycin-sorbitol (1.5 gm neomycin and 50 ml sorbitol syrup qid) and lactulose (50 ml every 1–2 hours orally) were comparable in improving mental status in patients with acute nitrogenous portal-systemic encephalopathy and underlying cirrhosis.

Breen KJ, et al. Neomycin absorption in man: Studies of oral and enema administration and effect of intestinal ulceration. Ann Intern Med 1972; 76:211–218.

The authors studied neomycin absorption in patients with normal intestinal mucosa and patients with ulcerated upper and lower gastrointestinal mucosa (peptic ulcer disease, Crohn's disease, ulcerative colitis). They found no significant differences in urine or serum neomycin levels between the two groups.

Conn HO, Lieberthal MM. *The Hepatic Coma Syndromes and Lactulose.* Baltimore: Williams & Wilkins, 1979. Pp 317–319.

A comprehensive and detailed monograph by the pioneer author and researcher in this field.

Conn HO, et al. Comparison of lactulose and neomycin in the treatment of chronic portal-systemic encephalopathy. Gastroenterology 1977; 72:573–583.

A randomized, double-blind clinical comparison of neomycin and lactulose in 33 cirrhotic patients with chronic portal-systemic encephalopathy. Both are effective in the majority of patients (83 and 90%, respectively) in improving mental state, trail-making test results, electroencephalograms, and arterial ammonia levels.

Demeulenaere L, Van Waes L, Van Egmond J. Emergency treatment of acute portal-systemic encephalopathy (PSE) with lactulose enemas: A controlled study. Gastroenterology 1977; 72:A-151/1174.

Lactulose enemas (lactulose 300 ml—tap water 700 ml: retention 20 minutes) produce a rapid decrease in blood ammonia levels with a rapid reversal of mental status abnormalities. By contrast, cleansing tap water enemas do not produce any colonic acidification and they do not result in decreased blood ammonia levels or mental status improvement.

Fessel JM, Conn HO. Lactulose in the treatment of acute hepatic encephalopathy. Am J Med Sci 1973; 266: 103–110.

Another series demonstrating efficacy of lactulose and neomycin in the treatment of hepatic encephalopathy. The mean duration of encephalopathy after initiation of therapy was 2.2 days in the lactulose group and 3.7 days in the neomycin group, an advantage of lactulose therapy.

Kersh ES, Rifkin H. Lactulose enema. Ann Intern Med 1973; 78: 81–84.

An early report of efficacy of lactulose (4-o-β-D-galactopyranosyl-D-fructose) in the treatment of hepatic encephalopathy in four patients.

Mortensen PB. The effect of oral administered lactulose on colon nitrogen metabolism and excretion. Hepatology 1992; 16:1350–1356.

This study investigates and futher reconfirms the effect of increasing amounts of orally administered lactulose on fecal concentrations and excretion of ammonia. The findings show that colonic acidification enhances fecal ammonia excretion as a result of the breakdown of lactulose.

Nelson DC, McGrew WRG, Hoyumpa AM. Hypernatremia and lactulose therapy. JAMA 1983; 249:1295–1298.

The authors note that in 20 of 75 courses of lactulose treatment for portal-systemic encephalopathy, serum sodium level exceeded 145 mEq/liter. In the group with hypernatremia, mortality was 41 percent compared with 14 percent in those who remained eunatremic. The proposed mechanism of lactulose-induced hypernatremia is excess fecal water loss with resulting contraction of extracellular fluid volume.

Orlandi F, et al. Comparison between neomycin and lactulose in 1973 patients with hepatic encephalopathy: A randomized clinical study. Dig Dis Sci 1981; 26:498–506.

A large study complementing the work of Conn. Both studies conclude that lactulose and neomycin are efficacious in the treatment of hepatic encephalopathy.

Simmons I, Goldstein H, Boyle JD. A controlled clinical trial of lactulose in hepatic encephalopathy. Gastroenterology 1970; 59: 827–832.

An early Veterans Administration trial suggesting benefit of oral lactulose therapy in patients with hepatic encephalopathy.

Vince A, Killingby M, Wong OM. Effect of lactulose on ammonia production in a fecal incubation system. Gastroenterology 1978; 74:544-549.

An in vitro fecal incubation system was used to demonstrate that lactulose decreases fecal ammonia concentrations by (1) increasing bacterial assimilation of ammonia, (2) reducing deamination of nitrogenous compounds, and (3) reducing bacterial metabolism in general by decreasing colonic pH.

Weber FL Jr, et al. Nitrogen in fecal bacterial, fiber, and soluble fractions of patients with cirrhosis: Effects of lactulose and lactulose plus neomycin. J Lab Clin Med 1987; 3:259–263.

Lactulose administration increased fecal nitrogen content by 165 percent and decreased fecal urea production by 23 percent.

Gallstone Therapeutic Agents

Amy M. Tsuchida and Michael F. Lyons

Cholelithiasis is a major health problem in America today. Gallstones afflict 15 to 20 million Americans, and approximately 500,000 cholecystectomies are performed each year. The cost of medical and surgical management of cholelithiasis is probably over 1 billion dollars annually.

The high prevalence of cholelithiasis with its complications has led physicians for many years to search for a safe, easy method to dissolve the stones. The first successful report on a patient was in 1891, by John Walker, an English surgeon who dripped ether onto an impacted cystic duct stone through a cholecystocutaneous fistula. Since then, many have dreamed of duplicating his feat by the use of oral medications.

In the early 1970s, gallstone dissolution by chenodeoxycholic acid, an oral bile salt, was reported. Amid much excitement, the National Cooperative Gallstone Study was launched to examine the efficiency, safety, and optimal dose of the medication. The discouraging result amplified the difficulties facing medical dissolution therapy: Only 14 percent of patients had complete dissolution after 2 years, and a significant number experienced side effects. Subsequently, the 7-beta-hydroxy epimer of chenodeoxycholate known as ursodeoxycholate underwent clinical trials. Although there has been no distinct advantage in gallstone dissolution for either compound, ursodeoxycholate consistently had fewer side effects, dissolved stones more rapidly, and resulted in less hepatotoxicity. While other oral topical agents have been explored for the management of symptomatic gallstones, advances in anesthesia and laparoscopic surgery have made cholecystectomy—the standard by which medical therapy must be measured—a safe and effective procedure. Elective cholecystectomy in the low-risk patient provides a permanent remedy for the problem, with a near zero mortality in most series.

Litholytic Bile Acids

Chenodeoxycholic Acid

Chenodeoxycholic acid (CDCA, chenodiol, Chenix) was the first approved oral dissolution agent. It is a naturally occurring bile acid, comprising 20 to 30 percent of the total bile salt pool. Unlike cholic acid, the predominant bile salt, chenodeoxycholate is effective in decreasing bile cholesterol saturation and can dissolve cholesterol gallstones. However, because of its slow dissolution rate and high incidence of side effects, CDCA therapy requires a considerable commitment by both physician and patient.

PHARMACOLOGY

Chenodeoxycholic acid decreases cholesterol bile saturation by several mechanisms. It impairs endogenous cholesterol synthesis by decreasing the activity at HMG CoA reductase, the rate-limitin enzyme of cholesterol synthesis. It also suppresses bile acid synthesis. The decreased synthesis, along with the additional CDCA in the bile from oral administration, leads to a significant increase in the CDCA percentage of the bile and expansion of the total bile salt pool. Physicochemically, CDCA transports biliary cholesterol in micelles. These changes all favor the removal of cholesterol from the solid form of a gallstone into the bile solution, thus gradually dissolving the stone.

A portion of CDCA, whether given orally or synthesized by the liver, is 7-dehydroxylated by intestinal bacteria to lithocholic acid. Lithocholic acid is hepatotoxic and the small amount reabsorbed may account for the hepatotoxicity often seen in CDCA administration.

SIDE EFFECTS

The most common side effect is diarrhea, which occurs in as many as 40 percent of patients receiving a full dose of CDCA. The diarrhea is usually mild, improves with a decreased dose, and is rarely a threat to the patient or enough to cause cessation of the therapy.

Of more concern is the elevation of liver aminotransferases, seen in as many as 25 percent of patients, with significant elevation occurring in 5 to 10 percent. The elevations are generally reversible, but the enzymes should be carefully followed to avoid significant damage to the liver and the drug discontinued should the enzymes rise more than threefold.

Chenodeoxycholic acid also raises low-density lipoprotein cholesterol by 10 percent. High-density lipoprotein cholesterol is unaffected. The significance of this elevation for the 2 years of therapy is unknown.

Dyspepsia is an uncommon complaint and usually diminishes or disappears after 2 to 4 weeks of therapy.

DOSAGE

The key to initiating CDCA therapy is to start at a low dose and increase it gradually to the full dose of approximately 15 mg/kg/day to minimize the side effects. If the patient is unable to tolerate a full dose, then the chance for successful dissolution is significantly reduced. Therapy is initiated with 500 mg at night for 1 week, then increased to 750 mg nightly. If a higher dose is required, splitting the medications to twice a day is advised. If mild diarrhea occurs, withholding the drug for 1 day often alleviates the symptoms. For more severe diarrhea, dosage reduction by 250 mg for 1 week, with reinstitution at the higher dosage by gradually titrating upward over 2 weeks, may allow better tolerance. Diphenoxylate hydrochloride (Lomotil) or loperamide hydrochloride (Imodium) may help manage the diarrhea during therapy.

Ursodeoxycholic Acid

Ursodeoxycholate (UDCA, ursodiol, Actigall) is the 7-beta-hydroxy epimer of chenodeoxycholate and is normally present in only trace amounts in human bile. A Japanese drug manufacturer had marketed a combination of ursodeoxycholate and B vitamins as a general hepatic tonic for over 2 decades when, in 1974, reports of gallstone dissolution in patients medicating themselves with the combination drug appeared in the Japanese literature. Subsequent therapeutic trials in Japan and Europe demonstrated efficacy in gallstone dissolution, without the diarrhea or liver enzyme elevations seen with CDCA therapy. Ursodeoxycholic acid is now the leading dissolution agent in the world due to this improved side effect profile.

PHARMACOLOGY

Ursodeoxycholic acid is well absorbed after ingestion and passes into the portal circulation. Extraction by the liver is so efficient that only a small amount reaches the circulation. It is then conjugated with either glycine or taurine and excreted into the bile. Enterohepatic recirculation of ursodeoxycholate is quite efficient, yielding a prolonged half-life of 3.5 to 5.8 days.

On a full dose of the drug, UDCA constitutes 50 to 60 percent of the total bile salt pool. This is a lower percentage than in CDCA therapy, probably because bile salt synthesis is not suppressed by UDCA. Nonetheless, the net effect is the production of bile unsaturated in cholesterol.

Stone dissolution by UDCA is a complex physicochemical process. The drug surrounds stones with a cholesterol and phospholipid ionophase, which enhances cholesterol solubilization from the stone. Cholesterol is not transported in micelles, as with CDCA therapy, but in a liquid crystalline form. Cholesterol in lipid membranes is less disrupted by UDCA; this may explain the lack of both hepatotoxicity and diarrhea.

In clinical trials it does not appear to be significantly more effective than CDCA, but it consistently dissolves stones faster. The advantage of UDCA is the significantly lower incidence of side effects. Diarrhea and hepatotoxicity are extremely rare, serum cholesterol is unaffected, and triglycerides may fall. The chief disadvantage is expense: The cost of therapy is almost 5 times that of CDCA.

SIDE EFFECTS

Diarrhea is only a rare problem with UDCA, and liver enzyme or cholesterol elevation does not occur. Calcification of the gallstone surface occurs in 10 percent of patients during therapy and may interfere with further dissolution. This incidence may not be significantly greater than the native calcification rate.

DOSAGE

The drug should be taken with meals or milk since it dissolves more rapidly in the presence of bile and pancreatic juice. The total daily dose is 8 to 10 mg/kg divided into morning and evening doses (usually a 300-mg capsule with breakfast and dinner). Alternatively, a single nighttime dose may be given and is considered more effective by some investigators.

New Lipid-Lowering Agents

While data are presently sparse, newer HMG-CoA reductase inhibitors (lovastatin, pravastatin, simvastatin) have been shown to dissolve gallstones. In animal models, lovastatin had equal efficacy (28%) to UDCA in dissolution of gallstones, which improved to 56 percent when combined with UDCA. In a case report, pravastatin was successful in gallstone dissolution after 4 months in a hyperlipidemic patient. Simvastatin in combination with UDCA was successful in dissolving gallstones in a young woman. Further studies are warranted with these agents.

INDICATIONS FOR DISSOLUTION THERAPY

The majority of gallstones are asymptomatic and never progress to clinical symptoms. Most authorities believe such silent stones do not require therapy of any type. For patients who do have true biliary colic, the pain is usually severe enough that a rapid, reliable, and permanent solution is needed: cholecystectomy. Thus, oral dissolution therapy is reserved mainly for those patients who have symptomatic cholelithiasis and medical problems severe enough to make them a high operative risk. There are patients who have an irreconcilable fear of surgery and will not consent to the procedure under any circumstances. Dissolution therapy may be indicated in such patients, but only after the physician has carefully reassured and educated them about the safety of surgery and the limitations and side effects of dissolution therapy. Table 30-1 summarizes important issues the physicians should consider when counseling patients about the choice of therapy.

The success of dissolution therapy is dependent on patient selection. Factors that favor dissolution are listed in Table 30-2. Those who have nonfunctioning gallbladders (nonvisualization in oral cholecystogram) or calcium detectable in the stones in radiographs will

Table 30-1. Issues to consider before deciding on medical dissolution therapy

1. The presence, frequency, and severity of biliary symptoms
2. The size and location of stones
3. The probability that the stones are composed primarily of cholesterol
4. Concomitant problems caused by the stones, such as pancreatitis, jaundice, and cholangitis
5. The patient's age and operative risk
6. The patient's future accessibility to medical and surgical care of good quality
7. The presence of hepatic or intestinal problems that might be exacerbated by medical therapy
8. The patient's emotional set toward surgery versus taking long-term medications and repeated laboratory or radiographic studies to monitor drug toxicity, stone dissolution, or recurrence
9. The patient's feelings about living with the unpredictability of gallstones for several years
10. The need for repeat therapy should the stones dissolve and recur

Table 30-2. Radiographic criteria favoring stone dissolution

Radiolucent stones
Patent cystic duct
Stones < 2 cm in diameter, preferably < 5 mm
Floating stones on oral cholecystography

Table 30-3. Gallstone therapeutic agents: Pregnancy and breast-feeding

Agent	FDA pregnancy category	Risk vs benefit (by trimester)			Breast-feeding category
		1st	2nd	3rd	
Actigall	BI	?	?	?	IIIA

Food and Drug Administration (FDA) pregnancy categories:
A = Well-controlled studies fail to demonstrate risk to the fetus.
B1 = Animal studies fail to demonstrate risk to the fetus but no human studies are available.
B2 = Animal studies show some risk to the fetus but this is not confirmed in human studies.
C1 = Animal studies show risk to the fetus but no human studies are available.
C2 = Animal and human studies are unavailable.
D = Drug associated with birth defects but with potential benefits that may outweigh known risks.
X = Drug associated with birth defects and with potential risk that clearly outweighs potential benefit.
Risk vs benefit: R >> B = Proven or potential risk outweighs potential benefits.
B > R = Potential benefits outweigh potential risks.
R >> B? = Risks may be outweighed by benefits in some circumstances.
? = Risk-to-benefit ratio is unknown.
Breast-feeding categories:
I = Drug does not enter breast milk.
II = Drug enters breast milk but is not known to be harmful in therapeutic doses.
IIIA = Drug may or may not enter breast milk but no adverse effects are expected.
IIIB = Drug may or may not enter breast milk but drug is systemically absorbed.
IV = Drug enters breast milk and poses a potential risk to the neonate.

not have successful dissolution and are not candidates for medical therapy. When gallstones are larger than 2 cm, or when multiple stones nearly fill the gallbladder, dissolution therapy is unlikely to be successful and the indications for medical therapy should be reexamined. Overall, 40 to 80 percent of appropriately selected patients have at least partial dissolution within 2 years of treatment; about one-half of these (20–40% overall) will have full dissolution. Carefully selected patients with small, "floating" (on oral cholecystogram) stones, and patients with radiolucent stones who are able to take a full dose of dissolution therapy for 2 years have an 80 percent chance of complete dissolution. Unfortunately, only 10 to 15 percent of symptomatic patients meet these criteria. Patients who have existing hepatitis or hyperlipidemia are likely to have these problems exacerbated by CDCA and are not candidates for the drug. Pregnant women or those likely to become pregnant during the 2 years of therapy should not be treated since its safety during gestation has not been studied (Table 30-3).

Efficacy of dissolution should be monitored during therapy. Cholecystograms at 6 and 12 months are useful to look for partial dissolution. Partial dissolution is indicative of ultimate success if therapy is continued and helps reinforce patient compliance. If partial dissolution is not evident at 12 months, success is unlikely and treatment should be abandoned. Once full dissolution is achieved, this should be confirmed by ultrasound and therapy should be continued for an additional 3 months.

A significant problem is recurrence of the gallstones. Five years after therapy, 25 to 50 percent of patients again have cholelithiasis. Ultrasonography every 1 to 2 years is recommended to look for recurrences. These stones usually dissolve after another course of therapy if a cholecystogram again demonstrates good gallbladder function, a patent cystic duct, and radiolucent stones. Prophylaxis against recurrence has been reported with low-dose UDCA (300 mg/day), aspirin (1300 mg/day), and nonsteroidal anti-inflammatory drugs (NSAIDs). Another alternative is to alter the risk factors for gallstone formation, that is, obesity, diet, clofibrate therapy, or exogenous estrogens.

Several trials have studied the combination of lower doses of UDCA and CDCA together in an effort to avoid the side effects of CDCA and the expense of UDCA. Preliminary results show the combination to be as efficacious as either drug alone and without adverse effects on transaminases, lipids, or diarrhea. Many lithotripsy centers are using the combination successfully to solubilize the debris remaining after lithotriptic destruction of gallstones.

Contact Solvents

With access through T-tubes or nasobiliary stents, multiple solutions have been used to directly dissolve cholesterol gallstones, the most successful being organic solvents or dilute micellar solutions. In addition, the solution must be safe with regard to its effect in the bile ducts, liver, intestine, and patient as a whole. Because of the latter requirement, initially promising agents such as ether and chloroform have been abandoned. Monooctanoin, a medium-chain diglyceride, dissolved or "softened" stones to allow for successful extraction in over half the patients studied. However, side effects (abdominal pain, nausea, vomiting, diarrhea) occurred in a significant number of the patients studied, requiring discontinuation of therapy in 9 percent, according to one article. Advances in endoscopic, percutaneous, and surgical methods for extracting intraductal stones have made monooctanoin infusion uncommon.

Methyl tert-butyl ether (MTBE) rapidly dissolves gallstones, but infusion is limited to direct instillation into the gallbladder because of its toxicity if absorbed by the gut. MTBE may have a very limited role in patients at high risk for surgery who are not amenable to other forms of treatment. Ethylenediaminetetraacetic acid (EDTA) and polysorbate have demonstrated in vitro activity for pigmented calcium gallstones.

PEARLS AND PITFALLS

1. UDCA and CDCA have equal efficacy in dissolution of cholesterol stones, but UDCA is much better tolerated, with fewer side effects and biochemical abnormalities.
2. Small, radiolucent, floating stones have the best chance at dissolution with UDCA or CDCA.
3. Recurrence rates are high after treatment; prevention may be achieved with low-dose UDCA, NSAIDs, or aspirin.
4. People who are losing weight rapidly through a rigorous diet are at increased risk of developing gallstones. UDCA has been shown to reduce this risk.
5. With the advances in anesthesia, laparoscopic surgery, endoscopy, and radiology, the role for gallstone dissolution is diminishing.

Suggested Reading

Bachrach WH, Hofman AF. Ursodeoxycholic acid in the treatment of cholesterol cholelithiasis. Dig Dis Sci 1982; 27:737, 833.

An exhaustive review, in two parts, of ursodeoxycholic acid pharmacology efficacy, and side effects.

From H. Gallstone dissolution therapy. Gastroenterology 1986; 91: 1560.

An excellent review of the physiology of dissolution therapy.

Palmer HC, Carey MC. An optimistic view of the National Cooperative Gallstone Study. N Engl J Med 1982; 306:1171.

An opinion professing just what the title promises, for a study that could use an optimistic outlook.

Peine CJ. Gallstone-dissolving agents. Gastroenterol Clin North Am 1992; 21:715.

A recent review of dissolution agents.

Roehrkasse R, et al. Gallstone dissolution treatment with a combination chenodeoxycholic acid and ursodeoxycholic acids. Dig Dis Sci 1986; 31:1032.

A combination of the two agents is as efficacious as a full dose of either. It also avoids the side effects of chenodiol and reduces the expense of UDCA.

Talamini MA, Gadacz TR. Gallstone dissolution. Surg Clin North Am 1990; 70:1217.

A recent review of dissolution agents.

Pancrelipase

Michael S. Gurney and Rodger A. Sleven

Enzyme replacement therapy for pancreatic disease is generally used in two clinical situations: for steatorrhea from exocrine insufficiency and for pain from chronic pancreatitis. Therapy for steatorrhea is well established and reasonably effective, but enzyme use for relief of pain—while proven in the proper circumstances—remains somewhat problematic and controversial.

Malabsorption from pancreatic disease begins to occur when pancreatic function falls below 10 percent of normal secretory capacity. Patients then experience weight loss, a decreased sense of well-being, and steatorrhea. The most common causes of exocrine pancreatic insufficiency in the adult are chronic pancreatitis (usually due to alcohol), pancreatic resection, and pancreatic carcinoma. In children, cystic fibrosis or Schwachman's syndrome (congenital exocrine pancreatic insufficiency and neutropenia) is the usual cause. The therapy for exocrine insufficiency is simple in theory: Replace the missing pancreatic enzymes with oral supplements. In practice, unless therapy follows several principles of intestinal physiology, treatment can be less than rewarding for both the patient and physician.

PHARMACOLOGY

Pancreatic enzyme products are derived from hog pancreas and contain standardized enzyme activity, which varies in amount from product to product. Most products now are pancrelipase, an enzyme preparation with high lipase activity—the most important enzyme for the relief of steatorrhea. The various products' potencies for relief of steatorrhea are best judged on the basis of their lipase content.

The primary problem in enzyme replacement therapy is irreversible inactivation of the lipase by gastric acid below a pH of 4. Concomitant antacid therapy with sodium bicarbonate is usually enough to prevent this inactivation, but in gastric hypersecretors, this can still be a problem. Histamine 2(H_2)-receptor antagonists have not been as effective as sodium bicarbonate, but the combination of the two may be helpful. Omeprazole, with its significantly stronger acid inhibition, has shown good efficacy in improving bioavailability of enzyme preparations.

Enteric-coated tablets and coated microspheres in a capsule are also available. The enteric coating is designed to dissolve at pH 6, protecting the enzymes from acid degradation in the stomach. However, the enteric-coated tablets have been shown to have poor bioavailability. The microsphere preparations can be useful but are plagued by questions of gastric emptying of the spheres, premature release of the enzyme in the stomach if concomitant bicarbonate is given, and lack of release in the duodenum due to poor duodenal alkalinization from the diseased pancreas. Improved size of the microsphere preparations will soon be available. The microspheres are more convenient (higher lipase content, thus fewer pills or capsules per meal) and have shown good results in relief of steatorrhea.

INDICATIONS

Pancreatic enzyme replacement is indicated for the treatment of malabsorption due to pancreatic insufficiency. Enzyme replacement therapy does not help malabsorption from other causes, such as gluten-sensitive enteropathy or small-bowel overgrowth. Thus, a firm diagnosis of pancreatic insufficiency should be made before therapy is begun.

Toskes has shown that enzyme replacement therapy is also effective in alleviating the pain of chronic pancreatitis. This beneficial effect is believed to be due to feedback inhibition of the pancreas, chiefly through delivery of serine proteases (trypsin, chymotrypsin, and elastase) to the duodenum. The patients who seem to respond best are those with mild to moderate disease and nondilated ducts.

In patients with both pancreatic exocrine insufficiency and diabetes, the steatorrhea must be controlled before glucose control is attempted. Without control of the steatorrhea, such patients are very sensitive to any changes in insulin dose and often have a decreased glucagon reserve as well, making their response to hypoglycemia inadequate.

Pancreatic enzyme replacement is not indicated as a digestive aid, alone or in combination with bile salts, sedatives, or antiflatulents. Bile salts or proteolytic enzymes of plant origin (Papain) are of no benefit in pancreatic insufficiency.

CONTRAINDICATIONS AND SIDE EFFECTS

There are no absolute contraindications to enzyme replacement therapy, although it should be given with caution to patients allergic to pork. Large doses of pancreatic enzymes may cause nausea, bloating, or cramps. Large doses in children have also been associated with elevated serum uric acid levels and uricosuria.

There are reports from Europe of ascending colon strictures in pediatric cystic fibrosis patients taking high protease preparations. There have been no reports of similar problems in adults.

DOSAGE

Table 31-1 is a suggested regimen for pancreatic enzyme replacement. Lipase activity of at least 20,000 units is suggested as a starting dose, with further benefit often seen with up to 40,000 units

Table 31-1. Suggested regimen for pancreatic enzyme replacement

1. Begin with a preparation providing a total of 20,000 to 40,000 lipase units per meal.
2. Enteric-coated formulations work well for control of steatorrhea, but nonenteric-coated preparations release proteases better in the duodenum and are preferred for pain control.
3. Enzyme preparations should be taken at the beginning of a meal or throughout the meal. If the patient is being treated for pain control, a nighttime dose should also be given.
4. If nonenteric-coated enzymes are used and no clinical improvement occurs, add one 650-mg tablet of sodium bicarbonate before and after meals, and with any nighttime enzymes.
5. If there is still no improvement, consider:
   a. Adding a proton pump inhibitor or an H_2-blocker.
   b. Is the diagnosis correct?
   c. Small-bowel bacterial overgrowth may be present—a frequent problem in patients with pancreatic disease.

Table 31-2. Pancrelipase: Pregnancy and breast-feeding

Agent	FDA pregnancy category	Risk vs benefit (by trimester)			Breast-feeding category
		1st	2nd	3rd	
Omeprazole	B1	?	?	?	IV

Food and Drug Administration (FDA) pregnancy categories:
A = Well-controlled studies fail to demonstrate risk to the fetus.
B1 = Animal studies fail to demonstrate risk to the fetus but no human studies are available.
B2 = Animal studies show some risk to the fetus but this is not confirmed in human studies.
C1 = Animal studies show risk to the fetus but no human studies are available.
C2 = Animal and human studies are unavailable.
D = Drug associated with birth defects but with potential benefits that may outweigh known risks.
X = Drug associated with birth defects and with potential risk that clearly outweighs potential benefit.
Risk vs benefit: R >> B = Proven or potential risk outweighs potential benefits.
B > R = Potential benefits outweigh potential risks.
R >> B? = Risks may be outweighed by benefits in some circumstances.
? = Risk-to-benefit ratio is unknown.
Breast-feeding categories:
I = Drug does not enter breast milk.
II = Drug enters breast milk but is not known to be harmful in therapeutic doses.
IIIA = Drug may or may not enter breast milk but no adverse effects are expected.
IIIB = Drug may or may not enter breast milk but drug is systemically absorbed.
IV = Drug enters breast milk and poses a potential risk to the neonate.

per meal. Increases above this are less likely to be of benefit, are difficult for patients to comply with, and may cause side effects.

If no significant improvement occurs with the extract alone, acid inactivation of lipase may be the problem and bicarbonate should be added. If there is still no benefit seen, the patient may be a hypersecretor and an H_2-receptor antagonist or omeprazole will improve availability. Occasionally, a combination of enzyme tablets and enteric-coated microspheres yields improvement when either preparation alone is ineffective.

In children, microspheres may be mixed with food, and activity is maintained as long as the food is ingested within 30 minutes. Enzyme powder (Viokase) can be mixed with food, but low-pH foods such as applesauce should be avoided since the lipase will be inactivated. Table 31-2 summarizes enzyme use in pregnancy and breast feeding.

Response to enzyme replacement should be measured by fecal fat determination; patients' subjective impressions are often unreliable.

PEARLS AND PITFALLS

1. Treatment of steatorrhea is often effectively accomplished by use of high-lipase microsphere preparations. Therapy for pain relief is probably best accomplished by traditional uncoated preparations with high protease content and attention to good acid neutralization.
2. Postgastrectomy patients have rapid gastric emptying, making the bioavailability of enteric-coated microspheres uncertain and often less than optimal.
3. Patients with cystic fibrosis are often acid hypersecretors. This, combined with poor bicarbonate secretion from the diseased pancreas, makes acid neutralization especially important in these patients.
4. Small-bowel bacterial overgrowth is a frequent concomitant problem in patients with pancreatic insufficiency and is usually due to previous surgery or hypomotility from narcotics. If pancreatic enzyme replacement is not efficacious, a course of antibiotic treatment may result in significant improvement.
5. In patients with severe pancreatic insufficiency, enzyme replacement may not completely reverse steatorrhea. A low-fat diet is then often enough to give symptomatic improvement. Supplemental MCT oil (not dependent on lipase for absorption) can be given, if then needed, for caloric supplementation.
6. Do not routinely give bicarbonate to patients receiving enteric-coated microspheres. The bicarbonate may make the enteric coat dissolve prematurely, subjecting the enzymes to subsequent inactivation.
7. A high-fiber diet makes enzyme replacement therapy less effective and should be avoided if possible.
8. Wait for 3 to 4 weeks before measuring the response to therapy. Steatorrhea often gradually improves as malnutrition is corrected.
9. Remember that whatever regimen is arrived at, it is a regimen for the rest of the patient's life. Therefore, the number of tablets, the ease of compliance, and the cost are all important issues.
10. Do *not* give magnesium- or calcium-containing antacids to patients with pancreatic insufficiency. The magnesium or calcium forms soaps with free fatty acids, worsening steatorrhea.

Suggested Reading

Campbell D, et al. Alcoholic patients with chronic pancreatitis do not experience suppression of CCK levels or pain relief following treatment with enteric coated pancreatin. Gastroenterology 1992; 102:A259.

A well-done study that illustrates one of the reasons for the poor response of pain control in chronic pancreatitis: inconsistent delivery of proteases to the duodenum, especially with enteric coated preparations.

Guarner L, et al. Fate of oral enzymes in pancreatic insufficiency. Gut 1993; 34:708–712.

An elegant placebo-controlled study that showed that most of the lipase delivered by enteric-coated pancreatin was actually to the ileum. Nevertheless, good efficacy was demonstrated.

Heijerman H, et al. Improvement of fecal fat excretion after addition of omeprazole to pancrease in cystic fibrosis is related to residual exocrine function of the pancreas. Dig Dis Sci 1993; 38:1–6.

Addition of omeprazole improved fecal fat excretion, especially in patients who had some remaining pancreatic function.

Hendeles L, et al. Treatment failure after substitution of generic pancrelipase capsules. JAMA 1990; 263:2459–2461.

Standard pancreatic enzyme preparations have enough trouble with bioavailability that it is not surprising that generic preparations are even more problematic. Three case reports are presented, along with an analysis of the meager enzyme content of the capsules.

Maguire S, Goodchild M. Enzyme contents of pancreatic enzyme preparations: Are they optimal? Drugs 1992; 44:685–689.

Another critical look at enzyme preparations.

Oades PJ, et al. High strength pancreatic enzyme supplements and large bowel stricture in cystic fibrosis. Lancet 1994; 343:109.

The first report of a colon stricture in a pediatric patient receiving concentrated enzyme replacement. Several more reports followed this publication.

Pitchumoni CS, Toskes PP. Is there an effective nonsurgical treatment for pain in chronic pancreatitis? Am J Gastroenterol 1991; 86:26–29.

The pros and cons of surgical and medical control of pain in chronic pancreatitis are well argued in this discussion. Toskes makes his case, and concludes by saying, "If one wants to be successful in relieving the abdominal pain. . . . one must use the appropriate enzyme formulation in the appropriate dose in an appropriate patient."

Motility Disorder Drugs

The modern study of gastrointestinal motility began in earnest with the work of Cannon in the early 1900s. His classic monograph, entitled "The Mechanical Factors of Digestion," closes its introduction with the opinion that "some who think that nothing of importance happened the day before yesterday may be surprised by it." The ensuing 4 score years have supported that statement. The expansion of the study of gut motility since that time has been inexorable. We are now confronted monthly with a large and often bewildering or contradictory volume of data on gastrointestinal motility. Despite this, we are seemingly no closer today to a unifying theory of motility than we were in Cannon's time. Indeed, only now are we understanding the effects on normal emptying and transit of various hormones, neuropeptides, luminal elements, and the intrinsic and extrinsic nervous systems of the gut. When one considers the multiple endogenous regulators of gut motility, and the emotional, physical, and dietary stresses to which we subject our systems daily, it is a wonder that the majority of the population is able to maintain the regularity of bowel movements that it does.

The difficulty in understanding the physiology of normal subjects as well as the pathophysiology of abnormal conditions has slowed the development of drugs to treat gastrointestinal motility disorders. Clinicians and pharmacologists have had no other choice but to use drugs empirically, to relieve symptoms or alter definable abnormalities toward normal. Thus, the most significant progress in drugs for motility disorders has been in the discovery of the mechanism of action of drugs that have been in clinical use for years. For example, it used to be thought that most contact laxatives exerted their effect by irritating the intestinal mucosa, thereby stimulating contraction. We now know that these drugs alter the normal regulation of mucosal electrolyte and water transport, increasing colonic fluid content, leading to a shorter transit time and increased defecation. Only bisacodyl has been shown to actually stimulate colonic motility.

The past several years have not been without therapeutic breakthroughs. Domperidone and cisapride represent major therapeutic advances in the treatment of gastric emptying and intestinal dysmotility. These drugs are thoroughly discussed by Thomas Dorsey in Chap. 36. For the diarrhea disorders, somatostatin and its analogue, octreotide (Sandostatin), are major advances in the treatment of carcinoid and pancreatic islet cell tumors. They clearly have profound effects on intestinal motility, and only time and clinical experience will reveal their final clinical applications.

Although these drugs help in the management of motility disorders, the clinician is still faced with a significant challenge in the patient who complains of a chronic alteration in gastrointestinal motility such as diarrhea or constipation. These complaints can be the *forme fruste* of multiple diseases, and such patients can be among the most difficult diagnostic and therapeutic problems in clinical gastroenterology. At the minimum, these patients deserve a careful history and physical examination with basic laboratory studies. Stool Hemoccult and proctoscopy should also be performed. If the constipation is recent in onset, a barium enema is indicated. An important part of the history is the drug and dietary history. Many patients unintentionally or intentionally omit nonprescription drugs or food items that could explain their symptoms. The over-the-counter availability of many motility drugs has led to the misconception that they are free of adverse effects. The easy access to laxatives has led to their frequent abuse and the paradoxical worsening of the constipated state. Fordtran has also shown us the frequency with which cathartics are used to get attention by the mentally ill.

Two of the physician's primary duties to these patients are to educate them about their bowel habits and to explain how different medications may either aid or exacerbate their symptoms. I hope this part will help the physician in those tasks.

Michael S. Gurney

Suggested Reading

Burks TF. Actions of Drugs on Gastrointestinal Motility. In LR Johnson (ed), *Physiology of the Gastrointestinal Tract.* New York: Raven, 1981.

A thorough summary of drug effects on gastrointestinal motility. An excellent review.

Cannon AE. *The Mechanical Factors of Digestion* (1911). Science History Publications, Walton Publishing, 1986.

A reprint of the classic monograph on gastrointestinal motility.

Farrar JT. The effects of drugs on intestinal motility. Clin Gastroenterol 1982; 11:673.

Another good review of drug effects on intestinal motility.

Huizinga JD. Electrophysiology of human colonic motility in health and disease. Clin Gastroenterol 1986; 15:879.

A well-written summary of a difficult topic.

Antidiarrheal Agents

Richard D. Baertlein

Kaolin and Pectin

Absorbents and gels have been used for decades to manage the symptoms of diarrhea. The most common preparation now in use is Kaopectate, a combination of kaolin, a hydrated aluminum silicate clay, and pectin, a purified carbohydrate gel derived from apples and citrus fruit.

The Chinese have used kaolin as an antidiarrheal compound for centuries. In the 1920s, both Walker and Braafladt reported that it absorbed bacterial toxins, protected intestinal mucosa, and reduced mortality from cholera. However, in vitro and in vivo studies in the 1940s cast doubt on its effectiveness, and it has generally been abandoned as a single-agent therapy for diarrhea.

PHARMACOLOGY

Kaopectate is not absorbed and remains in the gut lumen after oral administration. It is a nonspecific absorbent: Nutrients, medications, enzymes, salt, and water are all absorbed in the lumen. Numerous commercial combinations of kaolin and pectin are marketed, varying in the content of the two ingredients, the viscosity, and the flavor. Aluminum hydroxide is occasionally included to increase the absorptive capacity. Neomycin may also be added as an antibacterial agent.

INDICATIONS

Kaopectate is used for the symptomatic relief of diarrhea. However, the efficacy of the preparation is doubtful. Portnoy and associates showed that Kaopectate given to children with acute infectious diarrhea did not decrease either stool frequency or stool water content when compared with either compound alone or with placebo. The only improvement was a tendency for the stools to be more formed. McClung and colleagues showed that stool losses of water, sodium, and potassium were actually increased with Kaopectate in an experimental model.

Thus, Kaopectate is only of subjective benefit in diarrhea. Since the cornerstone of diarrhea therapy is replacement of stool and electrolyte losses, McClung's work showed that Kaopectate may actually do more harm than good. Thus, its routine use for acute diarrhea is not recommended.

CONTRAINDICATIONS AND SIDE EFFECTS

Kaopectate should not be used in patients with suspected obstructive lesions of the bowel, or in children younger than 3 years of age. It may absorb concomitant medications, reducing their bioavailability. Kaolin can cause a pneumoconiosis in kaolin-factory workers (it is also commonly used in plastics, paint, and adhesives), but this is not a problem with the medication.

DOSAGE

The dosage is 15 to 30 ml administered 3 or more times a day, as indicated.

PEARLS AND PITFALLS

1. Kaopectate absorbs other drugs. Concomitant medications should be given 1 hour before or 3 hours after Kaopectate.
2. Sodium and potassium losses may be increased by Kaopectate. Electrolytes may need to be followed closely in severe diarrhea or with prolonged therapy.
3. Pectin is a form of dietary fiber. Improvement in postprandial insulin and glucose concentrations has been shown in diabetics given supplemental pectin.

Loperamide

Loperamide is a synthetic antidiarrheal agent for oral use in the treatment of both acute and chronic diarrheal conditions. It appears to have antisecretory effects in addition to prolonging gut transit time. Loperamide is also now available in nonprescription formula.

PHARMACODYNAMICS AND PHARMACOKINETICS

Loperamide is a member of the phenylpiperidine analgesic class, like meperidine and diphenoxylate, but without significant nervous system effects.

After oral ingestion, serum concentrations of loperamide peak at 4 hours, with an elimination half-life of 7 to 14 hours. The drug is incompletely absorbed after oral ingestion, with delays due to inhibition of gastrointestinal motility. The drug is poorly soluble in water. Large oral doses do not cause euphoria and inhibit withdrawal symptoms only modestly. The abuse potential of loperamide is low.

MECHANISM OF ACTION

Loperamide slows intestinal transit time. Basilisco and associates demonstrated delays in breath hydrogen excretion with loperamide during lactulose hydrogen breath testing, a delay antagonized by concurrent naloxone administration.

Loperamide exerts its effect by agonist activity on gut-associated mu-opiate receptors. It inhibits the action of calmodulin. This effect is greatest in the jejunum and ileum and is associated with higher frequency and lower duration of irregular motor activity. Loperamide accentuates segmental motor activity in the proximal colon.

Besides effects on motor activity, loperamide appears to affect intestinal secretory activity as well. Turnberg showed that loperamide inhibits mucosal secretion by a variety of known intestinal secretagogues. From research in children, Sandhu found a prompt and impressive decrease in secretory diarrhea during steady-state perfusion studies of the jejunum.

Loperamide does not increase the rate of absorption of water or electrolytes from the intestine. During steady-state total gut perfusion of normal volunteers, Schiller found identical volumes of rectal effluent with or without loperamide. However, loperamide did increase the intraluminal volume of the total gut (985 ml without loperamide, compared to 1764 ml with loperamide).

Loperamide appears to exert it effect by local tissue action. Topical application of the drug to the mucosa of the descending and sigmoid colon of volunteers decreases spike activity (the myoelectric equivalent of propulsive movements). No decrease in plasma prostaglandin F alpha, motilin, or amylase activity is demonstrable. Basal gastric acid output and bile salt production are unchanged by loperamide.

INDICATIONS

Loperamide is approved by the Food and Drug Administration for the treatment of chronic diarrhea associated with inflammatory bowel disease, acute nonspecific diarrhea, and high-volume ileostomy output.

Bergman studied the action of loperamide in 29 patients with chronic diarrhea after intestinal resection for Crohn's disease. In comparison to diphenoxylate, 19 of the 29 patients preferred the decrease in stool frequency and increase in stool consistency associated with loperamide. Only five preferred diphenoxylate, while five had no benefit from either agent. Wille-Jorgensen and associates found no patient preference for loperamide over diphenoxylate in a study of 27 patients with iatrogenic short gut (jejunoileal bypass for morbid obesity).

Loperamide serves as a useful adjunct in the treatment of acute nondysenteric diarrhea in children. Karrar and associates in Saudi Arabia, Gasbarrini in Italy, Singh in India, and Vesikar in Scandinavia all found decreases in stool volume and frequency, and more rapid weight gain with the use of loperamide (0.8 mg/kg/24 hours) in conjunction with an oral rehydration regimen. Vesikar did find that cholestyramine, 2 grams daily, was nearly 3 times more effective than loperamide in decreasing stool frequency and inducing weight gain.

Loperamide is also useful in treatment of postvagotomy diarrhea, although the daily doses required (12–24 mg) were higher than those used in other conditions. Loperamide may have a useful role in the subgroup of patients with irritable bowel syndrome troubled predominantly by diarrhea. Lavo and Cann both found amelioration of stool frequency, urgency, and pain in separate studies of patients with irritable bowel syndrome. Self-titration of dose and nighttime dosing were both safe and effective.

Although the welfare of adult patients with acute infectious diarrhea is not known to be improved by loperamide (Bergstrom et al.), Johnson and associates found this drug to be more efficacious than bismuth subsalicylate in the treatment of acute traveler's diarrhea. Diarrhea decreased within the first 4 hours of therapy.

ADMINISTRATION

The usual dosage is one to two 2-mg capsules with each liquid bowel movement, not to exceed eight capsules a day. The typical daily dosage ranges from 4 to 8 mg. The use of Loperamide in pregnant and breast feeding patients is summarized in Table 32-1.

SIDE EFFECTS

Constipation can occur with loperamide use and is documented to occur in about 10 percent of patients receiving the drug for both acute and chronic diarrheal disorders. Constipation is most likely to occur in the patient receiving loperamide for treatment of irritable bowel syndrome.

Table 32-1. Antidiarrheal agents: Pregnancy and breast-feeding

Agent	FDA pregnancy category	Risk vs benefit (by trimester)			Breast-feeding category
		1st	2nd	3rd	
Loperamide	C2	?	?	?	IV

Food and Drug Administration (FDA) pregnancy categories:
A = Well-controlled studies fail to demonstrate risk to the fetus.
B1 = Animal studies fail to demonstrate risk to the fetus but no human studies are available.
B2 = Animal studies show some risk to the fetus but this is not confirmed in human studies.
C1 = Animal studies show risk to the fetus but no human studies are available.
C2 = Animal and human studies are unavailable.
D = Drug associated with birth defects but with potential benefits that may outweigh known risks.
X = Drug associated with birth defects and with potential risk that clearly outweighs potential benefit.
Risk vs benefit: R >> B = Proven or potential risk outweighs potential benefits.
B > R = Potential benefits outweigh potential risks.
R >> B? = Risks may be outweighed by benefits in some circumstances.
? = Risk-to-benefit ratio is unknown.
Breast-feeding categories:
I = Drug does not enter breast milk.
II = Drug enters breast milk but is not known to be harmful in therapeutic doses.
IIIA = Drug may or may not enter breast milk but no adverse effects are expected.
IIIB = Drug may or may not enter breast milk but drug is systemically absorbed.
IV = Drug enters breast milk and poses a potential risk to the neonate.

Other gastrointestinal side effects include abdominal pain, abdominal distention, bloating, nausea, and vomiting. In higher daily doses (> 8 mg/day), central nervous system depression with drowsiness, dizziness, and fatigue can occur.

CONTRAINDICATIONS

The use of agents that inhibit gastrointestinal motility is associated with the development of toxic megacolon in patients suffering from pseudomembranous enterocolitis and acute ulcerative colitis.

PEARLS AND PITFALLS

1. The use of naloxone is indicated for the treatment of central nervous system depression and respiratory depression in acute loperamide overdose.
2. Loperamide is contraindicated in the treatment of pseudomembranous enterocolitis and acute ulcerative colitis, as it is associated with the development of toxic megacolon.
3. Loperamide, when combined with antibiotic therapy, appears to be safe in the treatment of traveler's diarrhea and bacillary dysentery. There is, however, conflicting evidence regarding its impact on the duration of diarrheal symptoms.
4. The use of loperamide in irritable bowel syndrome should be restricted to that subgroup plagued with severe urgency, diarrhea, and pain.

Diphenoxylate

Diphenoxylate, like loperamide, is a synthetic narcotic analogue used as adjunctive therapy in the treatment of acute and chronic diarrhea. It is commercially available only in combination with a subtherapeutic dose of atropine to discourage deliberate overdosage. Also, like loperamide, it appears to possess antisecretory activity in addition to prolonging intestinal transit time.

PHARMACOLOGY

Diphenoxylate is a synthetic opioid of the phenylpiperidine class, structurally similar to meperidine. Following oral administration, diphenoxylate is rapidly metabolized to difenoxin, an active metabolite, with peak concentrations occurring at 2 hours. Onset of action is typically within 1 hour, with a duration of action of 3 to 4 hours. Difenoxin has an elimination half-life of 12 to 14 hours.

Therapeutic doses produce minimal or no analgesic/opiate effects, but high doses (> 40 mg) can cause euphoria and inhibit opiate withdrawal symptoms. Due to the addition of atropine to available preparations, the abuse potential is relatively low.

MECHANISM OF ACTION

Diphenoxylate increases intestinal transit time by limiting peristalsis via inhibitory binding to mucosal receptors, subsequently diminishing the local mucosal peristaltic reflex. Van Wyk and associates demonstrated delayed hydrogen breath excretion using diphenoxylate during hydrogen breath testing. Diphenoxylate, like loperamide, appears to exert antidiarrheal action by its antisecretory properties. This appears to be mediated by enteric neurons. Zavecz and colleagues demonstrated a correlation between calmodulin binding of diphenoxylate and antidiarrheal activity.

Diphenoxylate inhibits net fluid secretion in VIP-induced diarrhea in the rat jejunum, an action blocked by naloxone administration.

INDICATIONS

Diphenoxylate is useful as adjunctive therapy in the management of acute and chronic diarrhea.

Schenker studied diphenoxylate in 220 patients with acute diarrhea and 41 patients with chronic diarrhea. He found it effective within a short time in more that 80 percent of acute cases and over 70 percent of chronic cases, with stool frequency and consistency returning to normal at a total daily dose of 15 mg. Harford and associates found diphenoxylate to be effective in treating patients with chronic diarrhea and fecal incontinence, reducing both average stool frequency and stool weight by nearly 50 percent.

In direct comparison studies with loperamide, diphenoxylate has generally been shown to be no more effective, with a less favorable side effect profile. Wille-Jorgensen and associates found no significant difference in either drug's effectiveness in treating jejuno-ileostomy–induced diarrhea, while Jaffe found the drugs to be equally efficacious in alleviating acute nonspecific diarrhea. Loperamide has been shown to be more effective in reducing stool frequency and improving stool consistency in chronic diarrhea, at a lower effective dose than diphenoxylate. Palmer and colleagues found loperamide more efficacious in producing a solid stool and reducing urgency in chronic diarrhea, with fewer side effects than diphenoxylate.

ADMINISTRATION

Diphenoxylate is available in both tablet and liquid preparations. Each tablet or 5 ml liquid contains 2.5 mg diphenoxylate and 0.025 mg atropine. The usual initial dosage is 5 mg every 12 hours until diarrhea is controlled, followed by reduction to the lower effective maintenance dose, typically 5 to 10 mg/day. A response is normally seen within 48 hours of administration.

SIDE EFFECTS AND CONTRAINDICATIONS

The routine use of diphenoxylate results in a relatively low incidence of adverse effects. Those reported include nausea, abdominal distention, rash, pancreatitis, sedation, and dizziness. Side effects of atropine generally occur only after overdosage and include tachycardia, urinary retention, flushing, keratoconjunctivitis sicca, and dryness of the skin.

Diphenoxylate is contraindicated in patients with acute ulcerative colitis and pseudomembranous colitis, as it may induce the development of toxic megacolon. Caution must be used in patients with jaundice or cirrhosis, as diphenoxylate may precipitate hepatic coma under these circumstances.

PEARLS AND PITFALLS

1. Children are more sensitive to the effects of diphenoxylate and atropine and also show a narrow margin of safety with these drugs. Therefore, they must be used with caution in this age group; their use is contraindicated in children under 2 years of age.
2. Because of its structural similarity with meperidine, diphenoxylate must be used with caution in patients who are taking mono-

amine oxidase inhibitors, as this combination may precipitate hypertensive crisis.
3. Treatment of diphenoxylate overdose leading to severe respiratory depression includes gastric lavage and naloxone administration.

Suggested Reading

KAOLIN AND PECTIN

Allen MD, et al. Effect of magnesium-aluminum hydroxide and kaolin-pectin on absorption of digoxin from tablets and capsules. J Clin Pharmacol 1981; 26:26–31.
Kaopectate reduced absorption of digoxin tablets.

Bucci AJ, et al. In vitro interaction of guanidine with kaolin and pectin. J Pharmacol Sci 1981; 70:999–1002.
Quinidine may be absorbed when administered with kaolin-pectin preparations.

Jenkins DJA, et al. Decrease in postprandial insulin and glucose concentrations by guar and pectin. Ann Intern Med 1977; 86: 20–26.
Pectin improved the postprandial insulin and glucose profiles in diabetics.

Juhl RP. Comparison of kaolin-pectin and activated charcoal for inhibition of aspirin absorption. Am J Hosp Pharmacol 1979; 36:1097.
Kaopectate reduced aspirin absorption but not as much as did activated charcoal.

McClung HJ, Beck RD, Powers P. The effect of a kaolin-pectin absorbent on stool losses of sodium, potassium, and fat during a lactose-intolerance diarrhea in rats. J Pediatr 1980; 96:769.
Kaopectate increased stool losses of sodium, potassium, and water in this experimental model.

Portnoy BL, et al. Antidiarrheal agents in the treatment of acute diarrhea in children. JAMA 1976; 236:844.
Kaopectate did not decrease stool water loss of stool frequency when compared with placebo in this clinical trial. It did improve stool consistency slightly.

LOPERAMIDE

Awouters F, et al. Loperamide. Survey of studies on mechanism of its antidiarrheal activity (review). Dig Dis Sci 1993; 38:977–995.
The antidiarrheal action of loperamide can be considered to be mu-opiate receptor mediated.

Basilisco G, et al. Effect of loperamide and naloxone on mouth-to-cecum transit time evaluated by lactulose hydrogen breath test. Gut 1985; 26:700–703.
Mouth-to-cecum transit time was significantly longer after loperamide treatment. This prolongation was antagonized by the concomitant administration of naloxone.

Bergstrom T, et al. Symptomatic treatment of acute infectious diarrhea: Loperamide versus placebo in a double-blind trial. J Infect 1986; 12:35–38.
Neither the duration of pathogen excretion nor the frequency or consistency of diarrheal stools was significantly altered by loperamide in this study of acute infectious diarrhea in adults.

Cann PA, et al. Role of loperamide and placebo in management of

irritable bowel syndrome (IBS). Dig Dis Sci 1984; 29:239–247.
Eighteen of 28 patients with IBS received symptomatic benefit from loperamide therapy, with significant improvement in diarrhea, urgency, and borborygmi.

Johnson PC, et al. Comparison of loperamide with bismuth subsalicylate for the treatment of acute traveler's diarrhea. JAMA 1986; 255:757–760.
People receiving loperamide passed fewer unformed stools during the first 4 hours of therapy, the first 24 hours of therapy, and the first 48 hours of therapy.

Karrar ZA, et al. Loperamide in acute diarrhea in childhood: Results of a double-blind placebo-controlled clinical trial. Ann Trop Paediatr 1987; 7:122–127.
Loperamide, 0.8 mg/kg/day, plus standard oral rehydration therapy. The use of loperamide was associated with faster recovery and quicker weight gain in the majority of children.

Lavo B, Stenstam M, Nielsen AL. Loperamide in treatment of irritable bowel syndrome—a double-blind, placebo-controlled study. Scand J Gastroenterol 1987; 130 (suppl):77–80.
Significant advantages of loperamide were found to be improvements in stool consistency, pain relief, and diminished urgency.

Mellstrand T. Loperamide–opiate receptor agonist with gastrointestinal motility effects. Scand J Gastroenterol 1987; 130 (suppl): 65–66.
Loperamide is an opiate agonist that inhibits the action of calmodulin.

Murphy GS, et al. Ciprofloxacin and loperamide in the treatment of bacillary dysentery. Ann Intern Med 1993; 118:582–586.
Loperamide decreased the number of unformed stools and shortened the duration of diarrhea in Shigella*-induced dysentery in adults treated with ciprofloxacin.*

O'Brian JD, et al. Effect of codeine and loperamide on upper intestinal transit and absorption in normal subjects and patients with postvagotomy diarrhea. Gut 1988; 29:312–318.
Loperamide delayed transit and improved symptoms, but the doses required for this effect (12–24 mg) were higher than are usually considered necessary in secretory diarrhea.

Petrucelli BP, et al. Treatment of traveler's diarrhea with ciprofloxacin and loperamide. J Infect Dis 1992; 165:557–560.
Loperamide appears safe for the treatment of nonenterotoxigenic Escherichia coli *causes of traveler's diarrhea, although it does not offer a significant therapeutic benefit.*

Press AG, et al. Effect of loperamide on jejunal electrolyte and water transport, prostaglandin E_2–induced secretion and intestinal transit time in man. Eur J Clin Pharmacol 1991; 41:239–243.
Loperamide has a dual effect on intestinal activities, stimulating absorption and prolonging intestinal transit time.

Taylor DN, et al. Treatment of traveler's diarrhea: Ciprofloxacin plus loperamide compared with ciprofloxacin alone. A placebo-controlled, randomized trial. Ann Intern Med 1991; 114:731–734.
Loperamide appeared to have some benefit in the first 24 hours of treatment in patients with diarrhea secondary to enterotoxigenic E. coli.

DIPHENOXYLATE

Bergman L, Djarv L. A comparative study of loperamide and diphenoxylate in the treatment of chronic diarrhea caused by intestinal resection. Ann Clin Res 1981; 13:402–405.

Loperamide was statistically superior to diphenoxylate in reducing the number of stools and improving fecal consistency in 29 patients who had intestinal resection for Crohn's disease.

Harford WV, et al. Acute effect of diphenoxylate with atropine (Lomotil) in patients with chronic diarrhea and fecal incontinence. Gastroenterology 1980; 78:440–443.

Lomotil reduced average stool frequency and stool weight in 15 patients with chronic diarrhea.

Mader TH, Stulting RD. Keratoconjunctivitis sicca caused by diphenoxylate hydrochloride with atropine sulfate (Lomotil) [letter]. Am J Ophthalmol 1991; 111:377–378.

Case study demonstrating that diphenoxylate with atropine may cause keratoconjunctivitis sicca in susceptible patients.

McCallon MM, et al. Diphenoxylate-atropine (Lomotil) overdose in children: An update. Pediatrics 1991; 87:694–700.

A thorough review of the recent literature regarding Lomotil overdose in children.

Palmer KE, et al. Double-blind cross-over study comparing loperamide, codeine and diphenoxylate in the treatment of chronic diarrhea. Gastroenterology 1980; 79:1272–1275.

Diphenoxylate was less effective than loperamide in producing solid stool in patients with chronic diarrhea.

Van Wyk M, et al. Evaluation of gastrointestinal motility using the hydrogen breath test. Br J Clin Pharmacol 1985; 20:479–481.

Diphenoxylate caused a significant increase in small-bowel transit time as determined by breath hydrogen concentration after lactulose ingestion.

Wille-Jorgensen P, et al. Diarrhea following jejuno-ileostomy for morbid obesity. A randomized trial of loperamide and diphenoxylate. Acta Chir Scand 1982; 148:157–158.

Both loperamide and diphenoxylate had a significant effect on diarrhea when compared with no treatment, but no significant difference was found between the two drugs.

Zavecz JH, et al. Relationship between anti-diarrheal activity and binding to calmodulin. Eur J Pharmacol 1982; 78:375–377.

A positive correlation between calmodulin binding and antidiarrheal activity was seen with both diphenoxylate and loperamide.

Bile Salt Binders

Michael S. Gurney

Bile salts are normally reabsorbed in the terminal ileum. However, in the occasional patient, inappropriate passage of bile acids into the colon results in the clinical entity of bile acid diarrhea: a chronic, watery, secretory diarrhea. Such patients typically have frequent bowel movements after meals but not at night. The stool weight is only mildly increased, and significant steatorrhea is rarely present. The diarrhea is usually more bothersome than debilitating; dehydration and electrolyte abnormalities are uncommon. We now know that the dehydroxy bile acids cause this syndrome by stimulation of colonic cyclic AMP, with secondary secretion of water and electrolytes. The bile salt–binding agents, cholestyramine and colestipol, have been employed with great success in such patients, and their use has earned physicians many grateful patients for the relief they provide. The two resins are very similar and are discussed together.

PHARMACOLOGY AND MECHANISM OF ACTION

The resins are high-molecular-weight anion-exchange resins. Cholestyramine has quaternary ammonium groups on the resin, whereas colestipol contains secondary and tertiary amines. Both are protonated with chloride.

Following oral administration, both resins release their chloride ions and absorb bile acids in the small intestine. An insoluble, nonabsorbable complex is formed and excreted unchanged in the feces. In vitro, each gram of cholestyramine binds about 1100 μmoles taurocholate and 913 μmoles glycocholate. Colestipol binds 938 μmoles taurocholate and 825 μmoles glycocholate. Since both drugs are nonspecific anion-exchange resins, other compounds and drugs, especially those with an acid pH, are bound.

INDICATIONS

Bile acid diarrhea is divided on the basis of etiology into three groups. Type I is probably the most common form and is caused by ileal disease, resection, or bypass. The bile acids, which only have receptors in the terminal ileum, are unable to be reabsorbed and pass into the colon, causing secretory diarrhea. Type II is less common and seems to be due to a selective ileal transport defect of bile acids. Type III occurs after surgical truncal vagotomy or, more commonly, postcholecystectomy. The exact mechanism is unknown. Cholestyramine and colestipol are indicated in the treatment of all three types and are extremely effective. However, it must be remembered that patients with more than 100 cm of ileum resected do not actually have bile acid diarrhea. Their diarrhea is caused by a reduced bile salt pool from significant chronic intestinal loss. The lack of bile salts causes poor fat micelle formation in the small intestine and subsequent malabsorption and steatorrhea. Bile acid binders actually worsen the diarrhea in such patients.

Both colestipol and cholestyramine have been shown to bind the toxin of *Clostridium difficile*. In vitro, colestipol binds four times the amount of toxin that cholestyramine does. However, the two have not been tested against each other in a clinical study. Thus, mild *C. difficile*–induced pseudomembranous colitis responds to treatment with either resin. Moderate to severe disease, however, does not improve significantly with resin therapy and is better treated with antibiotics.

Chronic cholestatic liver disease, such as primary biliary cirrhosis and sclerosing cholangitis, is often complicated by chronic pruritus. The pruritus is thought to be due to elevated serum levels of bile acids and other pruritogens. This very bothersome complaint is usually improved with bile salt binders.

SIDE EFFECTS

There are no absolute contraindications to the use of either colestipol or cholestyramine. In patients with intestinal strictures, however, the drugs must be used carefully, in reduced amounts, since there are reports of obstruction caused by the resins. Use of colestipol and cholestyramine in pregnant and lactating patients is summarized in Table 33-1.

The most common side effects are gastrointestinal, especially with high doses and in patients older than 60 years of age. Constipation is the most frequent complaint in patients taking the drugs for lipid disorders; this is, of course, less of a problem when treating diarrhea illnesses. Bloating, abdominal pain, belching, flatulence, nausea, and vomiting are other less common intestinal side effects.

Of more practical concern is the resin binding of concomitant medications. Table 33-2 is a list of medications absorbed by colestipol and cholestyramine. All drugs, and especially those on the list, should be given either 1 hour before or 4 hours after the resins are taken. Occasionally, a rebound effect, such as prolonged anticoagulation with warfarin (Coumadin), is noted when resin therapy is stopped abruptly.

Cholestyramine and colestipol occasionally interfere with the absorption of fat. Deficiency of the fat-soluble vitamins (A, E, and K) may occur with long-term therapy and thus supplementation may be needed. Folate deficiency has also been reported with chronic therapy, and folate supplements should be given, especially in children.

There is a report of loss of dental enamel in a patient who swished the cholestyramine solution in his mouth for several minutes before swallowing. The suspension's acidic pH was the presumed cause. Patients should be cautioned about such activity.

DOSAGE

The starting dose for colestipol (Colestid) is one 5-gm packet 3 times a day, just before meals. The dose may be increased up to 30 gm/day if needed. The starting dosage for cholestyramine (Questran) is one 4-gm packet 3 times a day, just before meals. It may be increased to 24 gm/day if needed. Both resins should be mixed with at least 120 ml of a liquid. After the mixture is ingested, the glass should be rinsed with additional liquid and drunk to ensure that the entire dose has been taken. The resins should not be taken in the dry form, since this is associated with esophageal irritation or obstruction. Alternatively, either resin may be mixed with a soup or a pulpy fruit with a high moisture content, such as crushed pineapple or applesauce.

Cholestyramine is now available as Questran Light, which is sweetened with aspartame instead of sugar. Patient acceptance is markedly improved. Similarly, colestipol is now available

Table 33-1. Bile salt binders: Pregnancy and breast-feeding

Agent	FDA pregnancy category	Risk vs benefit (by trimester)			Breast-feeding category
		1st	2nd	3rd	
Cholestyramine	C1	B>R	B>R	B>R	IIIA
Colestipol	C1	B>R	B>R	B>R	IIIA

Food and Drug Administration (FDA) pregnancy categories: A = Well-controlled studies fail to demonstrate risk to the fetus.
B1 = Animal studies fail to demonstrate risk to the fetus but no human studies are available.
B2 = Animal studies show some risk to the fetus but this is not confirmed in human studies.
C1 = Animal studies show risk to the fetus but no human studies are available.
C2 = Animal and human studies are unavailable.
D = Drugs associated with birth defects but with potential benefits that may outweigh known risks.
X = Drugs associated with birth defects and with potential risk that clearly outweighs potential benefit.
Risk vs benefit: R> >B = Proven or potential risk outweighs potential benefits.
B>R = Potential benefits outweigh potential risks.
R> >B? = Risks may be outweighed by benefits in some circumstances.
? = Risk-to-benefit ratio is unknown.
Breast-feeding categories:
I = Drug does not enter breast milk.
II = Drug enters breast milk but is not known to be harmful in therapeutic doses.
IIIA = Drug may or may not enter breast milk but no adverse effects are expected.
IIIB = Drug may or may not enter breast milk but drug is systemically absorbed.
IV = Drug enters breast milk and poses a potential risk to the neonate.

Table 33-2. Medications commonly absorbed by cholestyramine or colestipol

Digoxin
Corticosteroids
Warfarin (Coumadin)
Iron
Penicillin
Phenobarbital
Phenylbutazone
Tetracycline
Thiazide diuretics
Thyroid hormone
Vitamin D

Flavored Colestid Granules, which also use aspartame and has added flavoring in addition to being more finely milled than regular Colestid.

For pseudomembranous colitis, the resins should be given 4 times a day initially, and the dose may later be reduced if needed. When given to patients with pruritus, improvement is usually noted in 1 to 3 weeks.

Once the desired clinical response has been achieved, the dose can be reduced. When reducing the dose, it should be remembered that the most important dose is the morning dose, since the gallbladder is then filled with bile from the overnight fast. Often, only a breakfast dose is ultimately needed for the control of symptoms.

PEARLS AND PITFALLS

1. Cholestyramine has been shown to reduce lower esophageal sphincter pressure, probably by stimulating cholecystokinin (CCK) release. Some patients' reflux symptoms might increase after administration.
2. In ileal dysfunction from Crohn's disease, one morning dose is often enough to relieve the bile salt diarrhea.
3. Some patients with idiopathic diarrhea have a bile salt transport defect and secondary bile salt diarrhea. Since this condition is difficult to diagnose, an empiric trial of colestipol can be rewarding in these challenging patients.
4. The binding resins should not be used in patients with partial small intestinal obstruction, since they can precipitate total obstruction.
5. Other medications should be given either 1 hour before or 4 hours after resins. If the evening dose of cholestyramine or colestipol is stopped as the dose is reduced, this is a convenient time to give other medications.
6. Fat-soluble vitamin and folate supplementation may be needed for patients on long-term resin therapy. This is especially important for patients receiving resins for cholestatic liver disease such as primary biliary cirrhosis.
7. Patients taking both warfarin and a binding resin may have a significant increase in their prothrombin time if the binding resin is stopped.

Suggested Reading

Aldini R, et al. Bile acid malabsorption and bile acid diarrhea in intestinal resection. Dig Dis Sci 1982; 27:495.

Aldini and associates studied patients with large and small ileal resections and colectomy versus normal control subjects, and found that stool pH and free fatty acids were as important as bile salts in causing diarrhea. This may explain why patients with large ileal resections usually respond well to low-fat diets.

Chang TW, Onderdonk AB, Bartlett JG. Anion-exchange resins in antibiotic-associated colitis. Lancet 1978; 2:258–259.

Both colestipol and cholestyramine were mixed in vitro with C. difficile *toxin. Both resins bound the toxin, but colestipol was four times more effective on a weight basis.*

Fromm H, Malavolti M. Bile acid–induced diarrhea. Clin Gastroenterol 1986; 15:567.

An excellent discussion of bile acid diarrhea and its pathophysiology.

Hoogwerf BJ, et al. Effects of long term cholestyramine administration on vitamin D and parathormone levels in middle-aged men with hypercholesterolemia. J Lab Clin Med 1992; 4:407–411.

Vitamin D and calcium metabolism were studied in 268 men who took either cholestyramine or placebo for nearly 10 years. No difference was seen between the groups in calcium, phosphorus, albumin, or hormone levels.

Merrick MV, Eastwood MA, Ford MJ. Is bile acid malabsorption underdiagnosed? An evaluation of accuracy of diagnosis by measurement of SeHCAT retention. Br Med J 1985; 280:665.
The investigators used a radiolabeled synthetic bile acid to study ileal function. They found that 5 of 42 patients with diarrhea and the irritable bowel syndrome actually had bile acid malabsorption. Cholestyramine relieved their symptoms.

Shakir KMM, et al. The use of bile acid sequestrants to lower serum thyroid hormones in iatrogenic hyperthyroidism. Ann Intern Med 1993; 118:112–113.
Cholestyramine was used to decrease thyroid hormone levels in iatrogenic hyperthyroidism, taking advantage of binding both the ingested and enterohepatically recirculated hormone. Cholestyramine has been shown in other studies to be potentially helpful in binding digoxin and organophosphates as well.

Zhu XX, Brown GR, St Pierre LE. Polymeric sorbents for bile acids. Comparison between cholestyramine and colestipol. J Pharmacol Sci 1992; 81:65–69.
An elegant physicochemical comparison of bile salt binding by the two resins.

Anticonstipation Agents

Michael Carboni and Michael S. Gurney

Constipation is the most common digestive complaint in America: Sonnenberg and Koch reported that this complaint alone leads to over 2.5 million physician visits each year. This is a particular problem for elderly patients; 20 percent of the population over 65 suffer from the problem, and 20 to 30 percent of this age group use laxatives frequently or chronically.

Fiber therapy remains the cornerstone of most treatment regimens, but some new agents and innovative uses of older preparations are finding niches of their own. Indeed, more effort is being directed at attempts to correct the pathophysiologic defects in individual patients.

Bulk-Forming Agents

The average American gets only 15 to 20 gm dietary fiber a day, when 20 to 50 gm is needed for normal bowel function. In order to normalize bowel function, bulk-forming agents are used as dietary fiber supplements. This chapter discusses and compares the more commonly used bulking agents: Citrucel, Fiberall, Metamucil, and Perdiem.

DIETARY FIBER

Dietary fiber is that portion of the plant cell wall that escapes digestion and is composed of lignins and polysaccharides (i.e., cellulose, hemicellulose, pectin, gums, and mucilage). These components exercise a variety of important mechanistic and metabolic functions and influence bacterial flora in the large intestine. Different sources of dietary fiber (i.e., brans, grains, fruits, and vegetables) vary in their fiber content and composition, as do the different bulk-forming agents. The differences in composition account for the differences in the water-holding capacity and mechanism of action of bulking agents.

COMPOSITION AND FORMULATION

Bulk-forming agents are more refined and concentrated than the usual dietary sources of fiber and are generally more effective. Most bulk-forming agents are composed of one of three major components of dietary fiber—psyllium, semisynthetic cellulose, or synthetic polycarbophil—in varying proportions.

1. Psyllium hydrophilic colloid (Metamucil, Fiberall, and Perdiem). The refined colloid obtained from psyllium seeds is rich in mucilage. This mucilloid preparation forms a gelatinous mass when mixed with water. Metamucil does contain dextrose as a dispersing agent, but sugar-free preparations are available. Various flavors can also be found. Powders are the usual form of psyllium preparations, but Perdiem is formulated as psyllium granules. The sodium content varies with each individual preparation.
2. Carboxymethylcellulose and methylcellulose (Citrucel). The indi-

gestible and nonabsorbable semisynthetic derivatives of cellulose form a bulky, hydrophilic colloid when mixed with water. The carboxymethyl preparation contains high amounts of sodium, which may lead to fluid retention and should be avoided in patients on sodium restrictions. Citrucel is available as a powder in regular and orange flavors. Forms of other preparations include liquids, capsules, and tablets.

3. Polycarbophil and calcium polycarbophil (Mitrolan, Equalactin, and FiberCon). The polycarbophils are synthetic polyacrylic resins that are nonabsorbable, indigestible, and metabolically inert. They have more water-binding activity than the other two types of agent, absorbing 60 to 100 times their weight in water. The sodium content is lower, but free calcium is released in the intestine and they should therefore be avoided in patients who are on calcium restriction or are using tetracyclines. Conversely, those who need calcium supplementation are able to have two problems addressed with one preparation. Tablets are the most common form used.

MECHANISM OF ACTION

The hydrophilic properties of dietary fiber in bulk-forming agents add weight and provide bulk to the stool through the absorption of water. This increase in water content normalizes transit time through the intestine, prevents overabsorption of water by the colon, and keeps the feces soft and bulky. In addition, dietary fiber components are digested by and stimulate the growth of colonic bacteria, thus adding to fecal mass. Movement of soft stools through the colon requires less pressure, thereby decreasing the colonic intraluminal pressures important in the treatment of diverticular disease. Bulk-forming agents usually take effect within 12 to 24 hours and with repeated administration a maximal effect can be reached in a few days.

In addition, bulk-forming agents have been shown to possess certain important metabolic properties. For example, water-soluble fibers (i.e., mucilages and pectins) are known to delay gastric emptying, to slow the absorption of glucose from the intestine, and to substantially reduce postprandial hyperglycemia. These properties are important in the management of diabetes and other conditions associated with the rapid breakdown of carbohydrates.

Cholesterol metabolism is also affected by soluble fibers, which bind bile acids and increase bile acid excretion in the feces. Decreased bile acid reuptake causes an increase in bile acid synthesis from cholesterol precursors, thus decreasing the plasma cholesterol concentration of low-density lipoproteins (LDLs). Water-insoluble fibers such as cellulose are not associated with the lowering of cholesterol levels.

INDICATIONS

1. Constipation. One of the most widely accepted therapeutic uses of bulk-forming agents is for the management of constipation. Constipation results from excessive absorption of water from fecal material due to slow passage through the colon. Bulk-forming agents absorb water, increase fecal bulk, alter stool consistency, and activate propulsive motility, preventing constipation. They are used for the treatment and prevention of constipation in the elderly, pre- and postpartum women, chronically bedridden or

immobilized patients, postoperative patients, patients receiving narcotics, and fiber-deficient patients.

2. Diverticular disease. Constipation is the number one cause of increased pressure in the colon. By preventing constipation, one of the most common causes of diverticular disease can be avoided. Preexisting diverticulae cannot be eliminated, but further diverticula formation and symptoms of diverticulosis can be prevented through the use of bulk-forming agents. The addition of dietary fiber decreases intestinal transit time, increases fecal weight, and decreases intracolonic pressures, which are all important factors in the treatment of diverticular disease.
3. Irritable bowel syndrome (IBS). Dietary fiber supplements can normalize bowel transit times and ameliorate the symptoms of diarrhea or constipation associated with IBS. Because each IBS patient has different symptoms, the dose of bulk-forming agents should be prescribed to meet individual needs. With prolonged treatment and dose adjustment, the IBS patient's symptoms should be well controlled.
4. Hemorrhoids, anal fissures, and anal surgical patients. Because bulk-forming agents act as stool softeners, patients who need to resist straining or to soften their stools are recommended to use bulking agents.
5. Diarrhea. Bulk-forming agents, especially methylcellulose and polycarbophil, are useful in the symptomatic relief of acute and chronic watery diarrhea by increasing bulk and consistency of the stool. They are also helpful in reducing the number of evacuations in the patient with an ileostomy or colostomy. However, bulk agents can increase losses of sodium, potassium, and water in these patients.
6. Diabetes. Since the water-soluble fiber components slow gastric emptying and the absorption of glucose, bulk-forming agents add an attractive dimension to the treatment of diabetics. Postprandial blood sugars have been lowered in patients receiving dietary fiber supplements, reducing their need for insulin. Although the exact mechanisms remain a mystery, the advantages of increased soluble fiber in the diabetic patient have been well documented.

DOSAGE AND ADMINISTRATION

The dosages and general information for some of the more common bulk-forming agents are presented in Table 34-1. The grams of dietary fiber in each dose are compared, as well as sodium content, sugar content, and calories.

It is important to remember that each oral dose of any bulk-forming agent must be taken concurrently with one or more glasses of water or juice to ensure that an obstruction does not develop from an improperly hydrated bolus.

Doses are usually taken with meals, in the morning or evening, or both, when taking two doses a day. The number of doses per day is determined by the patient's symptoms and their response to therapy.

CONTRAINDICATIONS AND SIDE EFFECTS

Since no systemic side effects occur with the use of bulk-forming agents, prolonged therapy is not a risk. Also, unlike other laxatives and cathartics, no dependence can develop, allowing for long-term therapy with bulking agents. In addition, children's doses are avail-

Table 34-1. Common bulk-forming agents

Product	Preparation	Oral dose (gm)	Dietary fiber (gm/dose)	Sodium (mg/dose)	Carbohydrate (gm/dose)	Calories (dose)
Citrucel	Regular	19 (1 Tbsp)	2	3	15	60
	Orange	19 (1 Tbsp)	2	3	15	60
Fiberall	Sugar-free	5 (1 tsp)	3.4	10		6
Metamucil	Regular	7 (1 tsp)	3.4	1	3.5	14
	Orange	11 (1 Tbsp)	3.4	1	7.1	30
	Sugar-free Regular	3.7 (1 tsp)	3.4	1	0.3	1
	Sugar-free Orange	4.3 (1 tsp)	3.4	1	0.6	2
	Instant Mix	1 pkt (0.19 oz)	3.4	2		1
Perdiem Fiber		6 (1 tsp)	4.03	1.8		4
Perdiem		6 (1 tsp)	3.25	1.8		4

able when indicated, with no major risks. Use of bulk-forming agents in pregnant and lactating patients is summarized in Table 34-2.

A caution should be given to phenylketonurics, as Sugar-Free Metamucil contains phenylalanine.

Contraindications for the administration of bulk-forming agents include any suspicion of bowel obstruction or impaction, an undiagnosed change in bowel habits, or an acute abdomen.

Fecal impaction or intestinal obstruction can occur in any condition that stops the progression of the bulk-forming agent through the intestine, including stenoses, ulceration with fibrosis, or obstructing adhesions of the alimentary canal. Water is reabsorbed from the bulking agent and the bolus can become inspissated within the bowel lumen. Thus, any narrowing of the intestinal lumen represents a risk. Obstruction can also occur within the esophagus and intestine if too little water is taken with the bulk-forming agent.

Allergic reactions (urticaria, rhinitis, dermatitis, and bronchial asthma) to bulk-forming agents are rare but possible. Workers involved in the production of psyllium powder can become sensitized from chronic exposure and may experience asthmatic symptoms on inhalation of the powder. The sugar added to some preparations can be hazardous if used by diabetics.

Cellulose can bind cardiac glycosides, salicylates, and nitrofurantoin and decreases their intestinal absorption. These interactions are not usually clinically significant. However, psyllium preparations may bind coumarin derivatives, with adverse clinical effect. Information on this interaction is sparse, but the potential effects are serious enough that close monitoring of prothrombin times in the care of patients taking coumarin is important.

Carboxymethylcellulose and some psyllium colloids may contain significant quantities of sodium and should not be used when sodium and water retention present a problem.

PEARLS AND PITFALLS

1. Citrucel and Regular Metamucil may be more palatable when mixed with juice.
2. Sugar-Free Metamucil has fewer calories and comes in assorted flavors.
3. Perdiem requires large amounts of water to prevent the formation of bezoars.
4. Mitrolan, Equalactin, and FiberCon contain calcium, which can be either a disadvantage or an advantage, depending on the individual patient.

Contact Laxatives

Contact (stimulant) laxatives are nonprescription preparations that usually promote a bowel movement within 6 to 12 hours. This rapid response is appealing to many in the general population, who are in search of an easy, inexpensive "quick fix" to the problem of constipation. The availability, low cost, rapid onset of action, and constant promotion of these products have led to their status as one of the most frequently used, misused, and least understood of all the classes of drugs in our therapeutic armamentarium. These laxatives are generally thought of as stimulants, under the common misconception that they cause propulsive peristaltic activity either through local irritation of the mucosa or a selective stimulation of colonic intra-

Table 34-2. Anticonstipation agents: Pregnancy and breast-feeding

Agent	FDA pregnancy category	Risk vs benefit (by trimester)			Breast-feeding category
		1st	2nd	3rd	
Aloe	C2	R>>B	R>>B	R>>B	IV
Anthraquinones (cascara)	C2	R>>B	R>>B	R>>B	IV
Bisacodyl	C2	R>>B	R>>B	R>>B	IV
Citrucel	B1	B>R	B>R	B>R	I
Docusate	C2	R>>B	R>>B	R>>B	IV
Fiberall	B1	B>R	B>R	B>R	I
Metamucil	B1	B>R	B>R	B>R	I
Mineral oil	C2	R>>B	R>>B	R>>B	IV
Mitrolan	B1	B>R	B>R	B>R	I
Perdiem Fiber	B1	B>R	B>R	B>R	I

Perdiem (senna)	C2	R>>B	R>>B	R>>B	IV
Phenolphthalein	C2	R>>B	R>>B	R>>B	IV
Ricinoleic acid	C2	R>>B	R>>B	R>>B	IV

Food and Drug Administration (FDA) pregnancy categories:
A = Well-controlled studies fail to demonstrate risk to the fetus.
B1 = Animal studies fail to demonstrate risk to the fetus but no human studies are available.
B2 = Animal studies show some risk to the fetus but this is not confirmed in human studies.
C1 = Animal studies show risk to the fetus but no human studies are available.
C2 = Animal and human studies are unavailable.
D = Drugs associated with birth defects but with potential benefits that may outweigh known risks.
X = Drugs associated with birth defects and with potential risk that clearly outweighs potential benefit.
Risk vs benefit: R>>B = Proven or potential risk outweighs potential benefits.
B>R = Potential benefits outweigh potential risks.
R>>B? = Risks may be outweighed by benefits in some circumstances.
? = Risk-to-benefit ratio is unknown.

Breast-feeding categories:
I = Drug does not enter breast milk.
II = Drug enters breast milk but is not known to be harmful in therapeutic doses.
IIIA = Drug may or may not enter breast milk but no adverse effects are expected.
IIIB = Drug may or may not enter breast milk but drug is systemically absorbed.
IV = Drug enters breast milk and poses a potential risk to the neonate.

cosal nerve plexus. Actually, most contact laxatives have no such peristaltic actions. In addition, there is a lack of awareness among the population of the potential complications of these medications.

The contact laxatives can be divided into several classes, based on their structure and mechanism of action. The classes include the anthraquinones, the diphenylmethanes, ricinoleic acid (castor oil), and docusate.

INDICATIONS

Contact laxatives are not indicated for chronic use, and their use in children should only be with the greatest discretion. Failure to heed these warnings can result in laxative-dependent constipation. Situations for which their use is indicated are

1. To ease the pain of defecation in patients with painful episiotomies, thrombosed hemorrhoids, anal fissures, or perianal abscesses
2. To decrease the need to administer the Valsalva maneuver to patients with abdominal wall or diaphragmatic hernias, anal stenosis, and aneurysms or other diseases of the cerebral or coronary arteries
3. To relieve constipation during puerperium
4. In geriatric patients with poor abdominal and perineal tone
5. For the temporary alteration of bowel motility due to other drugs
6. To prepare the colon for radiologic or endoscopic examination
7. To provide a fresh stool for ova and parasite analysis
8. For the relief of temporary constipation in a healthy patient

Anthraquinones

Anthraquinones are among the most used and abused of the contact laxatives. Most produce a soft or formed stool within 6 to 12 hours. The preparations range from the mildest (senna) to those that are quite strong and often cause colic (aloe, aloin, or rhubarb).

Aloe is the dried latex of the leaves of various species of the *Aloe* plant, found in Africa and the West Indies. The drug has a bitter taste and a disagreeable odor. Aloin is a microcrystalline powder that consists of a mixture of active ingredients extracted from aloe. Cascara sagrada is the dried bark of the buckthorn tree. The active ingredients are four anthraquinone glycosides (cascarasides A through D). Senna is the dried leaflet of the *Cassia* plant, and the active ingredients are sennosides A and B, another two anthraquinone glycosides.

The anthraquinones are poorly absorbed from the small intestine and hydrolyzed by colonic bacteria to the pharmacologically active free anthraquinones. Any absorbed anthraquinones are metabolized by the liver and then secreted into the bile or urine. Low levels may be excreted in breast milk. Table 34-2 summarizes use of laxatives in pregnant and breast-feeding patients.

MECHANISM OF ACTION

The anthraquinones' actions are restricted to the distal ileum and colon. The compounds stimulate fluid and electrolyte secretion and impair sodium absorption. These actions may be mediated by cyclic AMP, which is increased in colonic mucosal cells after anthraquinone administration. Contrary to popular belief, there is no good evidence for any action on the colonic nerve plexus or colonic motility.

CONTRAINDICATIONS AND SIDE EFFECTS

All laxatives are contraindicated in patients with acute or undiagnosed abdominal pain, nausea, or vomiting. Stimulant cathartics are contraindicated in intestinal obstruction.

Anthraquinone derivatives used chronically (more than 4 months) may cause melanosis coli, an accumulation of dark pigment in the mucosa of the cecum and rectum. There does not appear to be a problem with the accumulation of the pigment alone. The condition resolves in 3 to 6 months after discontinuation of the drug.

Other consequences of chronic use of stimulant laxatives include "cathartic colon" and metabolic alkalosis or acidosis. Cathartic colon occurs after many years of use and is defined as colonic dilatation and poor motor function. Such patients require colon stimulants for defecation or a prolonged colon retraining program.

All stimulant cathartics can result in severe cramping and diarrhea after ingestion.

DOSAGE

Table 34-3 shows the usual dosage of the various drugs. The dose should be reduced by half in geriatric and obstetric patients, and in children who weigh over 27 kg.

Diphenylmethane Derivatives

This family of contact laxatives consists of the bisacodyl preparations (Dulcolax, Fleet's Bisacodyl) and the phenolphthaleins (Modane, Phillips' LaxCaps, Prulet, Correctol, Doxidan, Ex-Lax, Feen-A-Mint, Yellolax). Both types of preparation produce a bowel movement within 6 to 8 hours after ingestion.

Bisacodyl is only minimally absorbed after oral administration, but 15 percent of oral phenolphthalein is absorbed and enters the enterohepatic circulation. Small amounts are excreted in the urine and breast milk (see Table 34-2).

Both the diphenylmethanes and the phenolphthaleins stimulate colonic fluid and electrolyte secretion, similar to the anthraquinones. Bisacodyl also causes stimulation of the submucosal neural plexus, increasing peristalsis. Phenolphthalein may interfere with fluid and electrolyte conservation in the small intestine.

CONTRAINDICATIONS AND SIDE EFFECTS

The contraindications and side effects mentioned under the heading Anthraquinones also apply to use of the diphenylmethanes.

Phenolphthalein can cause dermatologic reactions in sensitive patients. Fixed drug eruptions, pruritus, burning, and pigmentation have all been reported. Phenolphthalein also imparts a pink color to alkaline urine or feces, and patients should be forewarned. Because of a prolonged enterohepatic circulation, phenolphthalein's action may last for several days after only a single dose in sensitive patients.

Although bisacodyl usually produces soft stools with little or no colic, an enteric coating is required to minimize gastric irritation. The suppository preparation may cause stinging, tenesmus, and

Table 34-3. Contact laxatives*

Agent	Brand names	Adult dosage
Anthraquinones		
Cascara	Generic: 325-mg tablets	200–400 mg
	Fluid extract	0.5–1.5 ml
	Aromatic fluid extract	5 ml
Senna	Senokot: Tablets	2–4 tablets/day
	Granules	1–2 tsp bid
Bisacodyl	Dulcolax: Tablets (5 mg) Suppositories (10 mg) Fleet Bisacodyl: Tablets (5 mg) Suppositories (10 mg)	5–15 mg orally or 10 mg rectally
Castor oil	Generic liquid Emulsoil Neoloid Purge Concentrate	15–60 ml
Docusate	Sodium: Colace, 50 & 100 mg Regutol, 100 mg Modane Soft, 100 mg Potassium: Dialose, 100 mg Kasof, 240 mg Calcium: Surfak, 240 mg	50–400 mg/day
Phenolphthalein	Ex-Lax, 90-mg tablets Feen-A-Mint Gum, 97-mg chewable tablets Modane, Mild, 60-mg tablets Prulet, 60-mg tablets Yellolax	30–270 mg/day

*Combination preparations are not listed.

mild proctitis in a few patients. If the oral form is chewed and the enteric coating disrupted, oral and gastric irritation may result.

DOSAGE

See Table 34-3 for adult dosages. Children 6 years and older may receive either bisacodyl (5 mg orally or 10 mg by suppository) or phenolphthalein (30–60 mg orally).

Ricinoleic Acid

Castor oil is hydrolyzed in the small intestine to ricinoleic acid, a long-chain fatty acid. Castor oil produces one or more copious, watery evacuations 2 to 6 hours after ingestion. The colon is emptied so completely that passage of normal stool afterward may be delayed for 2 days or more. Because of its strong action, castor oil is principally used to prepare patients for radiologic examination. It should not be used to treat common constipation.

MECHANISM OF ACTION

Ricinoleic acid stimulates anion secretion in the small intestine and causes net accumulation of fluid and electrolytes. Some studies have shown that it may erode villous tips, disorganize the microvillous surface, and increase mucosal permeability to molecules with molecular weights as large as 16,000.

CONTRAINDICATIONS AND SIDE EFFECTS

Castor oil has the same general contraindications and side effects as other contact cathartics. In addition, because of its strong action, it is more likely to cause cramping, dehydration, and electrolyte disturbances.

DOSAGE

Table 34-3 states the usual dosage for castor oil. Palatability is improved by administering chilled castor oil along with fruit juice, or with a carbonated beverage afterwards. Neoloid is a flavored emulsion of castor oil and is more palatable.

Docusate (Dioctyl Sulfosuccinate)

The docusate salts—calcium (Surfak), potassium (Dialose, Kasof), and sodium (Colace, Regutol, Modane Soft)—are anionic surfactants promoted as stool-softening agents. It is now known that, in addition to their emollient properties, these drugs are also mild contact laxatives. They appear to be absorbed to some extent in the duodenum and jejunum and subsequently excreted in the bile. These drugs produce a softer bowel movement within 3 to 5 days of administration.

CONTRAINDICATIONS AND SIDE EFFECTS

The docusate salts are so mild that many of the side effects of other contact laxatives are not a problem. However, docusate does increase intestinal permeability, and other laxatives or mineral oil should not be given concomitantly. Increased toxicity, including hepatotoxicity, has been reported in such cases. Diarrhea and morphologic intestinal mucosal changes have also been reported.

DOSAGE

See Table 34-3 for dosage. It is recommended that 240 to 340 ml of water be taken with each dose.

Saline Cathartics

Magnesium, sodium, and potassium salts all have cathartic properties. They will generally produce a soft or watery bowel movement within 2 to 6 hours of administration, depending on the dose given.

Saline cathartics are popular for bowel preparation before endoscopic, radiographic, or surgical procedures. Fleet Phospho-Soda has become especially popular for colonoscopy preparation in lieu of polyethylene glycol purgatives. These preparations are also useful to eliminate parasites after therapy, or to collect stool samples for diagnosis. The watery diarrhea that occurs after administration of these drugs does not destroy the sensitive trophozoites of *Entamoeba histolytica* or *Giardia lamblia*.

MECHANISM OF ACTION

These preparations stimulate gut fluid secretion and increase contractility. Laxatives that contain magnesium also cause cholecystokinin release from the small-bowel mucosa; thus, increased colonic contractility may also contribute to the cathartic effect.

CONTRAINDICATIONS AND SIDE EFFECTS

Sodium salts should be avoided in patients with congestive heart failure and edema, and in those on sodium restriction. Magnesium and potassium salts are contraindicated in patients who have renal insufficiency. Overdose of any of these preparations can cause significant electrolyte disturbances. Care must be taken to assure adequate fluid intake during and after administration of these laxatives, or dehydration may occur. Efficacy is also improved with good fluid intake.

DOSAGE

See Table 34-3 for proper dosage. Each dose should be supplemented with 12 to 16 oz water.

PEARLS AND PITFALLS

1. An enema or suppository 20 minutes after breakfast or dinner, followed by 30 minutes on the toilet, can psychologically and physiologically (via the gastrocolic reflex) help a constipated patient return to normal bowel habits.
2. Contact laxatives should be avoided in children; too-frequent use can result in dependence. A key task is to educate their parents about the normal variability in bowel habits.
3. Laxatives confer no benefit for weight loss, contrary to popular belief.
4. Exercise, a high-fiber diet, generous fluid intake, abdominal strengthening exercises, and education by physicians are of more benefit for chronic constipation than are contact laxatives.
5. A patient who is taking laxatives chronically should have the drugs discontinued gradually. Stopping the laxatives abruptly results in a flare of the constipation and possible impaction.
6. Some elderly patients have difficulty with defecation because of weak abdominal muscles. Elevating the feet on a stepstool while sitting on the toilet increases the pelvic tilt and improves defecation.
7. Surreptitious abuse of phenolphthalein laxatives can be detected by alkalinizing the stool. The proper method is to add one drop of 1N sodium hydroxide to 3 ml stool supernatant or urine. If a pink or red color develops, check for absorption in a spectrophotometer at 550 to 555 μm to confirm the presence of phenolphthalein. Also, further alkalinization with 10N sodium hydroxide should cause the color to disappear at higher pH levels.

Lubricants

The general population is preoccupied by the idea of constipation. An important cause of this preoccupation is the misconception that lack of a regular, daily bowel movement is associated with the accumulation of toxins and leads to various disquieting somatic complaints. The public frequently turns to over-the-counter preparations in an effort to avoid this dreaded condition. A time-honored, simple, and seemingly innocuous drug used quite often is the lubricant laxative—primarily mineral oil. In 1982, use of mineral oil accounted for 15 percent of all over-the-counter laxatives, at a total cost of over 55 million dollars.

Mineral oil is a complex mixture of saturated hydrocarbons derived from crude petroleum. It is a colorless, transparent, oily liquid with a specific gravity of 0.818 to 0.880 and is insoluble in water or alcohol. The palatability, and possibly the effectiveness, is improved when it is emulsified with acacia. It is also often combined with milk of magnesia, bulk agents, or contact laxatives.

PHARMACOLOGY

Absorption of mineral oil is negligible after rectal administration, but as much as 30 percent may be absorbed after an oral dose. Absorbed mineral oil is distributed to the intestinal mucosa, mesenteric lymph nodes, liver, and spleen.

Mineral oil coats the feces in the colonic lumen, decreasing water reabsorption. The increased water content adds to the bulk of the stool and softens it significantly. Emulsified mineral oil reportedly has better wetting properties than does nonemulsified mineral oil, and penetration of the feces may thus be enhanced. Enemas of mineral oil exert their effect by lubrication of the stool, penetration and softening of the stool, and simple physical distention of the rectum.

INDICATIONS

Mineral oil is indicated for softening of the stool and easing defecation. It should generally be used only for short periods of time. Ideal patients are postoperative or postpartum patients, or those for whom straining at stool should be avoided, such as patients who have had a myocardial infarction. Oral or rectal mineral oil is also the laxative of choice for fecal impaction.

Mineral oil has also been shown by Sondheimer to be effective in the management of chronic functional constipation in children. At the other end of the spectrum, Mulinos showed that an emulsion of equal parts of mineral oil and milk of magnesia was effective in chronic constipation of the elderly. However, there is some concern about the toxicity of chronic use, and therefore other laxatives, such as fiber supplements or osmotic agents, should be used for these long-term indications if possible.

CONTRAINDICATIONS AND SIDE EFFECTS

Pulmonary aspiration of mineral oil causes a lipoid pneumonia that can be severe or even fatal. Thus, it is contraindicated in debilitated patients who are at risk for aspiration, in patients with poor esophageal emptying (such as Zenker's diverticulum), and in those with gastroesophageal reflux disease.

Chronic mineral oil ingestion leads to lipogranulomas in the mesenteric lymph nodes, liver, and spleen. The clinical importance of these granulomas is uncertain, but rare cases of organ failure, possibly caused by mineral oil, have been reported.

A common complaint of patients taking mineral oil is anal leakage and secondary pruritus. This usually improves with a decrease in dosage and reportedly is less common with emulsion preparations. Chronic mineral oil use can also cause malabsorption of the fat-soluble vitamins.

DOSAGE

The adult dose is 15 to 45 ml mineral oil orally, or 60 to 150 ml rectally. Children over 6 years of age may take 10 to 15 ml orally, or 60 ml per rectum. The onset of action is usually within 6 to 8 hours after an oral dose.

For fecal impaction, give 30 ml mineral oil orally every hour while the patient is awake, until the oil begins to seep from the anus (usually within 24–48 hours). Mineral oil retention enemas can also be given, to soften the mass. At this point, digital disimpaction with 5% lidocaine jelly is safer, more comfortable, and more successful. Saline enemas and oral cathartics can then expel the remainder. Careful attention to good hydration is important. The risk of mineral oil aspiration can be minimized by keeping the patient upright and avoiding administration of doses within 2 hours of sleep.

PEARLS AND PITFALLS

1. Stool softeners such as calcium or sodium docusate should not be given with mineral oil. The stool softeners enhance mineral oil absorption.
2. Since mineral oil primarily acts by increasing the stool water content, good oral hydration is important and increases the efficacy of therapy.
3. To reduce the risk of mineral oil aspiration, it should not be given within 2 hours of bedtime.
4. Mineral oil should not be given chronically to pregnant patients (see Table 34-2). Administration for prolonged periods during gestation has been associated with vitamin K malabsorption and subsequent hypoprothrombinemia and hemorrhagic disease of the newborn.

Miscellaneous Agents

Several agents discussed in other chapters of this book are useful in the management of chronic constipation.

Polyethylene glycol–electrolyte preparations (see Chap. 38) have been used in several trials to effectively manage constipation. Daily doses of 250 to 500 ml have resulted in increased defecation without the side effects seen with the large volumes used for colonoscopy preparation. Since these preparations are osmotically balanced and do not result in absorption of sodium or other electrolytes, they are especially useful in patients with congestive heart failure and renal failure. Palatability is a problem, but can be improved by chilling and addition of flavored drink powders.

Cisapride (Propulsid) is the first promotility drug (see Chap. 36) that has efficacy in the colon. It increases colonic contractility by increasing slow-wave activity and duration of spike activity. Several trials have shown good results in constipated patients, without an overshoot into diarrhea. Parkinsonian patients, with their common problem of refractory constipation, and children with encopresis both have shown good improvement on cisapride. Tolerability was excellent in all studies.

Finally, lactulose has long held a place in the armamentarium of hepatologists for therapy of hepatic encephalopathy (see Chap. 29). The unabsorbable sugar is split in the colon by bacteria, thereby causing an osmotic catharsis that has proved useful in treatment of chronic constipation. In fact, along with fiber, lactulose is the optimal drug for long-term management because of its lack of systemic absorption. However, the price has been prohibitively high—fifty dollars to the pharmacist per 960-ml bottle. Lederle and associates showed in a recent double-blind study that the similarly nonabsorbable sugar sorbitol is as efficacious as lactulose, yet only costs five dollars for an equal quantity. Patients tended to have less nausea with sorbitol; bloating and flatulence were the same with both drugs.

PEARLS AND PITFALLS

1. Addition of Crystal Light to GoLYTELY, then chilling it, improves the palatability considerably.
2. Flatulence and bloating are common complaints with lactulose and sorbitol but will generally improve after several weeks of therapy.
3. Cimetidine will reduce the bioavailability of cisapride.

Suggested Reading

BULK-FORMING AGENTS

Almy TP. Dietary fiber: Current role in therapy and preventive medicine. Drug Ther 1984; 14:51–59.
A comprehensive review of dietary fiber's role in therapy and preventive medicine.

Almy TP, Howell DA. Medical progress: Diverticular disease of the colon. N Engl J Med 1980; 302:324–331.
An in-depth look at diverticular disease, its etiology, and its treatment.

Anderson JW. Dietary Fiber and Diabetics. In GV Vanhouny, D Kritchevsky (eds), *Dietary Fiber in Health and Disease.* New York: Plenum, 1982. Pp 151–165.
An excellent chapter on dietary fiber's effect on diabetes.

Burkitt DP. Dietary fiber: Is it really helpful? Geriatrics 1982; 1: 119–126.
A discussion on how fiber-rich diets can protect against large-bowel cancer, diabetes, and other diseases.

Burkitt DP. Fiber as protection against gastrointestinal diseases. Am J Gastroenterol 1984; 79:249–252.
A discussion of the importance of fiber in the prevention of gastrointestinal disease.

Burkitt DP, Meisner P. How to manage constipation with high-fiber diet. Geriatrics 1979; 2:33–40.
Valuable information on the treatment of constipation with high-fiber diets.

McClung HJ, et al. Is combination therapy for encopresis nutritionally safe? Pediatrics 1993; 91:591–594.
Children with encopresis are perhaps the most difficult to manage of all constipated patients. Combination therapy, with fiber, laxatives, and lubricants (mineral oil), is often employed, but had nev

been studied with regard to nutrition. In this paper, growth rates, serum chemistries, and vitamin levels were not affected over a 6-month course of treatment. Efficacy was excellent: 75 percent of patients had resolution of encopresis and were able to discontinue laxatives. Suprisingly, psychopathology was not a significant problem. Acceptance of fiber preparations required frequent changes in commercial and nutritional sources—a lesson we could use in the adult population.

Rouse M, et al. An open randomized, parallel group study of lactulose vs isphagul in the treatment of chronic constipation in adults. Br J Clin Pract 1991; 45:28–30.

A trial of osmotic versus fiber laxatives, showing that they were equally effective. Lactulose was judged slightly more tolerable (certainly it sounds better) but was more expensive.

Stephen AM, Cummings JH. Mechanism of action of dietary fiber in the human colon. Nature 1980; 284:283–284.

An excellent explanation of the effects of dietary fiber on the colon.

Talley NJ, et al. Gastroenterology 1991; 101:927–934.

An excellent study of colonic symptoms in 1021 residents of Olmstead County, Minnesota. This is one of the best overviews of colonic symptoms in the general U.S. population.

Tedesco FJ, et al. Laxative use in constipation. Am J Gastroenterol 1985; 80:303–309.

A paper by the American College of Gastroenterology's Committee on FDA-Related Matters reviewing laxatives and their use in the treatment of constipation.

CONTACT LAXATIVES

Castle SC, et al. Constipation prevention: Empiric use of stool softeners questioned. Geriatrics 1991; 46:84–86.

Home care patients were randomized in a double-blind crossover fashion to docusate or placebo. No difference was seen in symptoms or additional laxatives used.

Donowitz M, Binder HJ. Effect of dioctyl sodium sulfosuccinate on colonic fluid and electrolyte movement. Gastroenterology 1975; 69:941.

This study demonstrated that so-called stool softeners were actually mild contact laxatives, with fluid and electrolyte secretion mediated by cyclic AMP.

Smooth-Muscle Relaxants

C. Samuel Ledford and D. Michael Jones

Smooth-muscle relaxants are frequently used in the treatment of disorders of the gastrointestinal tract. Smooth muscle comprises the major muscular component of the upper and lower gastrointestinal tract. Therefore, these drugs would seem ideal for the treatment of symptoms related to increased tone or spasticity of the gastrointestinal tract. Gastrointestinal disorders treated with these agents include the disorders of esophageal motility, irritable bowel syndromes (IBS), and biliary dyskinesia.

Nitrates

Nitroglycerin, first compounded in 1846, has been used sublingually for angina pectoris for many years. Since the mid-1970s, it has been used for symptomatic improvement in patients with esophageal motility disorders.

MECHANISM OF ACTION

Nitroglycerin and other nitrate-containing compounds activate guanylate cyclase, increasing the synthesis of cyclic GMP (guanosine-3′,5′-monophosphate) in smooth muscle. The protein kinase produced by the interaction of guanylate cyclase with nitric acid alters the phosphorylation process in smooth muscle, resulting in dephosphorylation of the light chain of myosin and inhibition of the normal contractile process of smooth muscle.

INDICATIONS

Current use of nitrates in gastrointestinal disease includes treatment of patients with esophageal motility disorders and biliary tract dyskinesia (including spasm of the sphincter of Oddi), and relief of elevated biliary pressure in patients with T tubes. Gelfond and associates found that use in patients with achalasia leads to a maximum fall in the lower esophageal sphincter (LES) pressure up to 63.5 percent. This reduction in LES pressure led to improved esophageal emptying and decreased food retention within the middle and distal esophagus (documented by radionuclide cine studies). The most notable finding of this study was symptomatic relief of dysphagia in 86 percent (13 of 15) of the patients.

Swamy demonstrated prompt relief of symptoms and normalization of motility patterns after the sublingual administration of nitroglycerin in patients with diffuse esophageal spasm (DES) without associated gastroesophageal reflux. In follow-up ranging to 4 years' duration, patients remained symptom-free when managed on long-acting nitrates. In patients with DES and associated reflux, response to nitrates was found to be unpredictable. In these patients nitrates may serve as an adjunct to antireflux therapy.

A trial of nitrates should be considered in the treatment of sphincter of Oddi dysfunction. Bar-Meir and associates demonstrated that medical therapy for papillary dysfunction may be an alternative to endoscopic sphincterotomy. They studied a patient with an elevated basal sphincter pressure of 43 mm Hg and a phasic sphincter pressure of 158 mm Hg. Following administration of 0.65 mg nitroglycerin sublingually, the basal and phasic sphincter pressures dropped to zero within 90 seconds. Long-term treatment with long-acting nitrates led to resolution of the patient's symptoms and persistent reduction of the basal and phasic sphincter pressures to the normal range.

DOSAGE AND ADMINISTRATION

Isosorbide dinitrate (Isordil) is dispensed in sublingual and oral formulations. Sublingual therapy yields maximum plasma concentration in 6 minutes but has a rapid decay. Orally administered Isordil provides prolonged therapeutic effect, likely due to isosorbide-2-mononitrate and isosorbide-5-mononitrate, because these compounds have longer half-lives (2–5 hours).

Dosing Guidelines

Nitroglycerin	Sublingual: 0.4 mg at mealtime and as needed
	Spray: 0.8 mg at mealtime and as needed
Isordil	Sublingual: 5–10 mg before meals
	Oral: 10–30 mg 30 minutes before meals
Erythrityl tetranitrate (Cardilate)	Oral: 10–15 mg 30 minutes before meals

SIDE EFFECTS

The primary dose-limiting side effect of nitrates is headache, which may be severe. However, headache may improve with continued treatment and often resolves after 1 to 2 weeks of therapy. Unfortunately, decreasing the nitrate dosage in order to alleviate headache frequently leads to recurrence of symptoms. Other less common side effects include dizziness, weakness, and flushing. Orthostatic hypotension occurs and is accentuated by alcohol usage. See Table 35-1 for effects in pregnancy and breast-feeding.

PEARLS AND PITFALLS

1. Nitrates are not often given over the long term because (1) as many as two-thirds of patients discontinue their use because of side effects, (2) symptoms often recur even without dosage reduction, and (3) the sporadic nature of symptoms promotes noncompliance with the 3- to 4-times-a-day regimen.
2. Controversy exists regarding the efficacy of oral therapy in achalasia because prolonged esophageal transit is likely, resulting in delayed gastric absorption. If oral treatment fails, sublingual administration may be attempted before nitrate therapy is abandoned.
3. If a patient with sphincter of Oddi dysfunction fails to respond to sublingual nitrates, the etiology may be sphincter stenosis rather than a hyperdynamic sphincter.

Calcium Channel-Blocking Agents

Numerous clinical trials suggest that calcium channel-blocking agents may be effective in the treatment of disorders of gastrointestinal motility. These drugs effect a decrease in the contractility of

Table 35-1. Smooth-muscle relaxants: Pregnancy and breast-feeding

Agent	FDA pregnancy category	Risk vs benefit (by trimester)			Breast-feeding category
		1st	2nd	3rd	
Belladonna	C1	?	?	?	IIIB
Dicyclomine	D	?	?	?	IIIB
Nitroglycerin	D	?	?	?	IIIB

Food and Drug Administration (FDA) pregnancy categories:
A = Well-controlled studies fail to demonstrate risk to the fetus.
B1 = Animal studies fail to demonstrate risk to the fetus but no human studies are available.
B2 = Animal studies show some risk to the fetus but this is not confirmed in human studies.
C1 = Animal studies show risk to the fetus but no human studies are available.
C2 = Animal and human studies are unavailable.
D = Drugs associated with birth defects but with potential benefits that may outweigh known risks.
X = Drugs associated with birth defects and with potential risk that clearly outweighs potential benefit.
Risk vs benefit: R >> B = Proven or potential risk outweighs potential benefits.
B > R = Potential benefits outweigh potential risks.
R >> B? = Risks may be outweighed by benefits in some circumstances.
? = Risk-to-benefit ratio is unknown.
Breast-feeding categories:
I = Drug does not enter breast milk.
II = Drug enters breast milk but is not known to be harmful in therapeutic doses.
IIIA = Drug may or may not enter breast milk but no adverse effects are expected.
IIIB = Drug may or may not enter breast milk but drug is systemically absorbed.
IV = Drug enters breast milk and poses a potential risk to the neonate.

smooth muscle leading to (1) decreased amplitude of peristalsis, (2) decreased lower esophageal pressure, and (3) a significant reduction in the amplitude of esophageal contractions.

MECHANISM OF ACTION

Normal smooth-muscle contraction is dependent on calcium binding to calmodulin. This complex then activates myosin light-chain kinase, which results in phosphorylation of light-chain myosin. Phosphorylation promotes actin-myosin interaction, leading to smooth-muscle contraction. The blockade of calcium-ion influx during membrane depolarization by these agents leads to smooth-muscle relaxation.

INDICATIONS

Calcium channel blockers have been studied and are frequently used in the disorders of esophageal motility. Although few studies exist to document their efficacy, these agents have also been used in the treatment of sphincter of Oddi dysfunction.

Richter and associates reported the effects of nifedipine and diltiazem in the treatment of nutcracker esophagus. In a 14-week crossover study, 20 patients received oral nifedipine or placebo. A significant decrease in the amplitude of esophageal contraction was noted with nifedipine compared to placebo. However, nifedipine was no more effective than placebo in the relief of symptoms. In another study of 10 patients, diltiazem was associated with a significant decrease in the duration and amplitude of peristaltic contractions; in these patients, an 8-week uncontrolled trial of oral diltiazem demonstrated significant improvement in chest pain and dysphagia. Cattau and colleagues reported similar results with diltiazem in a randomized, double-blind crossover trial of 14 patients with nutcracker esophagus.

In a small group of patients with achalasia, Bortolotti and associates documented a significant reduction in lower esophageal sphincter pressure and relief of dysphagia after administration of sublingual nifedipine. Gelfond and colleagues reported good results in a study of 15 achalasia patients treated with sublingual nifedipine 30 minutes before mealtime; 53 percent reported improvement in dysphagia and chest pain symptoms.

Blackwell and associates documented that oral nifedipine decreased the amplitude and frequency of nonperistaltic contractions in patients with diffuse esophageal spasm, and decreased frequency of symptoms in 50 percent of patients. Thomas and colleagues demonstrated improvement in symptoms of dysphagia in patients with diffuse esophageal spasm treated with nifedipine before meals.

Guelrud and associates studied the effect of calcium channel blockers on the sphincter of Oddi. In patients with elevated basal sphincter pressure, sublingual nifedipine produced a marked decrease in basal pressure. Sand and colleagues conducted a 16-week, double-blind crossover trial of nifedipine in patients with suspected type II sphincter of Oddi dyskinesia; nifedipine produced a significant reduction in the number of painful days and need for analgesics.

Calcium channel blockers may have a role in the treatment of IBS. Blume and associates found that oral nifedipine significantly diminished the abnormal colonic motor response to distention seen in patients with IBS.

The use of these agents in long-acting/sustained-release preparations for the treatment of gastrointestinal disorders has not been studied.

DOSAGE AND ADMINISTRATION

Nifedipine is supplied as 10-mg capsules. It can be given orally or sublingually; the sublingual route is preferred for patients with achalasia. Therapy should begin with 10 mg 3 times a day for several days, with dose titration to relief of symptoms versus tolerance of side effects. Diltiazem is supplied in 30-, 60-, and 90-mg tablets; initial therapy is 30 mg 4 times a day, increased as necessary for symptom relief and as side effects allow. Maximum suggested daily diltiazem dose is 360 mg.

SIDE EFFECTS

The dose-limiting side effect of nifedipine results from vasodilation. In 10 percent of patients, peripheral edema, dizziness, flushing, paresthesias, nausea, vomiting, and sedation develop. Orthostatic hypotension (5%), headache (8%), palpitations (2%), and syncope (1%) may also occur. Contraindications to nifedipine include aortic stenosis (due to the potential for coronary steal syndrome secondary to vasodilation), hypotension, and known hypersensitivity to the drug.

Diltiazem has no effect on the peripheral vasculature, but significant atrioventricular conduction defects are possible. It is contraindicated in patients with sick sinus syndrome, second- or third-degree heart block, digitalis toxicity, and known diltiazem hypersensitivity.

PEARLS AND PITFALLS

1. The overall response rate for diltiazem and nifedipine in the treatment of diffuse esophageal spasm, achalasia, and nutcracker esophagus is approximately 40 to 50 percent.
2. Nifedipine is more effective for esophageal pain and dysphagia associated with achalasia. Diltiazem is more effective for the treatment of nutcracker esophagus.
3. Hypertensive lower esophageal sphincter syndrome, in combination with nutcracker esophagus, responds very well to nifedipine. Nifedipine (10–30 mg sublingually 30 minutes before eating) used with an anticholinergic such as propantheline (15 mg 30 minutes after meals and again at bedtime) for the treatment of diffuse esophageal spasm leads to an additive reduction in esophageal contraction amplitude and an almost additive reduction in the lower esophageal sphincter pressure.
4. The side effect profiles of diltiazem and nifedipine are very different. McCallum advocates combination drug therapy to avoid side effects that might occur with higher doses of either drug alone.

Dicyclomine Hydrochloride

Dicyclomine hydrochloride (Bentyl), the prototypical anticholinergic agent, has been used for the treatment of irritable bowel syndromes for many years.

MECHANISM OF ACTION

Bentyl is a nonspecific smooth-muscle relaxant. It reduces gastrointestinal tract smooth-muscle spasm by decreasing spontaneous smooth-muscle activity. Page and Dirnberger have demonstrated the antagonism of Bentyl for the stimulant effect of agonists such as bradykinin that act directly on smooth muscle.

INDICATIONS

Bentyl is indicated for the symptomatic treatment of the "spastic" component of irritable bowel syndromes. It is commonly used for the temporary relief of pain in symptomatic cholelithiasis, although this is not an approved indication.

In one controlled, double-blind, randomized trial involving 71 patients, Page and Dirnberger demonstrated that 84 percent of Bentyl-treated (and 54% of placebo-treated) patients reported a reduction in abdominal tenderness and pain associated with improved bowel habits. Six percent of patients taking Bentyl (compared to 35% of the placebo group) complained of an exacerbation of abdominal pain by the second week of the trial.

The response of esophageal motility disorders to anticholinergic therapy has been disappointing. However, some authors still recommend a trial of antispasmodics as the initial pharmacologic intervention for esophageal motility disorders.

The abdominal pain and cramping of Crohn's disease may respond to low-dose anticholinergic therapy. Confusion may arise should bowel obstruction occur during anticholinergic therapy; therefore, careful counseling is necessary if anticholinergic agents are used for symptomatic treatment of Crohn's disease.

DOSAGE AND ADMINISTRATION

Bentyl is available as 10- and 20-mg tablets, as a syrup concentrate, and in an injectable form. For irritable bowel syndromes, treatment should begin with 10 to 20 mg at bedtime and can be titrated to 4 times per day if necessary. Spasmolytic drugs will complicate constipation and should be avoided until the constipation component of the irritable bowel is corrected. In cases in which higher doses of Bentyl are required, the clinician should remember that the oral dosage form is most efficacious in alleviation of irritable bowel symptoms if given 30 to 60 minutes before meals and at bedtime on a daily basis (rather than sporadically). Intramuscular Bentyl is indicated only for short-term management of patients who can be given nothing by mouth. Injectable dosages should be reduced to half the usual oral dosage because of the increased bioavailability of the injectable form.

SIDE EFFECTS

The most common side effects are dry mouth, blurred vision, and dizziness, which occur in up to one-third of patients. Less frequently seen are decreased gastric secretions, urinary retention, and exacerbation of glaucoma. Forty-four percent of the patients in one study were able to tolerate the side effects without decreasing the dosage; between 10 and 15 percent of patients discontinue therapy because of side effects. Contraindications to dicyclomine therapy include obstructive uropathy, mechanical or nonmechanical bowel obstruction, hemodynamic instability, severe flares of ulcerative colitis with or without toxic megacolon, glaucoma, or myasthenia gravis.

Belladonna and Similar Antimuscarinics

Belladonna and its related compounds (atropine, Bellergal, etc.) are agents that inhibit the effects of acetylcholine on autonomic effectors innervated by postganglionic nerves and on smooth muscle that lacks cholinergic innervation. They antagonize the muscarinic effects of acetylcholine. Antimuscarinics are useful adjuncts in the treatment of peptic ulcer disease and as antispasmodics in hypermotility syndromes. They may play a role in the treatment of biliary dyskinesia in the near future.

The specific effects of the antimuscarinics vary, depending on the organ system discussed. Small doses decrease sweating, salivation, and bronchial secretions; modest doses cause pupillary dilation and increases in heart rate. Larger doses block parasympathetic control of the urinary bladder and gastrointestinal tract, leading to inhibition of micturition and decreased tone and motility of the gut. Even larger doses are required to inhibit gastric secretions and motility. Reduction in tone, amplitude, and frequency of peristaltic contractions in the stomach, duodenum, jejunum, ileum, and colon occurs when therapeutic doses of antimuscarinics are used. However, multiple side effects common to lower doses are often too severe to permit long-term use and result in poor patient compliance.

INDICATIONS

When used alone, antimuscarinics (e.g., atropine, 0.4–0.6 mg before meals sublingually) inhibit gastric acid secretion by 15 to 25 percent. When used with H_2-antagonists these agents greatly enhance the effectiveness of the H_2-antagonist. Unfortunately, at these higher doses adverse side effects such as pupillary dilation, tachycardia, gastric retention, urinary retention, and aggravation of glaucoma preclude widespread use. Conversely, pepsin secretion is blocked at relatively small doses. Agents in this class were previously used as adjunctive therapy in the medical treatment of gastrinoma when gastric acid hypersecretion was not controlled by H_2-receptor antagonists alone. Schuster recommends using anticholinergics with more antisecretory activity than spasmolytic activity when treating dyspepsia in patients with irritable bowel syndromes.

Garrigues and associates compared the effects of atropine, 0.5 mg intravenously, and pirenzepine, 10 mg intravenously (an antimuscarinic) on sphincter of Oddi (SO) motility. Atropine did not modify the basal SO pressure; the amplitude of the phasic contractions decreased very slightly, but the frequency of phasic contractions decreased significantly within 1 to 2 minutes after drug administration. Pirenzepine significantly decreased the basal SO pressure and the amplitude and frequency of the phasic contractions within 2 minutes of drug injection. The effect of pirenzepine was maintained for 3 to 6 minutes after onset of action.

At the present time, no study supports the use of an antimuscarinic drug as the sole agent in the treatment of duodenal ulcer disease.

DOSAGE AND ADMINISTRATION

Tincture of belladonna is dosed at 10 drops 4 times a day, and the dosage is increased as symptoms warrant or side effects permit. The dose of propantheline (Pro-Banthine) is usually 15 mg before meals and 15 to 30 mg at bedtime.

In addition to belladonna, there are many similar agents, some combining several drugs to provide anticholinergic and antispasmodic effects. Donnatal, a combination of phenobarbital, atropine, and scopolamine, is dispensed in capsule (1–2 capsules 3–4 times a day) and elixir (1–2 tsp 3–4 times a day) forms. It is used extensively in the treatment of motor symptoms associated with irritable bowel syndromes. Bellergal-S, a sustained-release agent containing phenobarbital, ergotamine, and alkaloids of belladonna, is prescribed as one tablet twice a day. There are several other agents in this class; it is best to become familiar with a few agents and their particular dosage regimens.

SIDE EFFECTS

Major side effects include xerostomia, cycloplegia, mydriasis, constipation, urinary retention, palpitations, tachycardia, bloating, and dysphagia. The first four side effects are dose-dependent, whereas the remaining side effects may occur at any dosage. Contraindications to the use of antimuscarinics include glaucoma, obstructive uropathy, achalasia, pyloric stenosis, gastric outlet obstruction, ileus, severe ulcerative colitis with or without toxic megacolon, and myasthenia gravis.

PEARLS AND PITFALLS

The majority of disorders discussed in the belladonna section, with the exception of the irritable bowel syndromes, are best approached using other, more proven and effective medications. The antimuscarinics are best used as adjunctive agents, considering their high incidence of unpleasant side effects.

Suggested Reading

Achem SR, et al. Current medical therapy for esophageal motility disorders. Am J Med 1992; 92 (suppl 5a):98–105.
A review of current medical treatment alternatives for the esophageal motility disorders.

Bar-Meir S, et al. Nitrate therapy in a patient with papillary dysfunction. Am J Gastroenterol 1983; 78:94.
The authors advocate a trial of nitrates to distinguish functional versus obstructive sphincter of Oddi pathology, performing sphincterectomy only if nitrates are not efficacious.

Benjamin SB, et al. High amplitude, peristaltic esophageal contractions associated with chest pain and/or dysphagia. Gastroenterology 1979; 77:478–483.
Report on seven patients with high-pressure esophageal peristaltic waves and chest pain. The authors define "nutcracker esophagus" as a mean peristaltic amplitude of 111 torr for patients who present with esophageal pain or dysphagia, or both.

Blackwell JN, et al. Effect of nifedipine on esophageal motility and gastric emptying. Digestion 1981; 21:50–56.
Nifedipine (10, 20, 30 mg) decreased mean esophageal contractile pressure 17, 38, and 49 percent in both normal patients and those with nutcracker esophagus.

Blume M, et al. Effect of nifedipine on colonic motility in the irritable bowel syndrome (abstract). Gastroenterology 1983; 84:1109.

Bortolotti M, et al. Clinical and manometric effects of nifedipine in patients with esophageal achalasia. Gastroenterology 1981; 80: 39–44.
Significant reduction of lower esophageal sphincter pressure and improvement in symptoms with sublingual administration of nifedipine was documented in this study of 20 patients.

Castell DO. Chest pain of esophageal origin. Drug Ther 1983; November:129.
The medical and surgical options are discussed for treatment of esophageal disorders.

Castell DO. Calcium channel-blocking agents for gastrointestinal disorders. Am J Cardiol 1985; 55:210B.
A discussion of the pharmacologic effects of verapamil, diltiazem, and nifedipine on animal and human subjects.

Drossman DA, et al. The irritable bowel syndrome: Review and a graduated multicomponent treatment approach. Ann Intern Med 1992; 116:1009–1016.
A thorough review of the irritable bowel syndromes.

Garrigues V, et al. Effects of atropine and pirenzepine on sphincter of Oddi motility. J Hepatol 1986; 3:247.
This double-blind, randomized trial with 10 patients demonstrated a significant reduction in sphincter of Oddi basal pressure and phasic contractions due to pirenzepine. Atropine did not alter the basal pressure significantly.

Geenan JE, Venu RP. Sphincter of Oddi Dysfunction in Diseases of the Liver. In L Schiff, E Schiff (eds), *Diseases of the Liver* (6th ed.) Philadelphia: Lippincott, 1987. Pp 1427–1433.
The pathophysiology and manometric abnormalities seen in patients with sphincter of Oddi disease.

Gelfond M, et al. Isosorbide dinitrate and nifedipine treatment of achalasia: A clinical, manometric, and radionuclide evaluation. Gastroenterology 1982; 83:963.
The study involved 15 patients and correlated clinical response to radionuclide-documented esophageal emptying time. The authors favor the radionuclide test meal as the most objective way to evaluate drug therapy in patients with achalasia.

Guelrud M, et al. Effects of nifedipine on sphincter of Oddi motor function in humans. Studies in healthy volunteers and patients with biliary dyskinesia (abstract). Gastroenterology 1991; 92: 1418.

Kahn AA, Castell DO. Managing esophageal chest pain once a cardiac cause is ruled out. J Crit Ill 1987; July:61.
Criteria for diagnosis and management of esophageal dysmotility syndromes are discussed.

Lebovics E, et al. Sphincter of Oddi motility: Developments in physiology and clinical application. Am J Gastroenterol 1986; 81:736.
A review of sphincter of Oddi motility, the effects of various gastrointestinal hormones and drugs on sphincter of Oddi function, and clinical use of the manometric data obtained.

McCallum RW. The management of esophageal motility disorders. Hosp Pract 1988; February 15:131.
An extremely thorough and informative review of esophageal motility disorders.

Needleman P, et al. Drugs for the Treatment of Angina. In A Goodman (ed), *Goodman and Gilman's The Pharmacologic Basis of Therapeutics* (7th ed.) New York: Macmillan, 1985.

A review of the mechanisms of action of nitrates and calcium channel blockers.

Page JG, Dirnberger GM. Treatment of irritable bowel syndrome with Bentyl. J Clin Gastroenterol 1981; 3:153.

A 2-week, double-blind trial to compare Bentyl and placebo. Bentyl, 40 mg 4 times a day, was superior to placebo; however, 60 percent of patients taking Bentyl (160 mg/day) reported adverse effects.

Richter JE, et al. Nifedipine: A potent inhibitor of contractions in the body of the human esophagus. Gastroenterology 1985; 89:549.

A comparison of nifedipine and placebo effects on LES and amplitude of esophageal contractions in normal patients as well as those with nutcracker esophagus.

Richter JE, et al. Oral nifedipine in the treatment of noncardiac chest pain in patients with the nutcracker esophagus. Gastroenterology 1987; 93:21–28.

Sand J, et al. Nifedipine for suspected type II sphincter of Oddi dyskinesia. Am J Gastrenterol 1993; 88:530–535.

A 16-week, double-blind crossover study that demonstrated a significant decrease in biliary-type pain in patients given nifedipine.

Schuster MM. Irritable Bowel Syndrome. In T Bayless (ed), *Current Therapy in Gastroenterology and Liver Disease.* St. Louis: Mosby, 1986. P 342.

A complete review of the treatment modalities available to patients with irritable bowel syndromes.

Short TP, et al. An overview of the role of calcium antagonists in the treatment of achalasia and diffuse esophageal spasm. Drugs 1992; 43:177–84.

Swamy N. Esophageal spasm: Clinical and manometric response to nitroglycerine and long acting nitrites. Gastroenterology 1977; 72: 23–27.

A study of 12 patients with esophageal spasm, which documented an excellent response to nitrates (in the absence of associated gastroesophageal reflux).

Thomas E, et al. Nifedipine therapy for diffuse esophageal spasm. South Med J 1986; 79:847–849.

An uncontrolled trial of nifedipine, documenting symptom improvement in patients with DES.

Traube M, McCallum RW. Calcium channel blockers and the gastrointestinal tract. Am J Gastroenterol 1984; 79:892.

An excellent review of various gastrointestinal disorders in which calcium channel-blocker therapy may be attempted.

Weiner N. Atropine, Scopolamine, and Related Antimuscarinic Drugs. In A Goodman (ed), *Goodman and Gilman's The Pharmacologic Basis of Therapeutics* (7th ed). New York: Macmillan, 1985.

Prokinetic Agents

J. Thomas Dorsey III

Domperidone

Domperidone (Motilium) is a benzimidazole derivative related to the butyrophenones and was developed in 1974. It is a specific dopamine antagonist with upper tract prokinetic and antiemetic properties similar to those of metoclopramide but without the central side effects.

PHARMACOLOGY

Good plasma levels are achieved after oral, rectal, or intramuscular administration. Peak plasma levels are seen 15 to 30 minutes after oral or intramuscular administration and 1 to 2 hours after rectal administration. The bioavailability varies with route, achieving 90 percent after intramuscular administration, but only 13 to 17 percent after oral administration because of significant first-pass hepatic and gut-wall metabolism. Animal studies show levels 2 to 8 times those of plasma in most tissues, but minimal levels in brain, placenta, and breast milk (Table 36-1). Domperidone circulates in plasma more than 90 percent protein-bound. Metabolism is primarily hepatic via oxidative *N*-dealkylation and glucuronide conjugation. After oral administration, 7 percent is excreted unchanged in the stool and more than 60 percent appears in the stool as metabolites excreted in bile. About one-third of the dose is excreted as metabolites in the urine. Only 1.4 percent of the dose is excreted as unchanged drug in the urine. Its half-life is 7.5 hours.

MECHANISM OF ACTION

Domperidone has a high affinity for gut tissue, especially the esophagus, stomach, and small bowel. It acts on gastrointestinal smooth muscle by antagonizing the effects of dopamine.

In the esophagus, parenteral domperidone increased the lower esophageal sphincter pressure in healthy volunteers by 15 to 20 mm Hg. The effects of oral domperidone in normal individuals and patients with reflux are less clear, and higher doses may be required for effect.

In the stomach, there is no effect on serum gastrin or volume and pH of gastric secretions. It decreases adaptive relaxation in the fundus and increases the amplitude and duration of antral contractions. Pyloric dilatation has been noted endoscopically. Both antroduodenal coordination and the amplitude, frequency, and duration of duodenal contractions are improved. The net effect is increased solid- and liquid-phase gastric emptying.

There is no appreciable colonic effect.

Antiemetic activity is mediated by two mechanisms. First and most important, domperidone provides a central effect, as evidenced by its antagonism of apomorphine-induced emesis at the level of the chemoreceptor trigger zone. Peripherally, enhancement of gastric emptying plays a role in its antiemetic activity.

Table 36-1. Prokinetic agents: Pregnancy and breast-feeding

Agent	FDA pregnancy category	Risk vs benefit (by trimester)			Breast-feeding category
		1st	2nd	3rd	
Cisapride	B1	?	?	?	IV
Domperidone	B1	?	?	?	IV

Food and Drug Administration (FDA) pregnancy categories:
A = Well-controlled studies fail to demonstrate risk to the fetus.
B1 = Animal studies fail to demonstrate risk to the fetus but no human studies are available.
B2 = Animal studies show some risk to the fetus but this is not confirmed in human studies.
C1 = Animal studies show risk to the fetus but no human studies are available.
C2 = Animal and human studies are unavailable.
D = Drugs associated with birth defects but with potential benefits that may outweigh known risks.
X = Drugs associated with birth defects and with potential risk that clearly outweighs potential benefit.
Risk vs benefit: R >> B = Proven or potential risk outweighs potential benefits.
B > R = Potential benefits outweigh potential risks.
R >> B? = Risks may be outweighed by benefits in some circumstances.
? = Risk-to-benefit ratio is unknown.

Breast-feeding categories:
I = Drug does not enter breast milk.
II = Drug enters breast milk but is not known to be harmful in therapeutic doses.
IIIA = Drug may or may not enter breast milk but no adverse effects are expected.
IIIB = Drug may or may not enter breast milk but drug is systemically absorbed.
IV = Drug enters breast milk and poses a potential risk to the neonate.

INDICATIONS

Delayed Gastric Emptying

Domperidone has been reported to decrease symptoms of delayed gastric emptying in a number of settings, including scleroderma, pancreatitis, reflux esophagitis, anorexia nervosa, and postsurgical states (e.g., postvagotomy).

Diabetic gastroparesis is a common clinical problem, and domperidone has been effective in decreasing symptoms and increasing gastric emptying in the majority of patients. Although there may be a loss of benefit with solid food emptying when it is taken chronically, symptoms seldom return.

In idiopathic gastric stasis or idiopathic postprandial dyspepsia, domperidone is effective in improving gastric emptying and relieving symptoms such as belching, distention, fullness, burning, nausea, and vomiting.

Nausea and Vomiting

Domperidone has shown activity superior to that of placebo in nausea and vomiting associated with pancreatitis, radiotherapy, hemodialysis, dysmenorrhea, and head trauma. It decreases nausea and other symptoms associated with the use of levodopa, bromocriptine, and nonsteroidal anti-inflammatory drugs. In migraine headache it appears to abort attacks as well as relieve the nausea associated with acute attacks. Although ineffective prophylactically against postoperative nausea and vomiting, it decreases frequency after the first episode.

Perhaps its most important role will be in the therapy of nausea and vomiting due to antineoplastic chemotherapy. Multiple studies have shown it at least as effective as metoclopramide in both adults and children, but with a much lower incidence of side effects.

Gastroesophageal Reflux Disease

Results of current trials are conflicting, with some series reporting symptomatic, endoscopic, and histologic improvement and others failing to show benefit on some or all of these parameters. It appears possibly useful, but larger, well-controlled trials are necessary.

Miscellaneous Indications

Domperidone has been shown to decrease variceal blood flow without the hyperaldosteronism seen with metoclopramide. The clinical benefits of this action have not been demonstrated. There are reports of efficacy in healing of peptic ulcer disease. Domperidone has also been used as a premedication for endoscopy, to decrease postprocedure nausea.

SIDE EFFECTS

Acute and chronic use are well tolerated in the majority of patients, with side effects seen in only 7 percent (versus 20% with metoclopramide). As it does not cross the blood-brain barrier, the incidence of neurologic side effects such as tardive dyskinesia, acute dystonic reactions, and sedation, which can occur in 10 percent of patients treated with metoclopramide, are rare. Occasionally, headache and nervousness are reported.

Transient, minor problems include dry mouth, thirst, skin rash, pruritus, and diarrhea.

Elevation of serum prolactin is common (10–15%), but usually clinically silent, although gynecomastia, mastalgia, galactorrhea, and amenorrhea can be seen. Women are affected more often than men, although gynecomastia and impotence have been reported. Domperidone antagonizes the dopamine-induced suppression of prolactin release. It does not appear to further exacerbate the high levels seen with acromegaly or prolactinomas.

There have been no changes in hematologic or biochemical parameters, including growth hormone and the renin-angiotensin-aldosterone system, with acute or chronic use.

Initial studies have shown no effect on heart rate, blood pressure, or electrocardiogram, but several reports of sudden death after high doses (60–200 mg) of intravenous domperidone for chemotherapy-induced emesis prompted further investigation. High-dose parenteral therapy causes prolongation of the QT interval, which can be complicated by *torsades de pointes,* ventricular tachycardia, and ventricular fibrillation.

To date, drug interactions are limited to decreased bioavailability when used with cimetidine and with bicarbonate or other antacids.

Animal studies have shown low concentrations in the fetus (see Table 36-1) and no tetratogenic or carcinogenic potential. Human studies have shown low concentrations in breast milk.

There is no accumulation in mild to moderate renal insufficiency. Few data are available on use in liver disease.

DOSAGE AND ADMINISTRATION

Domperidone is available as a 10-mg tablet and a 1% solution (0.3 mg/ml). It is available in suppository form in Europe. Parenteral forms were discontinued in 1984. It should be given on an empty stomach 15 to 30 minutes before meals. Concurrent H_2-blockers or antacids should be avoided. An oral dose in adults is 20 to 40 mg orally 4 times a day before meals, and in children, 0.3 to 0.6 mg/kg 2 or 4 times a day. In adults a 60-mg suppository 2 or 4 times a day is recommended.

Cisapride

Cisapride (Propulsid) is a benzamide derivative with a mechanism of action different from that of the antidopaminergic agents, thus avoiding their side effects. In addition, it is the first prokinetic drug to show activity in the colon.

PHARMACOLOGY

The drug is well absorbed after oral or rectal administration (95%). Food increases bioavailability by 30 percent. The bioavailability after an oral dose is 35 to 40 percent, indicating significant first-pass metabolism. Peak plasma levels occur at 1.5 to 2.0 hours. Cisapride circulates 90 percent protein-bound. It is extensively metabolized by the liver via *N*-dealkylation, aromatic hydroxylation, and glucuronide conjugation. Fifty percent of a dose is excreted as metabolites into the feces via bile, and the remaining 50 percent is excreted in the urine as metabolites. Its half-life is 14.9 hours. Animal studies show specific gut uptake but low levels in the brain and placenta. In animal studies the drug is secreted in breast milk (see Table 36-1).

MECHANISM OF ACTION

Cisapride has no antidopaminergic effects (unlike domperidone and metoclopramide). Its primary action is facilitation of acetylcholine release via an indirect cholinergic mechanism mediated by 5-hydroxytryptamine (5-HT4) receptor. It does not activate muscarinic cholinergic receptors. In addition, it displays activity as a serotonin antagonist in guinea pig intestinal mucosa.

In the esophagus, it increases both the amplitude of contractions and the lower esophageal sphincter pressure in normal individuals and patients with reflux. In the stomach, it stimulates digestive and interdigestive antroduodenal motility and coordination. It decreases adaptive relaxation of the fundus. As with domperidone, the increase in gastric emptying is accomplished without effects on gastric secretion. In the small bowel, both jejunal and ileal activity are increased in amplitude and frequency. A unique action is induction of propulsive activity in the colon, with increased slow-wave activity and increased duration of spike activity. Clinically one sees increased solid and liquid gastric emptying, decreased mouth-to-cecum transit time, and decreased colonic transit time.

As cisapride lacks antidopaminergic activity, its antiemetic activity is less than domperidone's and results solely from increased gastric emptying.

INDICATIONS

Gastroesophageal Reflux Disease

Cisapride was approved for symptomatic reflux of nocturnal heartburn due to gastroesophageal reflux disease in the fall of 1993. Cisapride has been shown equivalent to H_2-receptor antagonists in symptomatic relief and healing of mild to moderate esophagitis. No trials have compared it to omeprazole. It is superior to placebo for maintenance of remission of mild (grade I), but less so for moderate (grade II or III), esophagitis healed by cisapride or H_2-receptor antagonists. Combination therapy with cisapride and H_2-receptor antagonist is more effective (and expensive) than either alone. Cucchiara and associates showed cisapride superior to placebo in a randomized, double-blind trial in 20 children with reflux esophagitis. Improvement was documented by pH monitoring, endoscopy, and histology.

Gastroparesis

Cisapride has been studied in double-blind placebo-controlled trials in diabetic and idiopathic gastroparesis, with demonstration of benefit in both objective parameters and symptoms. Two such trials using doses of 30 mg every day failed to show benefit. Smaller uncontrolled trials have shown benefit in postoperative gastroparesis and the delayed gastric emptying associated with anorexia nervosa, scleroderma, and cystic fibrosis.

Nonulcer Dyspepsia

In this heterogeneous population, cisapride is superior to placebo and comparable to metoclopramide and domperidone in symptom relief. A therapeutic trial of Propulsid may provide benefit in a subset of these patients.

Postoperative Ileus

Verlinden and associates studied 118 postoperative patients in a placebo-controlled trial of intravenous cisapride at doses of 2 to 8 mg. The 8-mg dose repeated at 1 hour showed a significant increase in motility as documented by passage of flatus. Boghaert and colleagues studied 53 postoperative patients in a double-blind, placebo-controlled trial of cisapride, 4 mg intravenously. When two 4-mg doses were given 1 hour apart, 50 percent of patients developed bowel sounds and 43 percent passed flatus within the next hour.

Chronic Constipation

Muller-Lissner, in a randomized, double-blind, placebo-controlled trial of 126 patients with chronic constipation, showed that cisapride, 20 mg orally twice a day, significantly increased spontaneous bowel movements and decreased laxative use compared to placebo.

Chronic Intestinal Pseudo-Obstruction

Camilleri and associates showed increased pylorus-to-cecum transit in eight patients treated with cisapride, 40 mg/day, and Cohen and colleagues reported a case of pseudo-obstruction in a child that responded to cisapride but had been unresponsive to all other therapy. Studies by the same group failed to show symptomatic improvement in longer-term follow-up reports.

Miscellaneous Indications

Reports have indicated that cisapride may be of use in selected patients with irritable bowel syndrome, particularly those with predominant constipation. Other conditions that may be benefited include bile reflux gastritis, bowel dysfunction associated with spinal cord injuries, and maintenance of duodenal ulcer healing.

SIDE EFFECTS

Initial studies in over 1600 patients, including geriatric and pediatric populations, have shown a low incidence of side effects. The most common adverse effects, occurring in 4 percent of patients, are abdominal cramping, diarrhea, and increased flatus. No genitourinary symptoms have been noted.

Major neurologic side effects such as tardive dyskinesia and acute dystonic reactions have not been noted, and neurologic side effects are limited to headache and mild fatigue. There have been no changes in psychomotor function. Caution is justified in patients with seizure disorder.

On chronic therapy (mean > 2 months), 200 patients manifested no hematologic or biochemical abnormalities. No changes were noted in gastrin, insulin, or prolactin levels. Acute therapy stimulates the release of pancreatic polypeptide and cholecystokinin (CCK) via atropine-sensitive mechanisms, while chronic use causes diminished CCK release by an unknown mechanism.

Although no electrocardiographic changes have been seen, slight but significant elevations of systolic blood pressure and heart rate are noted.

Drug interactions are few. Cimetidine, ranitidine, and omeprazole, but not antacids, decrease its bioavailability. No changes in digoxin, propranolol, or tolbutamide bioavailability or action have been discovered. No change in prothrombin time of patients receiving warfarin (Coumadin) has been noted. It does increase the absorption of alcohol, particularly in the fed state. It also decreases the bioavailability of slow-release compounds.

Animal studies indicate low placental levels but human data are lacking. Although animal studies suggest that cisapride is secreted in breast milk, human studies show only very low levels.

DOSAGE AND ADMINISTRATION

Cisapride is available as 10- and 20-mg tablets. Oral dosages of 10 to 20 mg 4 times a day before meals have been utilized. A suppository form is available in Europe.

PEARLS AND PITFALLS

1. Domperidone, like metoclopramide, acts via dopamine antagonism in the upper digestive tract and chemoreceptor trigger zone, but does not cross the blood-brain barrier and has a much lower incidence of side effects. Cisapride has a novel mechanism of action in its facilitation of acetylcholine release in the myenteric plexus. Unlike domperidone and metoclopramide, cisapride enhances colonic motility.
2. Major indications for domperidone will be in the therapy of gastric emptying disorders, most notably diabetic and idiopathic gastroparesis, and as an emetic in the setting of cancer chemotherapy. Cisapride has less antiemetic activity but appears to be as effective in gastric emptying disorders. In addition, it shows promise in the therapy of postoperative ileus, chronic intestinal pseudo-obstruction, and constipation.
3. Both are well tolerated acutely and chronically. Neither demonstrates the extrapyramidal effects associated with metoclopramide. Domperidone causes elevation of prolactin levels, especially in women, and this may cause clinical symptoms. Cisapride has no effect on prolactin levels. Its major side effects are abdominal cramping and diarrhea.
4. Domperidone should be given on an empty stomach; concomitant use of cimetidine and antacid decreases bioavailability. Cisapride bioavailability is not decreased with antacids but is decreased with cimetidine. Both show first-pass metabolism.
5. Use during pregnancy and in nursing mothers has yet to be fully explored. Caution in these settings is appropriate.

Suggested Readings

Abell TL, et al. Long term efficacy of oral cisapride in symptomatic upper gut dysmotility. Dig Dis Sci 1991; 36:616–620.
A useful new agent.

Blum A, et al. Effect of cisapride on relapse of esophagitis. Dig Dis Sci 1993; 38:551–560.
Heals mild reflux changes as well as H_2-receptor antagonists.

Boghaert A, et al. Placebo-controlled trial of cisapride in postoperative ileus. Acta Anaesthesiol Belg 1987; 38:195–199.
Cisapride increases bowel sounds and the passage of flatus.

Brogden RN, et al. Domperidone. Drugs 1982; 24:360–400.
A comprehensive review of the pharmacology and clinical use of domperidone.

Camilleri M, et al. Effect of six weeks of treatment with cisapride in gastroparesis and intestinal pseudo-obstruction. Gastroenterology 1989; 96:704–712.
Transit is speeded up by cisapride.

Champion MC, Hartnett M, Yen M. Domperidone, a new dopamine antagonist. Can Med Assoc J 1986; 135:457–461.
A recent review of the clinical indications for domperidone.

Cohen NP, et al. Successful management of idiopathic intestinal pseudo-obstruction with cisapride. J Pediatr Surg 1988; 23: 229–230.
A case report of cisapride's effectiveness in a pediatric patient.

Cucchiara S, et al. Cisapride for gastroesophageal reflux and peptic esophagitis. Arch Dis Child 1987; 62:454–457.
Cisapride showed benefit in children according to pH monitoring, endoscopy, and histology.

Deruyttere M, et al. Cisapride in the management of chronic functional dyspepsia. Clin Ther 1987; 10:44–51.
A randomized, double-blind trial showing symptomatic improvement in 75 percent of subjects.

Dreuth JPH, Engels LGJB. Diabetic gastroparesis. Drugs 1992; 44:537–553.
A current review.

D'Souza DP, Reyntjens A, Thornes RD. Domperidone in the prevention of nausea and vomiting induced by antineoplastic agents. Curr Ther Res 1980; 27:384–390.
Domperidone is as effective as metoclopramide in this setting, without major side effects.

First International Cisapride Investigators' Meeting. Digestion 1986; 34:137–160.
A collection of abstracts covering pharmacology and clinical uses.

Galmiche JP, et al. Double blind comparison of cisapride and cimetidine in treatment of reflux esophagitis. Dig Dis Sci 1990; 35: 649–655.
Mild gastroesophageal reflux disease (GERD) can be managed equally well by either agent.

Horowitz M, et al. Effect of cisapride on gastric and esophageal emptying in insulin-dependent diabetes mellitus. Gastroenterology 1987; 92:1899–1907.
Chronic cisapride therapy is effective in diabetic gastroparesis.

Horowitz M, et al. Acute and chronic effects of domperidone on gastric emptying in diabetic autonomic neuropathy. Dig Dis Sci 1988; 30:1–9.
A study of domperidone in diabetic gastroparesis.

McCallum RW. Review of the current status of prokinetic agents in gastroenterology. Am J Gastroenterol 1985; 80:1008–1016.
An excellent overview of a variety of prokinetics.

McCallum RW. Cisapride: A new class of prokinetic agent. Am J Gastroenterol 1991; 86:135–149.
The mechanism of action of cisapride is explored.

Muller-Lissner SA. Treatment of chronic constipation with cisapride and placebo. Gut 1987; 28:1033–1038.
A study showing decreased laxative use and increases in spontaneous bowel movements with cisapride.

Rosch W. Cisapride in nonulcer dyspepsia. Scand J Gastroenterol 1987; 22:161–164.
Cisapride decreases symptoms in nonulcer dyspepsia.

Talley NJ. Drug treatment of functional dyspepsia. Scand J Gastroenterol 1991; 26 (S182):47–60.
An extensive review.

Tytgat GNJ, et al. Effect of cisapride on relapse of reflux esophagitis healed with an antisecretory drug. Scand J Gastroenterol 1992; 27:175–183.
Cisapride decreases relapse rate.

Urbain JL, et al. Effect of cisapride on gastric emptying in dyspeptic patients. Dig Dis Sci 1988; 33:779–783.
A study showing symptomatic and imaging evidence of improvement.

Verlinden M, et al. Treatment of postoperative gastrointestinal atony. Br J Surg 1987; 74:614–617.
Intravenous cisapride decreases postoperative ileus.

Gastroenterology Procedure–Related Drugs

Gastrointestinal endoscopy as a discipline is barely 2 decades old. Fiberoptics, the technology that led to endoscopy, was born when Curtiss discovered that by coating a glass fiber with glass of a lower refractile index he could achieve nearly total internal reflection. The transmission of an image then became possible. The first modern endoscopes were subsequently developed in the late 1960s. From that beginning, endoscopy has rapidly flourished; over 1 million endoscopic procedures were performed in the United States in 1982. Today, the endoscopist can utilize laser, thermal coagulation, endoscopic ultrasound, and a variety of other new technologies. Even fiberoptics are now becoming obsolete as video endoscopy and its new capabilities take over the market.

Amid this abundance of technology, it is easy to forget that an endoscopic procedure is basically just an interaction between patient and physician. And, as every experienced endoscopist knows, the key to a successful procedure is a relaxed, cooperative patient. This is accomplished by a thorough, understandable explanation of the procedure; a confident, reassuring manner and technique; and effective use of adjunctive medications.

The application of drugs for endoscopic procedures is an art learned very much like endoscopy itself: by first observing their use by an experienced endoscopist, then by a gradual accumulation of one's own experience. Unfortunately for the trainee, it is difficult to find a thorough discussion of gastrointestinal procedure–related drugs, even in textbooks of gastroenterology or endoscopy. This part is intended to help the trainee bridge the gap between naivete and experience; the pharmacology, indications, contraindications, side effects, and dosage are discussed for each drug used during endoscopic procedures. Even the experienced endoscopist can find some unknown facts or pearls that may contribute to effective daily practice.

Michael S. Gurney

Antibiotic Prophylaxis

Barry E. Herman and D. Michael Jones

With the introduction of gastrointestinal endoscopy, there has been increasing interest in the role of antimicrobial prophylaxis. To date, much of the emphasis in the literature has been on preventing endocarditis. To the practicing endoscopist prophylaxis for individuals with noncardiac conditions, such as the leukopenic patient, the cirrhotic patient, and the patient with prosthetic devices, is of clinical interest. This chapter focuses on recommendations for antimicrobial prophylaxis for endocarditis and selected noncardiac situations.

While it is well accepted that susceptible individuals should receive prophylaxis before undergoing procedures that are likely to cause significant bacteremia, controlled clinical trials are lacking. Due to the large number of patients that would be required, it is unlikely that such a study will ever be conducted.

Documented cases of distant infectious complications resulting from presumed bacteremia following gastrointestinal procedures have been reported in the English literature. As of August 1993, an estimated 12 cases of endocarditis had been associated with gastrointestinal instrumentation. Endoscopy with therapeutic modalities, such as sclerotherapy, laser, and dilation, has been associated with bacterial peritonitis, sepsis, and central nervous system infections, respectively. A recent study reported a significant association of "clinically significant" bacteremia associated with immunoincompetent patients undergoing endoscopy.

Due to the the lack of clinical trials, there has been controversy among various groups such as the American Heart Association (AHA), the American Society of Gastrointestinal Endoscopy (ASGE), and the American Society of Colon and Rectal Surgeons (ASCRS) regarding antibiotic prophylaxis. Since the initial AHA recommendations in 1965, guidelines have become less stringent and more uniform. An ASGE update is pending.

The decision to use prophylaxis should be individualized by taking into consideration (1) the risk of the procedure for producing bacteremia, (2) the microbial species involved, and (3) the patient's inherent risk (cardiac lesion, immunosuppression, ascites, etc.). The effects of various antibiotics in pregnancy and breast-feeding are listed in Table 37-6.

Bacteremia

Bacteremia is the presence of bacteria in the bloodstream without any systemic signs such as fever or hypotension. The frequency of bacteremia has been evaluated in both diagnostic and interventional gastrointestinal procedures (Table 37-1). The most bacteremic procedures are endoscopic retrograde cholangiopancreatography (ERCP) in the setting of an obstructed biliary tract, dilation, laser therapy, percutaneous endoscopic gastrostomy tube placement, and sclerotherapy. Of note biopsy, fulguration, and polypectomy are not associated with an increased risk of bacteremia.

Table 37-1. Incidence of bacteremia with gastroenterologic procedures[a]

Procedure	Bacteremia (%)
ERCP with obstruction	50
Dilation	45
Laser: neoplasm[b]/colonic stenosis/arterio-venous malformations (AVMs)	33/19/0
Percutaneous endoscopic gastrostomy (PEG)	24
Sclerotherapy	20
Barium enema	10
Banding	6
Colonoscopy	5
ERCP	5
Rigid sigmoidoscopy	5
EGD	4
Digital examination	4

[a]Percentages were obtained from several sources and should be viewed as estimates. Most procedures have been reported to have wide ranges of associated bacteremia. The specific organisms isolated during bacteremia are variable with respect to their affinity for tissue adherence.
[b]Esophageal neoplasms. Bacteremia may be from the passage of the endoscope rather than from the laser treatment.

A few important points should be considered when evaluating the reported incidence of bacteremia resulting from gastrointestinal procedures. First, most bacteremic episodes associated with gastrointestinal manipulation are brief in duration with low levels of bacterial concentrations. Second, bacteria most likely to adhere to the endocardium are *Streptococcus viridans, Streptococcus fecalis* (enterococcus), and *Streptococcus bovis.* The majority of organisms isolated are commensal gut organisms that adhere poorly to the myocardium and are unlikely to cause endocarditis. Third, patients with obstructed biliary tracts frequently have cholangitis with bacteremia before manipulation. Fourth, bacteremia in and of itself is not always "clinically significant"; it has been known to occur with 4 percent of rectal examinations as well as with tooth brushing. Finally, antibiotic prophylaxis has been associated with pseudomembranous colitis and fatal anaphylaxis.

Endocarditis Prophylaxis

In December 1990, the American Heart Association Committee on Rheumatic Fever and Infectious Endocarditis issued its latest recommendations concerning antimicrobial prophylaxis for prevention of bacterial endocarditis. Table 37-2 lists cardiac conditions for which prophylaxis is and is not recommended. Patients with mitral valve prolapse without a murmur but with thickening or redundancy of the leaflets by echocardiography may be at increased risk for endocarditis, and prophylaxis should be considered.

Table 37-2. Cardiac conditions for which endocarditis prophylaxis is and is not recommended[a]

Recommended:
- Prosthetic cardiac valves, including bioprosthetic and homograft valves
- Previous bacterial endocarditis
- Most congenital cardiac malformations
- Rheumatic and other acquired valvular dysfunction
- Hypertrophic cardiomyopathy
- Mitral valve prolapse with valvular regurgitations

Not recommended:
- Isolated secundum atrial septal defect
- Surgical repair without residual beyond 6 mo of secundum atrial septal defect, ventricular septal defect, or patent ductus arteriosus
- Previous coronary artery bypass graft surgery
- Mitral valve prolapse without valvular regurgitation[b]
- Physiologic, functional, or innocent heart murmurs
- Previous Kawasaki disease without valvular dysfunction
- Previous rheumatic fever without valvular dysfunction
- Cardiac pacemakers and implanted defibrillators

[a]This table lists selected conditions but is not meant to be all-inclusive.
[b]Individuals who have a mitral valve prolapse associated with thickening and/or redundancy of the valve leaflets may be at increased risk for bacterial endocarditis, particularly men who are 45 years of age or older.
Modified from AS Dajani et al., Prevention of bacterial endocarditis: Recommendations by the American Heart Association. JAMA 1990; 264:2920. With permission.

Table 37-3. Gastrointestinal procedures for which endocarditis prophylaxis is and is not recommended[a]

Recommended:
- Sclerotherapy for esophageal varices
- Esophageal dilatation

Not recommended:[b]
- Endoscopy with or without gastrointestinal biopsy

[a]This table is not meant to be all-inclusive.
[b]For patients who have prosthetic heart valves, a previous history of endocarditis, or surgically constructed systemic pulmonary shunts or conduits, physicians may choose to administer prophylactic antibiotics, even for low-risk procedures.
Modified from AS Dajani et al., Prevention of bacterial endocarditis: Recommendations by the American Heart Association. JAMA 1990; 264:2920. With permission.

Table 37-3 lists the gastrointestinal procedures that the committee believed resulted in bacteremia requiring prophylaxis; these include sclerotherapy of esophageal varices and esophageal dilatation. Routine endoscopy with or without biopsy or polypectomy were removed from the list of procedures requiring endocarditis prophylaxis. However, in high-risk patients with prosthetic valves, previous endocarditis, or surgically constructed systemic pulmonary shunts, prophylaxis may be considered for routine endoscopy. Of note, several endoscopic procedures with "significant" bacteremia are not discussed in the AHA recommendations (see Table 37-1).

Table 37-4 outlines the antibiotic regimens for endocarditis prophylaxis when gastrointestinal procedures are performed. Amoxicillin is recommended rather than ampicillin, because it is better absorbed, providing higher and more sustained serum concentrations. A follow-up dose given 6 to 8 hours after the procedure is considered optional by some authorities and is usually one-half the initial dose.

Nonendocarditis Prophylaxis

Traditionally, antibiotic prophylaxis has focused on the prevention of infective endocarditis. It is apparent that other subsets of patients undergoing gastrointestinal procedures may benefit from prophylaxis (Table 37-5). Bianco and associates have reported a significant increase in "clinically significant" bacteremia following endoscopy in 19 percent of immunosuppressed patients. Although there are no good controlled trials, these patients may be considered at high risk and antibiotic prophylaxis seems reasonable.

In a retrospective review Schembre and Bjorkman showed that patients with cirrhosis and ascites are at increased risk of bacterial peritonitis following esophageal variceal sclerotherapy. Because cirrhotics are immunocompromised and the mortality associated with bacterial peritonitis is high (50%), administration of antibiotics before endoscopic procedures in these patients seems reasonable, especially for procedures with high bacteremic risk (see Table 37-1).

Jain and associates reported that a single 1-gm dose of cefazolin given 30 minutes before placement of a percutaneous endoscopic gastrostomy tube reduced the incidence of local skin infection by 75 percent.

The complications of cholangitis or pancreatitis/abscess are a major concern in patients undergoing endoscopic retrograde cholangiopancreatography, especially when obstruction exists in the biliary or pancreatic ducts. The incidence of cholangitis and sepsis is increased after ERCP in patients with biliary obstruction. Sphincterotomy and stent placement may further increase these infectious complications. Antibiotic prophylaxis in this setting is appropriate.

Nonvascular prostheses, shunts, intraocular lenses, and tissue augmentation materials have a very low risk of causing infection secondary to gastrointestinal instrumentation, and routine prophylaxis is not recommended. Vascular grafts put the patient at increased risk during the first year after placement, and prophylaxis is appropriate; however, prophylaxis beyond the first year after vascular grafting is not necessary.

The antibiotics selected under each of these circumstances should be based on coverage for the most likely organisms to cause bacteremia during the procedure performed. Follow-up doses are optional, except when the patient has an obstructed biliary tract that cannot be drained (see Table 37-5).

PEARLS AND PITFALLS

1. Appropriate cleaning and disinfection of endoscopes is paramount in reducing infectious complications.
2. Attention to good oral hygiene is important in reducing endocarditis risks, especially in those with high-risk lesions.

Table 37-4. Antibiotic regimens for gastrointestinal procedures

Drug	Dosage regimen
Ampicillin, gentamicin, and amoxicillin	Intravenous or intramuscular administration of ampicillin, 2.0 gm, plus gentamicin, 1.5 mg/kg (not to exceed 80 mg), 30 min before procedure; followed by amoxicillin, 1.5 gm orally 6 hr after initial dose; alternatively, the parenteral regimen may be repeated once 8 h after initial dose
Ampicillin/amoxicillin/penicillin-allergic patient regimen*	
Vancomycin and gentamicin	Intravenous administration of vancomycin, 1.0 gm, over 1 hr plus intravenous or intramuscular administration of gentamicin, 1.5 mg/kg (not to exceed 80 mg), 1 hr before procedure; may be repeated once 8 hr after initial dose
Alternative low-risk patient regimen	
Amoxicillin	3.0 gm orally 1 hr before procedure, then 1.5 gm 6 hr after initial dose

*If the patient is allergic to penicillin and vancomycin, one might consider ciprofloxacin.

Modified from AS Dajani et al., Prevention of bacterial endocarditis: Recommendations by the American Heart Association. JAMA 1990; 264:2921. With permission.

Table 37-5. Nonendocarditis prophylaxis[a, b]

Clinical scenario	Prophylaxis	Agents[c]
Leukopenia/immunosuppressed	Yes	AMP/GENT
Cirrhosis with ascites	Yes	AMP/SULB[d]
PEG	Yes	Cefazolin[e]
ERCP/nonobstructed biliary tree	No	N/A
ERCP/obstructed biliary tree[f]	Yes	Cefoxitin/GENT
Vascular graft within 1st yr[g]	Optional	AMP/GENT
Nonvascular prosthesis[h]	No	N/A

PEG = percutaneous endoscopic gastrostomy placement; ERCP = endoscopic retrograde cholangiopancreatography; AMP = ampicillin; GENT = gentamicin; SULB = sulbactam or other penicillinase inhibitor; N/A = not applicable.
[a]See Table 37-2 for endocarditis recommendations.
[b]This chart is by no means all-inclusive and should not be considered absolute.
[c]See Table 37-4 for dosages of AMP/GENT and regimens for penicillin-allergic patients.
[d]One should attempt to avoid aminoglycosides in the patient with end-stage cirrhosis.
[e]Cefazolin, 1 gm IV, 30 min before procedure.
[f]Continue antibiotics if unable to adequately decompress.
[g]Do not confuse this with a surgically constructed pulmonary systemic shunt.
[h]Vascular grafts after 1st yr CNS shunts, lenses, tissue augmentation.

3. The issue on mitral valve prolapse without a murmur is still unsettled. The examination can be variable, depending on the examiner or the position of the patient. Should everyone get an echocardiogram to look for valvular thickening and redundancy?
4. Norfloxacin is used at some liver transplant centers in those with ascites who are waiting for a donated organ. Gines and associates have shown that selective intestinal decontamination with norfloxacin, 400 mg/day, reduced the recurrence rate of spontaneous bacterial peritonitis from 35 percent in the placebo group to 12 percent in the study group (average follow-up 6.4 months).
5. Soriano and colleagues reported that prophylactic norfloxacin, 400 mg twice a day, reduced the infection rate of cirrhotics who were admitted and endoscoped for an upper gastrointestinal hemorrhage. Infections developed in 10 percent of 60 study patients versus 37 percent of 59 control subjects. Documented peritonitis occurred in 2 treated patients and 4 controls.
6. If vancomycin is administered intravenously it must be given slowly over 1 hour to avoid the “red man syndrome” with flushing and hypotension. This is not a “true” allergic reaction.
7. In those patients who are truly allergic to penicillin and vancomycin, one may have to consider oral or intravenous ciprofloxacin for coverage of enterococcus. Ciprofloxacin, 500 mg orally, is equivalent to 400 mg intravenously. Used in combination with gentamicin, ciprofloxacin, 400 mg intravenously before the procedure and 200 mg intravenously after the procedure (or the oral equivalent), appears to be a reasonable alternative for endocarditis prophylaxis in the patient who is allergic to penicillins and vancomycin.

Table 37-6. Antibiotic prophylaxis: Pregnancy and breast-feeding

Agent	FDA pregnancy category	Risk vs benefit (by trimester)			Breast-feeding category
		1st	2nd	3rd	
Amoxicillin	C2	?	?	?	IIIB
Ampicillin	C2	?	?	?	IIIB
Cefazolin	B1	?	?	?	II
Cefoxitin	B1	?	?	?	II
Ciprofloxacin	C1	R >> B?	R >> B?	R >> B	IV
Gentamicin	C2	?	?	?	IV
Norfloxacin	C1	?	?	?	IIIB
Sulbactam	B1	?	?	?	IIIB
Vancomycin	C2	?	?	?	IV

Food and Drug Administration (FDA) pregnancy categories:
A = Well-controlled studies fail to demonstrate risk to the fetus.
B1 = Animal studies fail to demonstrate risk to the fetus but no human studies are available.
B2 = Animal studies show some risk to the fetus but this is not confirmed in human studies.
C1 = Animal studies show risk to the fetus but no human studies are available.
C2 = Animal and human studies are unavailable.
D = Drugs associated with birth defects but with potential benefits that may outweigh known risks.
X = Drugs associated with birth defects and with potential risk that clearly outweighs potential benefit.
Risk vs benefit: R >> B = Proven or potential risk outweighs potential benefits.
B > R = Potential benefits outweigh potential risks.
R >> B? = Risks may be outweighed by benefits in some circumstances.
? = Risk-to-benefit ratio is unknown.
Breast-feeding categories:
I = Drug does not enter breast milk.
II = Drug enters breast milk but is not known to be harmful in therapeutic doses.
IIIA = Drug may or may not enter breast milk but no adverse effects are expected.
IIIB = Drug may or may not enter breast milk but drug is systemically absorbed.
IV = Drug enters breast milk and poses a potential risk to the neonate.

Suggested Reading

Bianco J, et al. Prevalence of clinically relevant bacteremia after upper gastrointestinal endoscopy in bone marrow transplant recipients. Am J Med 1990; 89:134–136.

A retrospective review of 47 immunosuppressed bone marrow transplant patients who required upper endoscopy. "Clinically significant" bacteremia, defined as hypotension, fever (> 38.5° C), and positive blood cultures within 24 hours after endoscopy, occurred in nine (19%). Most of these patients were receiving prednisone or had graft-versus-host disease, or both.

Dajani AS, et al. Prevention of bacterial endocarditis: Recommendations by the American Heart Association. JAMA 1990; 264: 2919–2922.

The American Heart Association's latest recommendations.

Durack DT, Kaplan EL, Bisno AL. Apparent failures of endocarditis prophylaxis: Analysis of 52 cases submitted to a national registry. JAMA 1983; 250:2318–2322.

The authors report on 52 cases of endocarditis prophylaxis failures reported to the American Heart Association (AHA). Most cases had mitral valve prolapse, were associated with dental procedures, involved viridans streptococci and received antibiotic prophylaxis that did not conform to the AHA recommendations.

Gines P, et al. Norfloxacin prevents spontaneous bacterial peritonitis recurrence in cirrhosis: Results of a double-blind, placebo controlled trial. Hepatology 1990; 12:716–724.

In a multicenter, double-blind trial, the recurrence rate of spontaneous bacterial peritonitis was reduced in cirrhotics given norfloxacin, 400 mg/day (see Pearls and Pitfalls).

Jain NK, et al. Antibiotic prophylaxis for percutaneous endoscopic gastrostomy. A prospective, randomized, double-blind clinical trial. Ann Intern Med 1987; 107:824–828.

The authors report that during PEG placement prophylactic cefazolin reduced the rate of wound infection. Of the prophylaxed patients, 2 of 27 (7.4%) developed wound infections compared to 9 of 28 (32%) of those who did not receive antibiotic prophylaxis. The authors concluded that cefazolin prophylaxis significantly reduced the risk for peristomal wound infection.

Keefe EB. Antibiotic prophylaxis: Who, when, and how? Gastrointest Endosc Clin North Am 1993; 3:431–445.

A nice review of the antibiotic prophylaxis issue from the gastrointestinal literature.

Kohler B, Riemann JF. Incidence of bacteremia after endoscopic laser treatment of stenosing processed in the upper gastrointestinal tract. Am J Gastroenterol 1987; 82:1026–1028.

The authors report a 34 percent (11 of 32) incidence of bacteremia associated with laser of esophageal stenosing lesions. Two patients developed sepsis, one of whom expired.

Kullman E, et al. Bacteremia following diagnostic and therapeutic ERCP. Gastrointest Endosc 1992; 38:444–449.

One hundred ninety-four ERCPs were performed. Bacteremia was reported in 19 of 126 (15%) of diagnostic procedures and 18 of 68 (27%) of therapeutic ERCPs. Complication rates did not differ between the two groups.

Neu HC, Fleischer D. Recommendations for antibiotic prophylaxis before endoscopy. Am J Gastroenterol 1989; 84:1488–1491.
The authors' individual views on the controversies surrounding the issue of antibiotic prophylaxis and endoscopy.

O'Connor HJ. Risk of sepsis in endoscopic procedures. Gastrointest Endosc Clin North Am 1993; 3:459–467.
A brief summary of serious infectious complications associated with diagnostic and therapeutic endoscopic procedures.

Schembre D, Bjorkman DJ. Post sclerotherapy bacterial peritonitis. Am J Gastroenterol 1991; 86:481–486.
A retrospective review of 213 sclerotherapy sessions for esophageal varices. Six cases of postprocedure peritonitis were noted (3%). No patients who received antibiotics during the procedure developed peritonitis.

Schembre D, Bjorkman DJ. Review article: Endoscopy related infections. Aliment Pharmacol Ther 1993; 7:347–355.
An excellent review of infections related to endoscopic procedures. Contains 115 references.

Scott NA, Tweedle DEF. Pyogenic arthritis of the knee following Nd:YAG laser destruction of esophageal cancer. Gastrointest Endosc 1990; 36:545–546.
A case report.

Shovoron PJ, et al. Gastrointestinal instrumentation, bacteremia, and endocarditis. Gut 1993; 24:1078–1093.
An extensive review of the literature for studies concerning the incidence of bacteremia and endocarditis associated with gastrointestinal procedures. The authors concluded that prophylaxis is a matter of individual judgment.

Shrake PD, Troiano F, Rex DK. Peritonitis following colonoscopy in a cirrhotic with ascites. Am J Gastroenterol 1989; 84:453–454.
A case report.

Sontheimer J, et al. Bacteremia following operative endoscopy of the upper gastrointestinal tract. Endoscopy 1991; 23:67–72.
The authors report the bacteremic rates for 160 patients undergoing surgical endoscopy of the upper gastrointestinal tract. They also include an excellent review of the literature.

Soriano G, et al. Norfloxacin prevents bacterial infection in cirrhotics with gastrointestinal hemorrhage. Gastroenterology 1992; 103: 1267–1272.
In a prospective randomized trial, the authors showed that selective intestinal decontamination prevented peritonitis and extraperitoneal infections in cirrhotic inpatients given norfloxacin, 400 mg/day.

Standards of Training and Practice Committee, American Society for Gastrointestinal Endoscopy. Infection control during gastrointestinal endoscopy: Guidelines for clinical application. Gastrointest Endosc 1988; 34 (suppl):37S–40S.

Standards Task Force, American Society of Colon and Rectal Surgeons. Practice parameters for antibiotic prophylaxis to prevent infective endocarditis or infected prosthesis during colon and rectal endoscopy. Dis Colon Rectum 1992; 35:277–285.
The ASCRS's latest antibiotic prophylaxis recommendations.

Wolf D, Fleischer D, Sivak MV. Incidence of bacteremia with selective upper gastrointestinal endoscopic laser therapy. Gastrointest Endosc 1985; 31:247–250.

Bacteremia was noted to occur during laser therapy of upper gastrointestinal lesions: neoplasms in 8 of 26 sessions (31%) and AVMs in 0 of 8 sessions (0%). The authors believed that the bacteremic episodes were related to mucosal disruption with passage of the endoscope rather than laser applications.

Purgatives

Thomas A. Dowgin

Polyethylene Glycol–Electrolyte Lavage Solutions

Early endoscopists adopted the standard bowel preparation devised by surgeons and radiologists, that is, 48 to 72 hours of clear liquids and laxatives, often followed by several enemas preprocedure. Patients complained of the inconvenience, dietary constraints, abdominal cramping, and anal irritation. Significant dehydration was a problem, especially in elderly patients. The preparation was occasionally inadequate, necessitating rescheduling of the study and repeat bowel prep.

In the late 1960s, oral whole-gut irrigation with high volumes (3–4 liters/hour) of isotonic solutions—the oral electrolyte-overload method—was introduced. This technique was very promising; rapid, effective colon cleansing was achieved. However, absorption of 1 to 2 liters of normal saline was common. Because of potential fluid volume and electrolyte changes, oral electrolyte-overload colon cleansing was not recommended for cardiac or renal patients.

In 1980, Davis and associates introduced a polyethylene glycol–electrolyte lavage solution (PEG-ELS). This preparation, with sulfate and polyethylene glycol added to create a nonabsorbable iso-osmotic solution, was capable of improved colonic cleansing in a shorter period of time, better patient tolerance, and minimal fluid or electrolyte shifts. Whether obtained commercially (GoLYTELY from Braintree in Braintree, MA, or Colyte from Reed & Carnrick in Piscataway, NJ) or made locally, PEG-ELS has become a preferred bowel preparation for colonoscopy, as well as for barium enema, intravenous pyelography, and colon surgery.

MECHANISM OF ACTION

Active absorption of sodium across the intestinal mucosa occurs when the accompanying anion is chloride. In designing a solution with sodium *sulfate* as the predominant salt, Davis and associates found that sodium absorption was markedly reduced, with the sulfate anion being very poorly absorbed. Isonatremic solutions of sodium sulfate, however, are hypo-osmotic to plasma because plasma anions are monovalent, whereas sulfate is divalent. Therefore, a nonabsorbable solute was added (mannitol initially) to create an iso-osmotic solution that, after ingestion, caused no net absorption or secretion of water. Mannitol presented a problem in that it is fermentable by colonic bacteria, with resultant production of hydrogen gas capable of exploding during colonoscopic cauterization. Polyethylene glycol, with negligible absorption and metabolism by colonic flora, was chosen to replace mannitol as the nonelectrolyte osmotic additive. Explosions after the use of PEG-ELS have not been reported. A study collecting colonic gas samples after PEG-ELS lavage found that the concentrations of explosive gases are well below hazardous levels.

In 1990, Fordtran and associates modified the standard PEG-ELS in an attempt to reduce the salty taste and thus improve palatability. They removed sodium sulfate, slightly increased the concentration of PEG, and made minor adjustments in the concentration of other ions (Table 38-1). This sulfate-free PEG solution (SF-ELS), marketed as NuLYTELY (Braintree), retains the advantage of negligible water or electrolyte absorption or secretion. The SF-ELS is as efficacious as the standard PEG-ELS with respect to colonic cleanliness and patient tolerance; its claim to improved palatability, however, is debatable. Although one study indicated a patient preference for the SF-ELS over the original solution, two well-designed Swiss studies refute this claim. They found no significant patient preference for one solution over the other; in fact, patients could not reliably distinguish which solution was low sodium.

DOSAGE AND ADMINISTRATION

PEG-ELS can be given orally or by nasogastric tube. It is usually given the afternoon before the examination, after a clear-liquid lunch. Patients should drink approximately 1 liter/hour (about 8 oz every 10 minutes), to a total of 4 liters or until the rectal effluent is clear and particle-free. The first bowel movement occurs about 1 hour after beginning lavage. Patients should be reminded to take nothing but clear liquids by mouth once the prep has started and until the study is completed. Alternatively, for patients who require close supervision or hospitalization, the lavage can be done the morning of the study, allowing at least a 1-hour postlavage waiting period before the procedure is performed.

Most manufacturers recommend against adding compounds (sweeteners, nutritional supplements) to the PEG-ELS. Sugars can result in increased electrolyte and fluid absorption; they can also allow for colonic fermentation with production of hydrogen and methane gas, negating the nonexplosive efficacy of PEG-ELS.

EFFICACY

Multiple clinical trials have shown PEG-ELS to be equal or superior to standard bowel preparations in colonic cleansing, with no significant changes in patient weight, or hematologic or biochemical parameters. It has been safely used in patients with congestive heart failure (CHF), renal failure, diabetes, cirrhosis, and pulmonary disease. Most studies show a clear patient preference for PEG-ELS over standard bowel preparations. Specifically, patients like the shorter prep, dietary freedom, and avoidance of enemas. However, about 10 percent will not tolerate PEG-ELS, either because of the taste or the volume of fluid that must be ingested.

Before PEG-ELS, early colonoscopy in the evaluation of acute hematochezia was technically limited by a poorly prepared colon. Rapid bowel cleansing by PEG-ELS is well tolerated in acute hematochezia and allows for adequate colonoscopy, with electrocautery if necessary.

It should be noted that, with respect to the histology of biopsy specimens, standard bowel preparations can flatten the surface epithelial cells and deplete goblet cells, whereas PEG-ELS preserves normal mucosal histology. Colonic mucosal tissue activity levels of ornithine decarboxylase (a possible marker for colonic neoplasia) are not affected by peroral PEG-ELS, whereas a twofold increase over baseline is seen after phosphate enema preparation. However,

Table 38-1. Composition of solutions

Solution	Na (mEq/liter)	K (mEq/liter)	Cl (mEq/liter)	HCO_4 (mEq/liter)	PEG		Osmolality (mOsm/kg)
					SO_4 (mEq/liter)	3350 (gm/liter)	
PEG-ELS	125	10	35	20	40	60	280
SF-ELS	65	5	53	17	0	105	288

PEG-ELS may interfere with the detection of tumor-associated antigens (via enzyme-linked immunosorbent assay) in colonic effluent. Interestingly, cytologic analysis of the clear rectal effluent after oral PEG-ELS has very high sensitivity and specificity for the diagnosis of colon cancer. The stool microflora is not affected by peroral PEG-ELS.

It is common to retain 0.5 to 1.0 liter of lavage fluid in the colon postprep. This residual fluid can usually be removed with endoscopic suction. There is less retained fluid when PEG-ELS is given the night before the procedure. This retained fluid interferes with mucosal coating during barium enema. Thus, PEG-ELS alone is not an adequate prep for barium enema, but the addition of bisacodyl (20 mg orally after PEG-ELS) makes oral lavage as good as the standard prep for barium enema. Post PEG-ELS bisacodyl has also been shown to improve colonoscopically judged bowel cleanliness. Furthermore, giving oral senna extract (or even bisacodyl) several hours before PEG-ELS has been shown to improve the prep and may result in less required volume of PEG-ELS for adequate cleaning.

Several small studies using PEG-ELS in children (10 months to 19 years old) have shown good tolerance, excellent bowel cleansing, and clinical safety. Slight, statistically significant, but clinically insignificant, changes in blood and urine chemistries were noted after PEG-ELS in one study. Vital signs were unchanged by administration of PEG-ELS to children. Encopretic children also tolerated it well. PEG-ELS is also efficacious in the elderly, although one study noted that patients over 75 years old tended to tolerate an enema-based preparation better than PEG-ELS.

SIDE EFFECTS AND CONTRAINDICATIONS

PEG-ELS is contraindicated in patients with ileus, bowel perforation, toxic colitis, and gastrointestinal obstruction. Two patients with large rectal carcinomas suffered colonic perforation with oral lavages.

Initial concern over the toxicity and possible carcinogenicity of absorbed PEG has not been borne out by clinical data. PEG 3350 is a mixture of different-sized molecules with a mean molecular weight between 3200 and 3700. The higher-molecular-weight PEGs (> 1000) have little or no gut absorption. Urinary excretion of PEG after oral lavage is minimal and is similar for normal individuals and patients with inflammatory bowel disease (IBD). Likewise, urinary sulfate excretion after lavage is not significantly changed from baseline. Thus, the potential toxicity from absorbed PEG or sulfate during PEG-ELS lavage is very low. Nevertheless, isolated cases of dermatitis and urticaria have occurred, as well as one case of PEG-ELS–related anaphylaxis. Therefore, the minimal gut absorption of the solution can, very rarely, be clinically significant.

Patients most commonly complain of nausea, abdominal fullness, and occasional abdominal cramps and vomiting. There have been several case reports of Mallory-Weiss tears precipitated by emesis during PEG-ELS lavage. In addition, two cases of Boerhaave syndrome have been reported following PEG-ELS–related emesis, though one occurred with too-rapid ingestion of the solution. In another report, two patients who complained of severe abdominal pain and emesis during peroral lavage were later found to have significant underlying gastroduodenal disease. Hence, beware of patients with a history of PEG-ELS–related emesis; it may indicate the presence of underlying upper gastrointestinal pathology, or it may predict patients at risk for emetogenic complications with subsequent lavage.

Lavage-induced pill malabsorption has been described. An elderly man took his procainamide tablet 1 hour before ingesting PEG-ELS. At colonoscopy 4 hours later, the intact tablet was found in the descending colon. Thus, patients should take essential medications more than 1 hour before starting colonic lavage.

There is a case report of reversible cardiac asystole occurring after a large bowel movement during 1-liter/hour PEG-ELS peroral colonic lavage in an elderly man presenting with massive hematochezia. The arrest was thought to be secondary to increased vagal tone in a patient with underlying sinoatrial node disease. This episode prompted a study in which 22 patients underwent continuous electrocardiographic (ECG) monitoring during a control period, during bowel preparation with chilled PEG-ELS, and during colonoscopy. In approximately half of the patients tested, an increase in ventricular ectopy was noted during the colonic lavage period. ECG changes included short runs of ventricular tachycardia (two patients) as well as complex ventricular ectopy without ventricular tachycardia, and significantly increased premature ventricular contractions (PVCs; Lown class IA in four patients, class II in one patient, and class IVA in four patients). All patients remained asymptomatic, and all were elderly. No electrolyte abnormalities were noted, and not all had documented heart disease. In patients with or without ischemic heart disease, the significance of this ectopy is unknown.

PEARLS AND PITFALLS

1. Supplemental simethicone, as a split oral dose before and after PEG-ELS, significantly reduces the amount of colonic foam noted on subsequent colonoscopy. The amount of residual stool is also reduced. The same results are obtained if the simethicone is added to the PEG-ELS (about 120 mg simethicone per 4 liters of PEG-ELS). Patients may also tolerate the lavage better with the addition of simethicone.
2. Patients, particularly the elderly, complain of difficulty ingesting a sufficient amount of PEG-ELS in the required time. This problem can usually be avoided by dividing the dose, giving one-half the evening before and the other half the morning of the study. No difference in bowel cleanliness has been seen between the single and split-dose regimens.
3. The salty taste of PEG-ELS may be disagreeable. The solution is made more palatable by chilling it before ingestion. Note that mild hypothermia developed in a 66-year-old man after he drank 5 liters of chilled PEG-ELS. During cold weather, sufficient care should be taken to minimize this potential complication.
4. Irrespective of manufacturers' recommendations, it has been shown that adding one tub (17 ml) of lemon-flavored Crystal Light Sugar-Free drink mix to 4 liters of PEG-ELS markedly improves palatability as compared to both plain PEG-ELS and SF-ELS. The addition of this flavoring does not affect the color of the colonic mucosa, the rectal effluent, or the quality of the colon prep. A pineapple-flavored solution is also available (Reed & Carnrick); its palatability has not been thoroughly studied.
5. The routine addition of enemas to PEG-ELS increases patient discomfort and does not improve colon preparation over PEG-

ELS alone. Supplementary precolonoscopy enemas may rarely be necessary after incomplete PEG-ELS ingestion or when significant diverticular disease results in retention of feculent debris.

Oral Sodium Phosphate Solution

In 1990, Vanner and associates first reported the safety and efficacy of an oral sodium phosphate (NaP) solution as a colonic purgative. The relatively small-volume solution was developed in an attempt to find an alternative to PEG-ELS for those patients who could not tolerate drinking a gallon of PEG fluid. The cathartic action of NaP is thought to occur primarily secondary to its osmotic effect. Marketed as Fleet Phospho-Soda, it contains 48 gm $Na(PO_4)_2$ plus 18 gm $NaHPO_4$/dl.

DOSAGE AND ADMINISTRATION

A clear-liquid diet is recommended on the day before the procedure; then, at 7 P.M., the patient drinks 45 ml of the NaP solution diluted with one-half glass of water to 90 ml. This is followed by ingestion of at least three 8-oz glasses of water before retiring. Only clear liquids are allowed until the procedure is completed. The following morning (examination day), at 6 A.M., another 90 ml of diluted NaP solution is ingested.

EFFICACY

In a trial of 102 inpatient colonoscopies, Vanner and associates found that patients clearly preferred NaP solution over PEG-ELS. No differences were seen in lavage-related symptoms or palatability; patients apparently preferred NaP because of the smaller volume of fluid ingested. Colonoscopists judged the cleanliness of the colon to be superior in the NaP group as compared to the PEG-ELS group. However, there was more retained colonic fluid after the NaP preparation. An asymptomatic increase in the serum phosphate by 3.5 mg/dl was noted a few hours after the second dose of NaP. The serum phosphate returned to normal within 24 hours. No concomitant change occurred in the serum calcium level, and there were no clinically significant changes in hemodynamic parameters, body weight, or other biochemical parameters with the NaP solution. Interpretation of colonic mucosal histology was not affected by the NaP purge.

Another well-designed study (Kolts et al.) confirmed the superiority of NaP over PEG-ELS with respect to patient acceptance and colonic cleanliness. However, Marshall and associates, in another large trial, found no difference in the overall quality of the bowel preparation between NaP and PEG-ELS, although, again, patients found the NaP prep easier to tolerate.

SIDE EFFECTS AND CONTRAINDICATIONS

Oral NaP solution is not recommended for use in patients with renal insufficiency (serum creatinine > 2.0 mg/dl), CHF, ascites, bowel obstruction, or ileus. Also, it should not be used in pregnant or breast-feeding women (Table 38-2). There is no information available on its use in inflammatory bowel disease.

Beware, there is a case report of fatal hyperphosphatemia occurring in a 64-year-old man with colonic ileus and renal insuffi-

Table 38-2. Purgatives: Pregnancy and breast-feeding

Agent	FDA pregnancy category	Risk vs benefit (by trimester)			Breast-feeding category
		1st	2nd	3rd	
Polyethylene glycol purge	C2	?	?	?	IIIA
Fleet Phospho-Soda	C2	?	?	?	IIIA

Food and Drug Administration (FDA) pregnancy categories:
A = Well-controlled studies fail to demonstrate risk to the fetus.
B1 = Animal studies fail to demonstrate risk to the fetus but no human studies are available.
B2 = Animal studies show some risk to the fetus but this is not confirmed in human studies.
C1 = Animal studies show risk to the fetus but no human studies are available.
C2 = Animal and human studies are unavailable.
D = Drugs associated with birth defects but with potential benefits that may outweigh known risks.
X = Drug associated with birth defects and with potential risk that clearly outweighs potential benefit.
Risk vs benefit: R >> B = Proven or potential risk outweighs potential benefits.
B > R = Potential benefits outweigh potential risks.
R >> B? = Risks may be outweighed by benefits in some circumstances.
? = Risk-to-benefit ratio is unknown.
Breast-feeding categories:
I = Drug does not enter breast milk.
II = Drug enters breast milk but is not known to be harmful in therapeutic doses.
IIIA = Drug may or may not enter breast milk but no adverse effects are expected.
IIIB = Drug may or may not enter breast milk but drug is systemically absorbed.
IV = Drug enters breast milk and poses a potential risk to the neonate.

ciency who was given over twice the recommended dose of NaP, along with 4 liters of PEG-ELS. This complication is easily avoidable if the above-noted contraindications are followed.

PEARLS AND PITFALLS

1. As efficacious as PEG-ELS is as a bowel preparation, NaP is considerably (at least 3 times) cheaper than PEG-ELS.
2. Avoid using NaP solution in patients with renal, heart, or liver insufficiency.
3. There may be a tendency toward hypovolemia with NaP; ensure adequate hydration during NaP catharsis.
4. It is recommended that 3 hours elapse after the morning dose of NaP before colonoscopy is performed. This may interfere with the scheduling of early-morning procedures, especially when accounting for patients who are waiting for the acute purgative effects to subside before traveling to the endoscopy unit.

Suggested Reading

POLYETHYLENE GLYCOL–ELECTROLYTE LAVAGE SOLUTIONS

Brady CE III, et al. Urinary excretion of PEG 3350 and sulfate after gut lavage with a PEG-ELS. Gastroenterology 1986; 6:1914.
A study showing that there is minimal absorption of these compounds after oral lavage in either normal individuals or patients with IBD.

Brinberg DE, Stein J. Mallory-Weiss tear with colonic lavage (letter). Ann Intern Med 1986; 6:894.
The first report of a PEG-ELS–associated Mallory-Weiss (MW) tear.

Caos A, et al. Colonoscopy after GoLYTELY preparation in acute rectal bleeding. J Clin Gastroenterol 1986; 1:46.
Urgent colonoscopy in 35 patients with acute hematochezia was well tolerated, with excellent mucosal visualization.

Clarkson WK, Smith OJ. The use of GoLYTELY and Dulcolax in combination in outpatient colonoscopy. J Clin Gastroenterol 1993; 2:146.
A large, double-blind, placebo-controlled trial showing that 15 mg oral bisacodyl given after PEG-ELS results in an improved prep with no increased symptoms.

Davis GR, et al. Development of a lavage solution associated with minimal water and electrolyte absorption or secretion. Gastroenterology 1980; 78:991.
The original article describing the development of PEG-ELS.

Dipalma JA, Marshall JB. Comparison of a new sulfate-free polyethylene glycol–electrolyte lavage solution versus a standard solution for colonoscopy cleansing. Gastrointest Endosc 1990; 3:285.
A large, prospective, randomized trial comparing PEG-ELS to SF-ELS. The solutions were comparable in colonic cleansing and patient tolerance. Patients preferred the taste of SF-ELS.

Fordtran JS, Santa Ana CA, Cleveland MB. A low sodium solution for gastrointestinal lavage. Gastroenterology 1990; 98:11.
The initial report describing the development of SF-ELS. The authors also noted that infusion of the solution at 0.9 liter/hour

resulted in an overall lesser volume required for colonic cleansing, though it took longer than the 1.8-liter/hour rate.

Froehlich F, et al. Palatability of a new solution compared with standard polyethylene glycol solution for gastrointestinal lavage. Gastrointest Endosc 1991; 3:325.
A double-blind randomized taste test comparing PEG-ELS to SF-ELS. No taste preference was found; subjects could not regularly distinguish the difference in salt concentration between the two solutions.

Froehlich F, et al. Low sodium solution for colonic cleansing: A double blind, controlled, randomized prospective study. Gastrointest Endosc 1992; 5:579.
A comparison of SF-ELS to PEG-ELS. No differences were found in taste, patient tolerance, or quality of bowel preparation.

Ingebo KB, Heyman MB. Polyethylene glycol–electrolyte solution for intestinal clearance in children with refractory encopresis. Am J Dis Child 1988; 142:340.
PEG-ELS is well tolerated in normal children as well as encopretics.

Lashner BA, Winans CS, Blackstone MO. Randomized clinical trial of two colonoscopy preparation methods for elderly patients. J Clin Gastroenterol 1990; 4:405.
A study of 124 patients over age 75. They seemed to tolerate an enema and oral bisacodyl preparation better than they tolerated PEG-ELS. Both groups were treated with oral citrate of magnesia the day before colonoscopy, at different dosages. The PEG group also received metoclopramide. Little difference in cleansing quality was seen between the two groups.

Lazzaroni M, et al. Efficacy and tolerability of polyethylene glycol–electrolyte lavage solution with and without simethicone in the preparation of patients with inflammatory bowel disease for colonoscopy. Aliment Pharmacol Ther 1993; 7:655.
A randomized, double-blind, placebo-controlled study of 115 patients with IBD. The addition of 120 mg simethicone to the PEG-ELS did not affect the overall efficacy of bowel cleansing, though it did significantly improve patient tolerance.

Lever EL, et al. Addition of enemas to oral lavage preparation for colonoscopy is not necessary. Gastrointest Endosc 1992; 3:369.
A prospective, randomized, observer-blinded study of 116 patients, comparing PEG-ELS alone to PEG-ELS plus tap-water enemas on the morning of the procedure. Adding enemas did not improve the quality of the bowel preparation.

Love R, et al. Colon ornithine decarboxylase activity following standard endoscopy preparation regimens. J Surg Oncol 1989; 42:150.
PEG-ELS did not affect mucosal levels of ornithine decarboxylase (ODC), whereas phosphate enemas increased biopsy-specimen ODC levels twofold over baseline.

Marsh WH, et al. Ventricular ectopy associated with peroral colonic lavage. Gastrointest Endosc 1986; 4:259.
Colonic lavage was associated with significantly increased complex ventricular ectopy. The clinical significance of this finding is unknown.

Matter SE, Rice PJ, Campbell DR. Colonic lavage solutions: Plain versus flavored. Am J Gastroenterol 1993; 1:49.
Adding one tub of lemon-flavored Crystal Light Sugar-Free drink mix to PEG-ELS significantly improved patient preference. None of the patients preferred SF-ELS (NuLYTELY).

McBride MA, Vanagunas A. Esophageal perforation associated with polyethylene glycol–electrolyte lavage solution (letter). Gastrointest Endosc 1993; 6:856.

Another report of PEG-ELS–associated MW tear.

McNally PR, Maydonovitch CL, Wong RKH. The effectiveness of simethicone in improving visibility during colonoscopy: A double-blind randomized study. Gastrointest Endosc 1988; 3:255.

Ninety-seven patients were studied; adding 80 mg simethicone to the PEG-ELS significantly lessened the amount of bubbles and haziness noted on colonoscopy.

Pham T, Porter T, Carroll G. A case report of Boerhaave's syndrome following colonoscopy preparation (letter). Med J Aust 1993; 159:708.

Esophageal perforation after emesis following ingestion of 2 liters of a PEG-ELS.

Raymond PL. Mallory-Weiss tear associated with polyethylene glycol–electrolyte lavage solution (letter). Gastrointest Endosc 1991; 3:410.

Another report of PEG-ELS–associated MW tear.

Rosman AS, Federman Q, Feinman L. Diagnosis of colon cancer by lavage cytology with an orally administered balanced electrolyte solution. Am J Gastroenterol 1994; 1:51.

A study of 33 patients with suspected colorectal cancer, 15 of whom turned out to have cancer. Colonic lavage cytology (of the clear anal effluent before colonoscopy) had a 93 percent sensitivity and 100 percent specificity for the diagnosis of adenocarcinoma.

Santoro MJ, Chen YK, Collen MJ. Polyethylene glycol–electrolyte lavage solution—induced Mallory-Weiss tears (letter). Am J Gastroenterol 1993; 8:1292.

Still more reports of PEG-ELS–associated MW tears.

Schuman E, Balsam PE. Probable anaphylactic reaction to polyethylene glycol–electrolyte lavage solution (letter). Gastrointest Endosc 1991; 3:411.

A 70-year-old man suffered an anaphylactic reaction after drinking his second glass of PEG-ELS. He was receiving no other medications.

Shaver WA, Storms P, Peterson WL. Improvement of oral colonic lavage with supplemental simethicone. Dig Dis Sci 1988; 2:185.

The addition of simethicone to PEG-ELS (15 ml/liter) decreased the amount of colonic foam and residual stool.

Strocchi A, et al. Colonic concentrations of hydrogen and methane following colonoscopic preparation with an oral lavage solution. Gastrointest Endosc 1990; 6:580.

The minimal explosive concentrations of hydrogen and methane are greater than 4 percent and greater than 5 percent, respectively. After PEG-ELS the highest measured levels of H_2 were 0.6 percent, and 0.7 percent of CH_4.

Ziegenhagen DJ, et al. Addition of senna improves colonoscopy preparation with lavage: A prospective randomized trial. Gastrointest Endosc 1991; 5:547.

A study of 120 patients, half of whom received 75 ml of X-Prep the afternoon before colonoscopy. All patients drank PEG-ELS the morning of the procedure. The patients who received senna had cleaner colons and required less PEG-ELS. Patient tolerance was equal in the two groups.

ORAL SODIUM PHOSPHATE SOLUTION

Fass R, Do S, Hixson LJ. Fatal hyperphosphatemia following Fleet Phospho-Soda in a patient with colonic ileus. Am J Gastroenterol 1993; 6:929.

A case report, with a tabulated review of other cases of enema and oral NaP-induced hyperphosphatemia.

Kolts BE, et al. A comparison of the effectiveness and patient tolerance of oral sodium phosphate, castor oil, and standard electrolyte lavage for colonoscopy or sigmoidoscopy preparation. Am J Gastroenterol 1993; 8:1218.

A prospective randomized trial of 113 outpatient colonoscopies. It concludes that NaP is better tolerated, more effective, and cheaper than PEG-ELS.

Marshall JB, et al. Prospective, randomized trial comparing sodium phosphate solution with polyethylene glycol–electrolyte lavage for colonoscopy preparation. Gastrointest Endosc 1993; 5:631.

Predominantly outpatient (N = 143) colonoscopies, finding equal colonic cleansing efficacy and no difference in the frequency of gastrointestinal intolerance between the two preparations. However, patients preferred NaP, probably because of the lesser volume of solution to ingest with it.

Vanner SJ, et al. A randomized prospective trial comparing oral sodium phosphate with standard polyethylene glycol–based lavage solution (GoLYTELY) in the preparation of patients for colonoscopy. Am J Gastroenterol 1990; 4:422.

The first study to document the safety and efficacy of oral NaP solution as a bowel preparation. A comprehensive analysis of 102 patients, it recommends NaP as the agent of choice for most patients.

Tranquilizers

Michael M. Van Ness

Benzodiazepines

Proper preparation of the patient for endoscopy is essential for achievement of optimal results. The patient should be relaxed and have minimal spasticity of the buccopharyngeal, esophageal, and gastric musculature without obliteration of peristaltic movements. This requires full confidence in the endoscopic team, adequate voluntary muscle relaxation, and a relative freedom from discomfort, pain, anxiety, and apprehension. This environment has been achieved by the use of benzodiazepines, primarily diazepam and midazolam, as premedicants for endoscopy. Chlordiazepoxide, the prototype of the benzodiazepines, was first synthesized but inadvertently set aside in 1955. It was rediscovered in 1957 during a laboratory cleaning operation at Hoffman–La Roche, Inc., and found to have sedative, muscle-relaxant, and anticonvulsant properties. Numerous analogues of chlordiazepoxide have been synthesized since that time. Diazepam and midazolam were synthesized in 1959 and 1976, respectively.

Diazepam

Diazepam (Valium) is a colorless, crystalline compound that is relatively lipid-soluble and water-insoluble. It is one of the most widely used drugs in clinical medicine. Approximately 55 million prescriptions for diazepam were filled at American retail pharmacies in 1972, and the number has progressively increased since that time.

PHARMACOLOGY

After oral administration, diazepam is rapidly and completely absorbed, reaching peak blood concentrations within 2 hours. Absorption of intramuscular diazepam is slow, erratic, and probably incomplete. This is not surprising since the drug is poorly water-soluble at physiologic pH. After intravenous administration, diazepam exhibits the redistribution kinetics typical of highly lipid-soluble agents. Initially it is rapidly distributed centrally (to the brain). Then the concentration in plasma declines rapidly because of redistribution, with an initial distribution half-life of 10 to 15 minutes. However, there is often a return of drowsiness with an increased concentration of diazepam in plasma after 6 to 8 hours. This is probably due to absorption from the gastrointestinal tract after excretion in bile. The injectable form is available as 5 mg diazepam per milliliter of organic solvent. The organic solvent is composed of 40 percent propylene glycol, 10 percent ethyl alcohol, 5 percent sodium benzoate, and 1.5 percent benzyl alcohol. The mixture is a viscous, oily substance with a pH of 6.8. Dilution with water or saline results in transient cloudiness from crystallization of small particles.

Metabolism of diazepam proceeds slowly in the liver, with an elimination half-life of between 20 and 40 hours in most patients.

The major metabolic product, desmethyldiazepam, is formed by a removal of the N-1 methyl group. This compound has appreciable sedative and anxiolytic activity, and is biotransformed even more slowly than diazepam. Hydroxylation of desmethyldiazepam at the 3 position yields oxazepam, also an effective sedative, which is rapidly glucuronidated and excreted in the urine as the major urinary metabolite of diazepam. Steady-state concentrations are reached after 5 to 10 days. Diazepam is 99 percent protein-bound.

Pharmacokinetic studies have shown that the plasma half-life of diazepam increases linearly with age. This is a result of an increase in the initial distribution space and volume of distribution at steady state. Elderly patients appear to have an increased nervous system sensitivity to diazepam, but this is independent of the increased plasma half-life. Patients with liver disease may have a more than twofold increase in plasma half-life as a result of a decrease in plasma clearance. There is no important change in the initial volume of distribution in cirrhosis, but the volume of distribution at steady state increases significantly. This is probably a reflection of decreased diazepam protein binding in cirrhosis.

MECHANISM OF ACTION

Most clinically important effects of benzodiazepines are mediated through the central nervous system. Specific benzodiazepine receptors have been found throughout the mammalian central nervous system, with the highest density of receptors in the cerebral cortex and limbic forebrain. The drugs appear to work by potentiating inhibitory interneurons mediated by gamma-aminobutyric acid that regulate excitatory input from collaterals in many areas of the central nervous system, and by interaction with glycine receptors in the brainstem and spinal cord. Interactions between gamma-aminobutyric acid receptors and benzodiazepine receptors have been shown at the molecular level. The benzodiazepine receptors are membrane proteins located in the immediate vicinity of gamma-aminobutyric acid synapses. They form part of a supramolecular complex of functionally related macromolecules, including the gamma-aminobutyric acid receptor, its associated chloride ionophore, and other proteins. The final result of the activation of benzodiazepine receptors appears to be an increase in the frequency of gamma-aminobutyric acid chloride channel opening, which results in potentiation of gamma-aminobutyric acid release, thus increasing the inhibitory activity of the neuron. The sedative properties of diazepam appear to result from this facilitation of gamma-aminobutyric acid neurotransmission in the cerebral cortex.

The antianxiety action of benzodiazepines has been localized to the limbic system. Electrical discharge from the amygdaloid nuclei and amygdalohippocampal transmission are inhibited by low doses that do not depress the rest of the brain. In essence, they appear to reduce anxiety by means of a pharmacologic amygdalectomy. Benzodiazepines also produce objective muscle relaxation in both healthy patients and patients with neuromuscular diseases. Multiple factors are believed to contribute to muscle relaxation, including facilitation of brainstem inhibitory neurons, influencing of interneuronal activity in the spinal cord, and direct depression of motor nerve and muscle function.

It has been proposed that memory consolidation requires neural perseveration in the hippocampus. Benzodiazepines may cause terograde amnesia by blocking this perseverative activity, which is indispensable to the generation of a memory trace.

INDICATIONS

The most common indication for diazepam is as an anxiolytic agent. Intravenous diazepam is extremely helpful in facilitating endoscopy, colonoscopy, peritoneoscopy, cytoscopy, and bronchoscopy by producing a light anesthesia. This is not a true anesthesia; it is created by sedation and an anterograde amnesia that produce the illusion of anesthesia. The anterograde amnesia is at its peak 2 to 3 minutes after intravenous injection of diazepam. Most patients are also given a parenteral opiate before their procedure. It is unclear whether this significantly enhances sedation or amnesia. It has been shown that 80 to 90 percent of patients given intravenous diazepam and meperidine for gastroscopy have good to excellent relaxation and resolution of apprehension and muscle tension. Administration of diazepam alone is not sufficient for performance of a successful examination, since suppression of the gag reflex is not obtained. This is generally achieved by administering a topical anesthetic or an opiate.

Diazepam has also been shown to be effective in relieving nonspecific muscle spasms in healthy patients as well as the pathologic muscle spasticity seen in neuromuscular diseases. Intravenous diazepam is the drug of choice when intractable, repetitive seizure activity mandates parenteral therapy. Diazepam is effective in suppressing the symptoms of alcoholic withdrawal. Its sedative and amnesic effects make it ideal to use as sedation for cardioversion, as a premedicant for surgical procedures, and as an induction agent before general anesthetic administration.

CONTRAINDICATIONS

Injectable diazepam is contraindicated in patients with a known hypersensitivity to the drug, acute narrow-angle glaucoma, and open-angle glaucoma unless patients are receiving appropriate therapy.

SIDE EFFECTS

Dose-related excessive central nervous system depression is the most common side effect of diazepam. It is more likely to occur in the elderly, in patients with liver disease, in those with low serum albumin, in neonates (because of an inability to biotransform diazepam into inactive metabolites), and in those who are taking other central nervous system depressants. Manifestations of central nervous system depression include drowsiness, somnolence, fatigue, muscle weakness, nystagmus, ataxia, dysarthria, and impairment of memory.

Injection-site complications occur in 3 to 10 percent of patients receiving parenteral diazepam. These range from transient local pain on injection to thrombophlebitis and thrombosis. They may be caused by inherent properties of the diazepam itself, the propylene glycol solvent, or both. Preventive measures that have been employed include using heparin flush or saline flush, use of larger veins, use of a different solvent (Cremophor-EL), use of dilutions, injecting slowly (5 mg/minute), and use of other benzodiazepines.

Diazepam has been shown to cause respiratory and circulatory depression. Overly rapid intravenous administration of diazepam may cause apnea, particularly in the setting of concomitant opiate use. Intravenous injection causes a decrease in tidal volume, PaO_2, and pH, and an increase in PCO_2. The decrease in tidal volume appears to be exclusively mediated by a decrease in the abdominal contribution to respiration. Intravenous diazepam may also result in a moderate (15–20%) decrease in systemic blood pressure and vascular resistance. Heart rate may show a slight decrease or a moderate increase. These effects are also potentiated by concomitant opiate use. Generally the respiratory and circulatory depression of diazepam is not clinically significant and requires no therapeutic intervention. However, means to administer respiratory and circulatory support should always be readily available when intravenous diazepam is given. Studies have shown that the respiratory changes do not necessarily correlate with the overt sedative effects of diazepam.

There is an increased risk of congenital malformations associated with diazepam use in the first trimester of pregnancy. Diazepam readily crosses the placenta and is associated with fetal sedation and respiratory distress at birth (Table 39-1). Its use should therefore be avoided during pregnancy.

Other adverse effects of diazepam include physiologic addiction, sleep disturbances (including hallucinations and nightmares), and paradoxical excitement, hostility, and rage.

DRUG INTERACTIONS

Diazepam produces additive central nervous system depression when administered concomitantly with other central nervous system depressants (opiates, barbiturates, alcohol, etc.). Benzodiazepines have been reported to enhance the activity of digoxin, possibly by decreasing its rate of renal excretion.

DOSAGE AND ADMINISTRATION

The dosage should be titrated to the patient's response. It must be stressed that no specific number of milligrams is important in dosing. Rather, the drug should be titrated to effect by the clinician. The usual recommended dose in adults is between 2 and 20 mg intravenously or intramuscularly, depending on the indication. Determinants of the intravenous dose required include age, prior chronic benzodiazepine use, weight, and liver disease. When used for conscious sedation during procedures such as endoscopy, 5 to 15 mg intravenously is recommended. Ten milligrams intramuscularly is recommended for use as a preoperative antianxiety agent. The intravenous solution should be injected slowly (5 mg/minute) into a large vein. It should not be mixed or diluted with other drugs in a syringe. Lower (2–5 mg) doses should be used in the elderly, debilitated patients, and patients who have received other premedications.

Midazolam

Midazolam, an imidazobenzodiazepine derivative, is a white to light-yellow crystalline compound whose hydrochloride salt is soluble in water. The unique chemical structure of midazolam confers a number of physicochemical properties that distinguish it from other benzodiazepines in terms of its pharmacologic and pharmacokinetic characteristics.

Table 39-1. Tranquilizers: Pregnancy and breast-feeding

Agent	FDA pregnancy category	Risk vs benefit (by trimester) 1st	2nd	3rd	Breast-feeding category
Diazepam	D	R>>B	R>>B	R>>B	IV
Midazolam	D	R>>B	R>>B	R>>B	IV
Flumazenil	D	R>>B	R>>B	R>>B	IV

Food and Drug Administration (FDA) pregnancy categories:
A = Well-controlled studies fail to demonstrate risk to the fetus.
B1 = Animal studies fail to demonstrate risk to the fetus but no human studies are available.
B2 = Animal studies show some risk to the fetus but this is not confirmed in human studies.
C1 = Animal studies show risk to the fetus but no human studies are available.
C2 = Animal and human studies are unavailable.
D = Drugs associated with birth defects but with potential benefits that may outweigh known risks.
X = Drugs associated with birth defects and with potential risk that clearly outweighs potential benefit.
Risk vs benefit: R>>B = Proven or potential risk outweighs potential benefits.
B>R = Potential benefits outweigh potential risks.
R>>B? = Risks may be outweighed by benefits in some circumstances.
? = Risk-to-benefit ratio is unknown.

Breast-feeding categories:
I = Drug does not enter breast milk.
II = Drug enters breast milk but is not known to be harmful in therapeutic doses.
IIIA = Drug may or may not enter breast milk but no adverse effects are expected.
IIIB = Drug may or may not enter breast milk but drug is systemically absorbed.
IV = Drug enters breast milk and poses a potential risk to the neonate.

PHARMACOLOGY

The principal difference between midazolam's structure and that of the older benzodiazepines is a fused imidazole ring. The imidazole ring accounts for the basicity (pK 6.15), stability in aqueous solution, and rapid metabolism. The basicity allows the preparation of salts that are stable in water solution. At a pH of less than 4, part of the drug in solution has an open benzodiazepine ring, imparting water solubility. At physiologic pH the drug is believed to be present in a closed-ring form that results in increased lipid solubility. It is available in an injectable form (intravenous or intramuscular) that is composed of 5 mg midazolam hydrochloride per milliliter of solvent. The solvent is composed of 0.8 percent sodium chloride, 0.01 percent disodium edetate, and 1 percent benzyl alcohol as a preservative. The pH is adjusted to approximately 3. The oral form of midazolam is not available in the United States.

The effects of midazolam on the central nervous system are dependent on the route of administration, the dose administered, and the presence or absence of other premedications. Sedation after intravenous injection is achieved in 3 to 5 minutes. After intravenous administration of midazolam to healthy young humans, disappearance of midazolam from plasma proceeds in two distinct phases. The initial phase of rapid disappearance is due principally to distribution of the drug, while the final and slower phase of disappearance is attributable mainly to biotransformation. The onset of sedative effects after intramuscular injection is seen in approximately 15 minutes, with peak sedation occurring in 30 to 60 minutes. The mean absolute bioavailability of midazolam after intramuscular injection is greater than 90 percent. Oral midazolam is absorbed very rapidly from the gastrointestinal tract, achieving peak plasma concentrations within 1 hour of ingestion. Only 40 to 50 percent of the drug reaches the systemic circulation in nonmetabolized form because of extensive and rapid first-pass hepatic clearance.

Metabolism of midazolam involves hydroxylation by hepatic microsomal oxidative mechanisms. Microsomal enzymes rapidly hydrolyze the fused imidazole ring. The principal metabolites are 1-hydroxymethylmidazolam (50–70%), 4-hydroxymethylmidazolam (3%), and 1,4-hydroxymethylmidazolam (1%). These metabolites are excreted in the urine in the form of glucuronide conjugates. Very little intact drug is excreted in the urine. The 1- and 4-hydroxymethylmidazolam metabolites have pharmacologic activity, although less than the parent compound. The elimination half-life of midazolam in healthy young humans ranges from 1.5 to 3.5 hours. It is prolonged in obese and elderly patients, patients with liver disease, and patients in shock. Midazolam is approximately 96 percent protein-bound. The free fraction of the drug is increased in patients with chronic renal failure.

MECHANISM OF ACTION

Midazolam appears to work in a manner similar to that of diazepam and other benzodiazepines, by facilitating gamma-aminobutyric acid inhibitory neurons and increasing glycine inhibitory neurotransmission. Midazolam's affinity for the benzodiazepine receptor is approximately two times that of diazepam.

Midazolam causes anterograde amnesia similar to that of other benzodiazepines. The incidence and duration of the amnesia is dose-related. The degree of amnesia does not always parallel the drowsi ness. The amnesic effect of midazolam may be more intense than that of diazepam.

Midazolam reduces the cerebral metabolic rate for oxygen and cerebral blood flow in a dose-related manner. These findings suggest that midazolam can protect against cerebral hypoxia and be useful for patients who have impaired intracranial compliance or increased intracranial pressure.

The behavioral and central nervous system electrophysiologic effects of midazolam are antagonized by the benzodiazepine agonist (flumazenil; Romazicon). The clinical effects of midazolam may also be nonspecifically reversed by physostigmine and glycopyrrolate in combination. Use of flumazenil in patients who are dependent or habituated to benzodiazepines can cause acute withdrawal seizures.

INDICATIONS

1. Intramuscular midazolam is indicated for preoperative sedation and to impair memory of perioperative events.
2. Intravenous midazolam is indicated for induction of general anesthesia, before administration of other anesthetic agents.
3. Intravenous midazolam is indicated as an agent for conscious sedation before short diagnostic or endoscopic procedures, such as gastroscopy, colonoscopy, bronchoscopy, cystoscopy, and cardiac catheterization, either alone or with an opiate. It is titrated to produce sleep or, more commonly, dysarthria. It results in mild sedation and amnesia. The onset of sedation is more rapid than with diazepam.

CONTRAINDICATIONS

As with other benzodiazepines, midazolam is contraindicated in patients with acute narrow-angle glaucoma and should only be used in open-angle glaucoma patients who are receiving appropriate therapy.

SIDE EFFECTS

Excessive central nervous system depression is commonly seen with midazolam. As with other benzodiazepines, this is dose-related. The central nervous system depression is potentiated when midazolam is used concomitantly with other central nervous system depressants. Paradoxical agitation, anxiety, argumentativeness, and sleep disturbances may also occur.

Midazolam causes a centrally mediated respiratory depression. It reduces the ventilatory and mouth occlusion-pressure response to carbon dioxide (as does diazepam). Intravenous midazolam decreases tidal volume and increases respiratory frequency without a change in minute ventilation. PCO_2 is increased and PaO_2 is decreased. As with diazepam, the fall in tidal volume is mediated by a reduction in the abdominal contribution to respiration. Midazolam causes apnea in a variable percentage of patients (0–77%). The incidence of apnea is related to the total dose and the rate of administration of midazolam. It is more likely to occur in patients who have been premedicated with opiates. Equipotent doses of midazolam and diazepam have approximately the same degree of respiratory depression. Respiratory depression is more marked and prolonged in patients with chronic obstructive pulmonary disease.

The cardiovascular effects of midazolam are more significant than those of diazepam. Intravenous midazolam decreases systolic and diastolic blood pressure by approximately 5 and 10 percent, respectively. Heart rate is increased. Systemic vascular resistance is decreased 15 to 33 percent. Midazolam is believed to decrease myocardial contractility by a direct effect. Other cardiovascular side effects include bigeminy, premature ventricular contractions, vasovagal episodes, and nodal rhythms.

The frequency of local venous complications with midazolam is much lower than with diazepam. However, there is still a low incidence of pain at the injection site (5%), local tenderness (2%), and phlebitis (0.4%). Intramuscular injection can result in local pain (3.7%), induration (0.5%), redness (0.5%), headaches, and muscle stiffness.

Midazolam crosses the placenta. It is not recommended for use during pregnancy. It is not known whether midazolam appears in human breast milk (see Table 39-1).

Other adverse reactions that have been reported with intravenous midazolam include hiccups, nausea, vomiting, coughing, and headaches.

DRUG INTERACTIONS

The sedative effect of midazolam is accentuated by opiates, barbiturates, and alcohol. Intravenous midazolam may potentiate the antihypertensive effect of beta-adrenoceptor–blocking drugs.

DOSAGE AND ADMINISTRATION

The dosage should be titrated to patient response. As a guide, midazolam, 0.05 to 0.07 mg/kg, is usually given for intravenous conscious sedation. The dose should be lowered in elderly, debilitated patients and patients who have received other premedications. Intravenous midazolam for conscious sedation should be administered slowly over 2 to 3 minutes. Rapid injection may cause respiratory depression or apnea. Injectable midazolam is compatible with 5% dextrose in water, 0.9% sodium chloride, and lactated Ringer's solution. It can be mixed in the same syringe with meperidine, morphine sulfate, scopolamine, and atropine. When intravenous midazolam is used, oxygen, resuscitative equipment, and personnel resources for the maintenance of a patent airway should be immediately available.

COMPARISON OF DIAZEPAM AND MIDAZOLAM

Compared with diazepam, midazolam is more potent and faster acting. There are fewer adverse reactions (e.g., pain on injection and thrombophlebitis) with midazolam. Randomized clinical trials have shown similar recovery times using the Trieger test and critical flicker fusion. Endoscopist and patient satisfaction with the agent have also been similar. Patients have generally preferred midazolam, primarily because of its significantly greater amnesic effect. The major differences in the pharmacokinetics of diazepam and midazolam are that the distribution half-life of midazolam is at least one-half that of diazepam, and that the elimination half-life of midazolam is about 10-fold slower. Disadvantages of diazepam include prolonged action, with a second peak effect at 6 to 8 hours, pain on injection, and a high incidence of thrombophlebitis. The primary disadvantage of midazolam is the need to give repeated doses to maintain sedation during prolonged procedures.

PEARLS AND PITFALLS

1. Midazolam is 1.5 to 2 times more potent than diazepam.
2. Benzodiazepines should be avoided during early pregnancy and during labor and delivery.
3. Neither drug has been shown to cause retrograde amnesia.
4. The sedative effects of both drugs are potentiated when other central nervous system depressants are used concomitantly.
5. Low-dose intravenous aminophylline has been shown to decrease recovery time from sedation with diazepam.
6. Apnea is associated with rapid intravenous injection of both drugs. It is dose-related. Patients with underlying lung disease are particularly sensitive to respiratory complications.
7. Injection-site complications with diazepam can be reduced by using larger veins, saline flush, heparin flush, and a different solvent, and by injecting slowly.
8. Oxygen, resuscitative equipment, and personnel to maintain a patent airway should be immediately available when either drug is used intravenously.
9. The elimination half-life of midazolam is increased in the elderly, the obese, and patients with liver disease. The half-life of diazepam may be doubled in the setting of liver disease and increases linearly with age.
10. The free fraction of midazolam is increased in patients with renal disease.
11. Both drugs are metabolized to psychopharmacologically active metabolites.
12. The elderly have an increased sensitivity to benzodiazepines that is independent of dose and pharmacokinetics.
13. A specific benzodiazepine agonist (flumazenil; Romazicon) is available.
14. The dose of midazolam should be titrated to dysarthria, not overt sedation.

Suggested Reading

Berggren I, et al. Changes in breathing pattern and chest-wall mechanics after benzodiazepines in combination with meperidine. Acta Anaesth Scand 1987; 31:381–386.
Benzodiazepines are shown to decrease tidal volume by decreasing the abdominal contribution to respiration.

Cole SG, Brozinsky S, Isenberg JI. Midazolam, a new more potent benzodiazepine, compared with diazepam: A randomized, double-blind study of pre-endoscopic sedatives. Gastrointest Endosc 1983; 3:219–222.
A randomized trial that found midazolam to be significantly more potent, faster acting, and associated with greater amnesia, compared with diazepam.

Dalen JE, et al. The hemodynamic and respiratory effects of diazepam. Anesthesiology 1969; 3:259–263.
The hemodynamic and respiratory effects seen in 15 patients given 5 to 10 mg diazepam intravenously for cardiac catheterization are discussed.

Dundee JW, et al. Midazolam: A review of its pharmacological properties and therapeutic use. Drugs 1984; 28:519–543.
A thorough review of all aspects of midazolam.

Foster PN. Low-dose aminophylline accelerates recovery from diazepam premedication for digestive endoscopy. Gastrointest Endosc 1987; 6:421–424.

A randomized trial of 110 patients given low-dose intravenous aminophylline, versus placebo, after sedation with diazepam. Low-dose aminophylline reduced recovery time.

Greenblatt DJ, Shader RI. Benzodiazepines I. N Engl J Med 1974; 19:1011–1015.

The first of a two-part review of benzodiazepines.

Greenblatt DJ, Shader RI. Benzodiazepines II. N Engl J Med 1974; 23:1239–1243.

The second of a two-part review of benzodiazepines.

Klotz U, et al. The effects of age and liver disease on the disposition and elimination of diazepam in adult man. J Clin Invest 1975; 55:347–359.

An excellent study of the effects of age and liver disease on the pharmacokinetics of diazepam.

Magni VC, et al. A randomized comparison of midazolam and diazepam for sedation in upper gastrointestinal endoscopy. Br J Anaesth 1983; 55:1095–1100.

A randomized trial concluding that midazolam produced a greater degree of amnesia and was generally preferred by patients.

Mitchell PF. Diazepam-associated thrombophlebitis: A review and discussion of possible prevention. JAMA 1980; 101:492–495.

A thorough review of the injection-site complications of diazepam.

Reves JG, et al. Midazolam: Pharmacology and uses. Anesthesiology 1985; 62:310–324.

An excellent review of midazolam's pharmacology, pharmacokinetics, and uses.

Richter JR. Current theories about the mechanisms of benzodiazepines and neuroleptic drugs. Anesthesiology 1981; 54:66–72.

An excellent discussion of the mechanisms of action of benzodiazepines.

Sclerosing and Hemostatic Agents

David A. Johnson

The initial application of injection therapy to gastrointestinal hemorrhage was for bleeding esophageal varices. Although the bulk of the now voluminous information regarding injection therapy of upper gastrointestinal hemorrhage pertains to variceal bleeding, there has been a more recent blossoming of interest in use of this technique in nonvariceal hemorrhage as well. The advantages of this latter application center around the simplicity, relatively low expense, and efficacy that is comparable to thermal therapy (electrocoagulation, heater probe laser). This method has also been used by several investigators for therapy of nonbleeding angiodysplastic lesions in both the upper and lower digestive tract. This chapter focuses on the agents currently available for injection therapy in the United States: sodium tetradecyl sulfate, sodium morrhuate, absolute alcohol, epinephrine, and vasopressin.

MECHANISM OF ACTION

The acute injury from the injection of sclerosants is characterized by thrombosis of the vessel and ulceration of the overlying tissue. A chronic reaction is also produced and is characterized by an evolution from granulation tissue to mature collagen, with an accompanying chronic inflammatory cellular infiltrate that becomes less prominent with time. Alcohol is a tissue desiccant and causes local dehydration and vasoconstriction. Vascular-wall and endothelial-cell destruction occur, with subsequent thrombogenesis.

Sodium Tetradecyl Sulfate

Sodium tetradecyl sulfate (STS) is a synthetic anion detergent approved for use in the treatment of small, uncomplicated varicose veins of the lower extremities. However, it is also in widespread use in many medical centers as a sclerotherapy agent for esophageal variceal hemorrhage. It is believed that the surface activity of the fatty acid anions of the soap accounts for the physical properties that lead to vessel thrombosis.

DOSAGE AND ADMINISTRATION

Sodium tetradecyl sulfate is available commercially as 1% and 3% solutions. Intravenous injection has been shown to be more effective than perivenous injection in producing vein occlusion. In general, a 1.5% solution of STS is used (mixed with 50% dextrose in water), is comparable to 95% ethanol and 5% ethanolamine, and is slightly more effective than 5% sodium morrhuate. It is recommended by most investigators that no more than 2 ml be given per injection, although occasionally larger varices require more. The volume required can be assessed by the degree of distention and blanching of the varix. The total volume of the solution injected during the first procedure is generally less than 25 ml, with progressively lesser amounts in subsequent procedures.

SIDE EFFECTS

This agent is a sclerosant that causes contact irritation, and care should be taken to protect the patient and endoscopy team from splash contact with the eyes. Allergic reactions are exceedingly rare but anaphylactic reactions have been reported. The effect of long-term esophageal variceal sclerotherapy using this agent has been evaluated, with no serious long- or short-term impairment of lung function with either the 1 or 3% solution. See Table 40-1 for effects in pregnancy and breast feeding.

Sodium Morrhuate

Sodium morrhuate is a mixture of unsaturated fatty acids found in cod liver oil. These fatty acids are capable of injuring endothelial cells and provoking thrombosis as a consequence.

DOSAGE AND ADMINISTRATION

This agent is available as a 5% mixture. Restrictions for total and per-injection volume are the same as with sodium tetradecyl sulfate. Efficacy as a sclerosant has been demonstrated in clinical trials, but in animal models Jensen has shown this to be a less effective agent than sodium tetradecyl sulfate or absolute alcohol. The drug is supplied in 5- and 30-mg ampules, with 50 mg/ml.

SIDE EFFECTS

The preparation of this agent can be nonuniform, and allergic reactions may be seen. Fever, chest pain, and pleural effusion are more common than with sodium tetradecyl sulfate. Also, since this agent has a higher incidence of deep sclerotherapy-induced ulceration, the complications of esophageal perforation such as bleeding and stricture are also more common. Acute respiratory distress syndrome has been reported in two patients within 24 hours of sclerotherapy with sodium morrhuate. Two of the fatty acids in sodium morrhuate (oleic and linoleic acids) are known to induce experimental pulmonary toxicity. A study of sodium morrhuate delivery to the lung during esophageal sclerotherapy showed that approximately 20 percent of the injected dose reached the pulmonary circulation via the azygos vein. In this study no change in diffusing capacity was noted.

CONTRAINDICATIONS

This drug is contraindicated in patients who have shown a previous hypersensitivity to the drug or the fatty acids of cod liver oil.

Absolute Alcohol

MECHANISM OF ACTION

This agent has been used for intravariceal injection of esophageal varices, but more recently for treatment of nonvariceal bleeding lesions. Alcohol is a tissue desiccant and causes local dehydration and vasoconstriction. Vascular-wall and endothelial-cell destruction then occur, with subsequent thrombogenesis. This thrombogenic effect has particular appeal in the treatment of bleeding nonvariceal lesions. In contrast to vasoconstrictors (e.g., epinephrine), the poten-

Table 40-1. Sclerosing and hemostatic agents: Pregnancy and breast-feeding

Agent	FDA pregnancy category	Risk vs benefit (by trimester)			Breast-feeding category
		1st	2nd	3rd	
Absolute alcohol	C2	?	?	?	IIIB
Epinephrine	B1	?	?	?	IIIB
Ethanolamine	C2	?	?	?	IIIB
Nitroglycerin	C2	?	?	?	IIIB
Sodium morrhuate	C2	?	?	?	IIIB
Sodium tetradecyl sulfate	C2	R >> B?	R >> B?	R >> B?	IIIB
Vasopressin	C2	?	?	?	IIIB

Food and Drug Administration (FDA) pregnancy categories:
A = Well-controlled studies fail to demonstrate risk to the fetus.
B1 = Animal studies fail to demonstrate risk to the fetus but no human studies are available.
B2 = Animal studies show some risk to the fetus but this is not confirmed in human studies.
C1 = Animal studies show risk to the fetus but no human studies are available.
C2 = Animal and human studies are unavailable.
D = Drugs associated with birth defects but with potential benefits that may outweigh known risks.
X = Drugs associated with birth defects and with potential risk that clearly outweighs potential benefit.
Risk vs benefit: R >> B = Proven or potential risk outweighs potential benefits.
B > R = Potential benefits outweigh potential risks.
R >> B? = Risks may be outweighed by benefits in some circumstances.
? = Risk-to-benefit ratio is unknown.
Breast-feeding categories:
I = Drug does not enter breast milk.
II = Drug enters breast milk but is not known to be harmful in therapeutic doses.
IIIA = Drug may or may not enter breast milk but no adverse effects are expected.
IIIB = Drug may or may not enter breast milk but drug is systemically absorbed.
IV = Drug enters breast milk and poses a potential risk to the neonate.

tial for a longer-lasting hemostasis seems more tenable if thrombosis is effected, rather than merely inducing a transient vasoconstriction. There are no prospective, controlled studies addressing comparative efficacy, however.

DOSAGE AND ADMINISTRATION

Desiccated alcohol (98%) should be used. Concentrations below 90% are not as effective. Most investigators recommend that the total volume injected be less than 1 ml. The alcohol is available in 1-ml ampules. Approximately 1.5 ml is needed to preload a standard sclerotherapy needle. Aliquots of 0.1 to 0.2 ml of this agent are then injected circumferentially around a bleeding or visible vessel, with the needle placed 1 to 2 mm away from the vessel.

SIDE EFFECTS

The ulcerogenic potential for this agent must be appreciated. Extension of the ulcer may occur, and perforation is reported in about 1 percent of cases.

Epinephrine

The vasoconstrictive effects of epinephrine have great advantage for dealing with ongoing hemorrhage. In particular, local injection of a 1 : 10,000 solution has been helpful in endoscopic therapy of nonvariceal bleeding lesions. Some investigators prefer to use epinephrine in conjunction with another therapy, such as thermal therapy, to allow for a more directed application once active bleeding slows. Leung and associates used endoscopic injection of epinephrine for treatment of bleeding peptic ulcers. These authors injected aliquots of 0.5 ml of 1 : 10,000 epinephrine around and into the bleeding point and the immediately adjacent area until the bleeding stopped. The total volume used ranged from 1.5 to 10 ml (mean, 4.1 ml). Local injection of adrenaline has several effects that can impose hemostasis. First, it causes vasoconstriction of the submucosal arterioles of the stomach. Submucosal injection can also cause a local tamponade effect. Furthermore, epinephrine causes platelet aggregation and may promote thrombogenesis.

Other investigators prefer to combine epinephrine with other agents. Hirao and associates have utilized the vasoconstrictive effects of epinephrine and the physicochemical properties of hypertonic sodium chloride as an injection to create the tissue effects of swelling, fibrinoid degeneration of the vascular wall, and consequent thrombosis of the vascular lumen. These authors used a solution of 0.005% epinephrine with 3.6% hypertonic saline for injection. In acute nonfibrotic bleeding ulcers, 3 ml of the first solution was injected at three to four sites around the base of the exposed vessel. In ulcers with extensive fibrosis (due to previous treatment), 1 ml of the second solution was injected in three to four sites around the base of the bleeding vessel. Combining their entire experience (which includes patients treated with only one injection before the “prophylactic” injections were begun), 94 percent of bleeding gastric ulcers and 80 percent of duodenal ulcers achieved permanent hemostasis. Rebleeding occurred in 3.5 percent of gastric ulcers and 13.3 percent of duodenal ulcers, but retreatment was successful in most instances.

Sohendra has used 5 to 10 ml epinephrine 1 : 10,000, delivered to the submucosa directly around the bleeding vessel, to create hemostasis by compression and vasoconstriction. Following this he injected 5 ml of a sclerosant (polidocanol) to provoke thrombosis. Spurting vessels in 16 of 22 patients were controlled with a single treatment, and retreatment was successful in the remaining 6.

SIDE EFFECTS

In that the injection of epinephrine in bleeding lesions is intended to be around and not into a vessel, systemic side effects should not develop. Since epinephrine is a sympathomimetic and acts on both alpha- and beta-receptors, all actions of the sympathetic nervous system conceivably can develop. Inadvertent venous injection may cause cerebrovascular hemorrhage, resulting from a sharp rise in blood pressure. Fatalities conceivably may also occur, resulting from pulmonary edema due to the peripheral constriction and cardiac stimulation produced. In addition, patients with atherosclerotic vascular disease are at increased risk for infarction secondary to decreased organ perfusion. If intravenous injection is used, immediate follow-up with vasodilators such as nitrates or alpha-blocking agents is recommended, to counteract the vasoconstriction and marked pressor effects of this agent. Also, this product contains sodium bisulfite (an antioxidant) and may cause an allergic-type reaction, including anaphylaxis, in certain susceptible individuals. Repeated local injections can result in necrosis at the injection sites due to the vascular constriction.

Vasopressin

Vasopressin is a naturally occurring nonapeptide produced by the posterior pituitary gland. Since its discovery, many studies have reported on the use of this agent in acute upper gastrointestinal tract hemorrhage. Trials assessing the efficacy of systemic infusion for nonvariceal hemorrhage have not been successful, although demonstration of the efficacy for selective infusion has had mixed results.

MECHANISM OF ACTION

This agent is a splanchnic vasoconstrictor, and the rationale for its use in variceal hemorrhage is based on the fact that it can reverse (to normal) the increased flow that is known to occur in portal hypertension. Two forms of vasopressin, differing by only one amino acid, are available for clinical use: lysine-vasopressin and arginine-vasopressin. The vasoconstrictive activity of both is similar. In the United States, clinical experience has developed from a mixture of arginine- and lysine-vasopressin (Pitressin). Vasopressin also has a potent antidiuretic effect, ascribed to increasing reabsorption of water by the renal tubules.

INDICATIONS

Although widely used in the treatment of gastrointestinal hemorrhage (in particular, variceal bleeding), Pitressin is only approved for use in the prevention and treatment of postoperative abdominal distention, to dispel interfering gas shadow on abdominal x-rays, and for the treatment of diabetes insipidus. Vasopressin has been used for the treatment of other sources of nonvariceal bleeding (i.e., vascular malformation, Mallory-Weiss tears, diverticular hemorrhage, and postpolypectomy bleeding), but this treatment usually requires mesenteric intraarterial infusion and often selective or subselective infusion into the vessel(s) directly supplying the bleeding site. Alcohol- or drug-induced diffuse hemorrhagic gastritis may also respond to vasopressin administration.

DOSAGE AND ADMINISTRATION

Vasopressin can be given intraarterially as well as intravenously. Since the intraarterial administration requires special skills and facilities and superimposes complications related to catheterization, continuous intravenous infusion is the route of choice for portal hypertensive bleeding. In addition, continuous intraarterial infusion has no proven hemodynamic advantage over continuous intravenous infusion at the same rate. Intravenous vasopressin infusion should be started at a dosage of 0.3 units/minute for at least 30 minutes and, if ineffective, increased at approximately 30- to 60-minute intervals to 0.6, 0.9, 1.2, and 1.5 units/minute. Intraarterial infusions are begun at 0.1 units/minute for at least 30 minutes and, if ineffective increased at approximately 30- to 60-minute intervals to 0.2, 0.3 0.4, and 0.5 units/minute. For intravenous use, dosages of up to 1.5 units/minute may be necessary for efficacy, but this significantly increases the potential for toxicity. Vasopressin is supplied in ampules containing 0.5 ml (10 pressor units). Twenty units of Pitressin mixed in 100 ml 5% dextrose in water (D/W) provides 0.2 units/ml thus, 1 ml/minute provides a dose of 0.2 units/minute. Tapering the dose before discontinuation appears to be unnecessary because vasopressin does not prevent rebleeding from varices.

SIDE EFFECTS AND CONTRAINDICATIONS

The list of potential adverse side effects is lengthy. Vasopressin produces increased gut motility, presumably by stimulation of smooth muscle, with attendant abdominal cramps and occasionally diarrhea. The vasoconstrictive effect may result in bowel ischemia with necrosis. An increase in cardiac afterload, baroreceptor-mediated bradycardia, decreased coronary blood flow, and direct impairment of cardiac contractility are factors responsible for the decreased cardiac output and myocardial performance observed with this agent. Severe arrhythmias and myocardial infarction have been reported with the use of vasopressin. Close supervision and cardiac monitoring are therefore advised during infusion. The drug is contraindicated in patients with known, severe coronary artery disease and should be used cautiously in alcoholics, who may have a subclinical cardiomyopathy. Vasopressin has also been associated with respiratory arrest and cerebral hemorrhage. Other dynamic effects include antidiuresis, which may result in hyponatremia. This should be treated with withdrawal of the vasopressin until polyuria occurs. If severe, induction of an osmotic diuresis with mannitol, hypertonic dextrose, or furosemide should be undertaken. Additional side effects include stimulation of endothelial release of plasminogen activator and factor VIII. Administration of vasopressin to nonbleeding patients with cirrhosis, however, has not been associated with chemical evidence of fibrinolysis.

VASOPRESSIN ANALOGUES

An investigational vasopressin analogue, triglycyl-vasopressin, has been studied and compared with vasopressin. Advantages claimed for triglycyl-vasopressin over vasopressin are mesenteric selectivity of action, lack of stimulation of plasminogen, lack of systemic hemodynamic activator release effects, and ease of intermittent bolus injection over continuous infusion. A comparative study of triglycyl-vasopressin (20 μg/kg) and vasopressin (2.8 mU/kg/minute) in dogs, however, reported equivalent changes in mean arterial pressure and reduction in cardiac output.

NITROGLYCERIN-VASOPRESSIN

Nitrates have been studied in conjunction with vasopressin therapy and may enhance the hemostatic potential and decrease the systemic toxic effects of vasopressin administration alone. As a potent venous and mild arterial dilator, nitroglycerin reverses the cardiotoxic effects of vasopressin. Furthermore, enhancement of portal hypotensive effects is accomplished by reducing the vasopressin-induced increase in portal venous resistance. Results from several clinical trials using this combination are encouraging. It is likely that the combination will become the treatment of choice for pharmacologic management of acutely bleeding varices due to portal hypertension. Nitroglycerin has been administered sublingually, transdermally, nd intravenously, although the transdermal route may have an npredictable absorption. A more rapid titration and control of syslic pressure are possible with intravenous administration, and in ost centers this is the route of choice. Dosages used in reported ials range from 40 to 400 μg/minute, with a median dose of 250 300 μg/minute.

ONTRAINDICATIONS

itroglycerin (intravenous) is contraindicated in the following situaons: hypersensitivity to nitroglycerin, idiosyncratic reactions to itrates, severe hypotension or uncorrected hypovolemia, increased ntracranial pressure (e.g., from head trauma or cerebral hemorhage), inadequate cerebral circulation, constrictive pericarditis, and pericardial tamponade.

DOSAGE AND ADMINISTRATION

Nitroglycerin must be diluted in a 5% dextrose or 0.9% sodium chloride solution before infusion. The fluid requirements of the patient as well as the expected duration of the infusion should be considered in selecting the appropriate dilution. To obtain a concentration of 500 μg/ml, add 5 mg nitroglycerin to 100 ml diluent, or 50 mg to 1 liter. For a concentration of 100 μg/ml, add 25 mg to 250 ml, or 100 mg to 1 liter. Initial infusion at this concentration should be 5 μg/minute (3 ml/hour), with titration of 5-μg/minute increments every 3 to 5 minutes until some response is noted. If no response is noted at 20 μg/minute, increases can be made with 10- to 20-μg/minute increments until a pressure effect is noted. The dosage used for sublingual administration in one study was 0.6 mg every 30 minutes for 6 hours.

Dosage is titrated to the level of hemodynamic function. Blood pressure, pulse rate, and other physiologic parameters must be monitored continuously to ensure maintenance of adequate systemic blood pressure for critical organ perfusion (target systolic pressure,

> 90 mm Hg). Since a fall in pulmonary capillary wedge pressure precedes the onset of arterial hypotension, wedge pressure can serve as a useful guide to safe titration of the drug. However, no studies to date have used dose titration to determine the optimal beneficial effect in an individual patient. It appears that a reduction in the hepatic venous pressure gradient is accompanied by a reduction in mean arterial pressure and cardiac index.

SIDE EFFECTS

Central nervous system complaints of headache are not uncommon. Apprehension, dizziness, restlessness, and muscle twitching have been described. Gastrointestinal side effects are rare but include nausea, vomiting, and abdominal pain. Patients with severely impaired hepatic or renal disease may be more sensitive to this drug and it should be used with great caution in such patients. Administration of exogenous thiols (e.g., *N*-acetylcysteine) enhances the nitrate vascular effects in the nontolerant state. Interestingly, higher concentrations of *N*-acetylcysteine are found in the urine of patients with chronic liver disease. This may explain the decreased tolerance for nitrates in patients with cirrhosis.

DRUG INTERACTIONS

Use with other vasodilators, antihypertensive agents, or alcohol increases the orthostatic hypotensive effect of nitroglycerin. A reduced effect of the following drugs has been noted when they are used concomitantly with nitroglycerin: acetylcholine, norepinephrine, histamine, and sympathomimetics.

PEARLS AND PITFALLS

1. The ulcerogenic potential of all agents used for injection therapy must be appreciated; in particular, even small volumes of etha can cause serositis and perforation. The sclerosis achieved is d pendent on the balance struck between thrombosis, necros and fibrosis.
2. Sodium morrhuate is thick, viscid, and passed with great difficult through a 25-gauge sclerotherapy needle.
3. Nitroglycerin is readily absorbed by many plastics. Glass intravenous bottles should be used to dilute and store the drug. Filters that absorb nitroglycerin should be avoided. Common administration sets made of polyvinyl chloride (PVC) can absorb 40 to 80 percent of the total nitroglycerin. Since the loss is neither constant nor self-limited, it cannot be simply calculated or corrected for. Published trials have used PVC tubing and the recommended doses (25 μg/minute or more to start, as is recommended for cardiac patients), but these doses may be too high if administration sets with nonabsorbable materials are used.
4. Paradoxical bradycardia may accompany nitroglycerin-induced hypotension.
5. Tachyphylaxis to nitrate preparations is well recognized in patients who receive nitrates for 18 hours or longer.

Suggested Reading

Brooks WS. Variceal sclerosing agents. Am J Gastroenterol 1984; 79:424–428.

This article discusses agents used in the United States and Europe: sodium morrhuate, tetradecyl sulfate, ethanolamine oleate, and polidocanol.

Goff JS. Gastroesophageal varices: Pathogenesis and therapy of acute bleeding. Gastroenterol Clin North Am 1993; 22:779–800.
Comprehensive summary of endoscopic therapies for variceal hemorrhage.

Groszman RJ. Drug therapy of portal hypertension. Am J Gastroenterol 1987; 82:107–113.
A review of the vasoconstrictors, vasodilators, and other miscellaneous agents that have shown potential use in the treatment of portal hypertension.

Jones AL, Hayes PC. Organic nitrates in portal hypertension. Am J Gastroenterol 1994; 89:7–14.
An update on the use of nitrates in treatment of variceal hemorrhage.

Laine L. Rolling review: Upper gastrointestinal bleeding. Aliment Pharmacol Ther 1993; 7:207–232.
An outstanding overview of endoscopic therapies for the various hemostatic techniques and agents.

Zuccaro G Jr. Bleeding peptic ulcer: Pathogenesis and endoscopic therapy. Gastroenterol Clin North Am 1993; 22:737–750.
Current summary of the endoscopic therapies including injection techniques for peptic bleeding.

Antimotility Agents

Richard D. Baertlein

Gastrointestinal endoscopy, long recognized as an excellent diagnostic study, has gained wide recognition for its therapeutic potential. Polypectomy has been widely accepted for over 2 decades. Sclerotherapy of esophageal varices and thermal treatment of nonvariceal bleeding have proved effective. The fields of biliary and pancreatic endoscopy are widely accepted for their diagnostic and therapeutic benefits.

The ability to suppress the natural motility of the gastrointestinal tract is of immense help in the exacting task of therapeutic endoscopy. Endoscopists have chiefly relied on two medications, atropine and glucagon, to stop peristalsis for these procedures. Investigators are now focusing attention on hyoscyamine, since it shows promise as a cheaper antimotility aid for endoscopy. Controlled trials and written guidelines for the use of these three drugs as antimotility agents are rare.

Atropine

Atropine competitively antagonizes acetylcholine at both M_1- and M_2-muscarinic receptor sites. It does not block transmission at either the neurosmucular junction or autonomic ganglia in clinical doses. This parasympatholytic effect decreases esophageal, gastric, and intestinal motility, and reduces lower esophageal sphincter pressure.

The antimotility effect is pronounced because the parasympathetic nerves almost exclusively supply the extrinsic nervous motor control of the gut. Atropine has a less potent effect on gastric secretion and the smooth muscle of the bile ducts, gallbladder, ureters, bladder, and myometrium.

Atropine is well absorbed after oral administration and can also be given by the subcutaneous, intramuscular, or intravenous routes. In addition, it is absorbed well when applied locally to any mucosal surface. The half-life is 2.5 hours, and most of the drug is renally excreted within 12 hours.

INDICATIONS

Atropine is rarely used now as a routine adjunct to gastrointestinal procedures. This decline in popularity is due to the high incidence of side effects and the emergence of glucagon as an equally effective but safer drug.

Atropine is very useful in decreasing the sialorrhea associated with esophageal obstruction from malignancy or tumor. It is also used to prevent vasovagal reactions during procedures such as peritoneoscopy, for which preprocedure sedation may be minimal.

Anticholinergics may be used as an effective adjunct to H_2-antagonists in the treatment of resistant peptic ulcers, but the advent of a selective anticholinergic such as pirenzepine has significantly reduced the use of atropine. The irritable bowel syndrome responds to anticholinergic drugs, but the systemic side effects of atropine limit its utility.

CONTRAINDICATIONS AND SIDE EFFECTS

Side effects noted with clinical doses of atropine include dryness of the mouth, anhidrosis, tachycardia, abdominal distention, and acute urinary retention. High doses may cause extreme dryness of the mouth, dysphagia, photophobia, fever, leukocytosis, vomiting, tachycardia, and hypotension or hypertension.

Ileus and toxic megacolon have occurred with atropine use in patients with inflammatory, ischemic, or amebic colitis. Its use in such conditions is generally contraindicated. Physostigmine may counteract these complications.

DOSAGE AND ADMINISTRATION

The usual dosage of atropine is 0.3 to 1.0 mg every 4 to 6 hours via the oral, subcutaneous, intramuscular, or intravenous route. Dryness of the mouth, along with the cardiac and cycloplegic effects of atropine, is often seen before gastrointestinal motility is reduced.

Glucagon

Glucagon is currently the agent of choice for reducing gastroduodenal motility for upper endoscopy. Compared to anticholinergics, glucagon is superior in effect, causes less patient discomfort, and has fewer contraindications. Because of its prompt and transient antimotility capability, glucagon has become widely used for radiologic examinations as well as endoscopy.

PHARMACOLOGY

Glucagon is a straight-chain polypeptide hormone that contains 29 amino acids, normally produced by the alpha cells of the pancreas. Following intravenous administration, glucagon's spasmolytic effect on the gut begins within 30 to 60 seconds and lasts about 7 minutes. Glucagon is extensively degraded in the liver, kidney, and plasma through enzymatic proteolysis. The elimination half-life is 3 to 6 minutes.

Glucagon inhibits gastric, duodenal, and colonic motility as well as gastric and pancreatic secretion. The mechanism by which glucagon induces a spasmolytic effect on the gut remains unexplained. Early studies showed that there was no relation between glucagon's effect on bowel motility and its metabolic effect on glucose and insulin release. It is postulated that glucagon's inhibitory effect on the motility of the smooth muscle of the gastrointestinal tract may not be due to a direct action on the muscle receptor, but its interference with intramural cholinergic neuronal transmission.

Glucagon's metabolic actions are antagonistic to those of insulin. Blood glucose is raised through increased glycogenolysis and gluconeogenesis.

INDICATIONS

Glucagon is indicated for the elective induction of temporary paralysis of the upper gastrointestinal tract in order to facilitate diagnostic or therapeutic procedures. It is particularly useful as an aid to ~nulation of the sphincter of Oddi, for gastric or duodenal polypectomy, and to coagulate difficult bleeding lesions. It is also the most widely used drug for barium studies of the gastrointestinal tract.

DOSAGE

Glucagon should be prepared in a solution with a concentration of 1 mg/ml and given in a dose of 0.1 to 0.5 mg intravenously. A total dose of 1 mg can usually be given without problem. Total doses of 1 to 2 mg are safe but result in an increased incidence of side effects.

CONTRAINDICATIONS AND SIDE EFFECTS

Glucagon is known to stimulate catecholamine and insulin release; therefore, absolute contraindications include pheochromocytoma and insulinoma. In pheochromocytoma, a sudden, clinically evident release of catecholamines is seen within minutes, but with insulinoma, the hypoglycemic effects may not be apparent for hours.

The incidence of side effects is markedly lower with glucagon than with anticholinergic agents. In early studies, in which relatively large doses were used (1–2 mg), nausea, vomiting, and headaches were relatively common. These side effects are seen infrequently with the above recommended dose. Interestingly, even with the early, larger doses, no significant effects on pulse or blood pressure were seen.

PEARLS AND PITFALLS

1. Glucagon is inactivated rapidly after the solution is prepared. It should be reconstituted only immediately before administration, or stored in a refrigerator.
2. Intravenous glucagon, 1 mg, can relieve the esophageal spasm associated with meat impaction and allow spontaneous passage of the food bolus.
3. Both atropine and glucagon can cause significant abdominal distention. Endoscopists should be judicious in their use of air durin procedures in which these medications are used.
4. Children are much more sensitive than adults to the effects o atropine. Explanation of expected side effects and use of the lowest doses may help avoid some problems.
5. Concomitant use of glucagon and atropine does not provide additional benefit, but does increase the incidence of side effects.
6. Atropine can be helpful for the reduction of sialorrhea in esophageal obstruction.

Hyoscyamine

Hyoscyamine is a naturally occurring belladonna alkaloid that is effective as adjunctive therapy in the treatment of irritable bowel syndrome and peptic ulcer. It has recently been employed to reduce duodenal motility in facilitating upper gastrointestinal radiologic procedures and endoscopic retrograde cholangiopancreatography (ERCP).

PHARMACOLOGY

Hyoscyamine (1-hyoscyamine) is the levorotatory isomer of atropine. It is an antimuscarinic, anticholinergic agent that specifically inhibits the actions of acetylcholine on structures innervated by postr

Table 41-1. Antimotility agents: Pregnancy and breast-feeding

Agent	FDA pregnancy category	Risk vs benefit (by trimester)			Breast-feeding category
		1st	2nd	3rd	
Atropine	C2	?	?	?	IV
Glucagon	C2	?	?	?	IIIB
Hyoscyamine	C2	?	?	?	II

Food and Drug Administration (FDA) pregnancy categories:
A = Well-controlled studies fail to demonstrate risk to the fetus.
B1 = Animal studies fail to demonstrate risk to the fetus but no human studies are available.
B2 = Animal studies show some risk to the fetus but this is not confirmed in human studies.
C1 = Animal studies show risk to the fetus but no human studies are available.
C2 = Animal and human studies are unavailable.
D = Drugs associated with birth defects but with potential benefits that may outweigh known risks.
X = Drugs associated with birth defects and with potential risk that clearly outweighs potential benefit.
Risk vs benefit: R >> B = Proven or potential risk outweighs potential benefits.
B > R = Potential benefits outweigh potential risks.
R >> B? = Risks may be outweighed by benefits in some circumstances.
? = Risk-to-benefit ratio is unknown.
Breast-feeding categories:
I = Drug does not enter breast milk.
II = Drug enters breast milk but is not known to be harmful in therapeutic doses.
IIIA = Drug may or may not enter breast milk but no adverse effects are expected.
IIIB = Drug may or may not enter breast milk but drug is systemically absorbed.
IV = Drug enters breast milk and poses a potential risk to the neonate.

glionic nerves and on smooth muscles that lack cholinergic innervation but nevertheless respond to acetylcholine.

Following intravenous administration, hyoscyamine has an onset of action of 2 to 3 minutes, peak effect within 15 to 30 minutes, and duration of action of up to 4 hours. Hyoscyamine is excreted in the urine as unchanged drug (30–50%) an hepatic metabolite, with an elimination half-life of $3^1/2$ hours.

INDICATIONS

Recent evidence suggests that hyoscyamine will prove to be an economical alternative to glucagon for temporary paralysis of the upper gastrointestinal tract. In a recent randomized trial, Hui and Ostroff found hyoscyamine to be as efficacious as glucagon in aiding performance of ERCP, with a higher incidence of dry mouth and minor tachycardia, but at one-third the cost. Of note, patients at high risk for development of significant anticholinergic complications were excluded from the study. Moeller and associates showed hyoscyamine to be as effective as glucagon in reducing duodenal motility to facilitate hypotonic duodenography. The side effect profile of the two drugs was similar, with hyoscyamine causing a higher incidence of dry mouth.

ADMINISTRATION

Hyoscyamine for parenteral administration is available in 1-ml ampules and 20-ml vials. The usual adult dose is 0.5 to 1.0 ml (0.25–0.5 mg) intravenously 5 to 10 minutes before the diagnostic procedure.

CONTRAINDICATIONS AND SIDE EFFECTS

The side effects of hyoscyamine are due to its anticholinergic properties. These include drowsiness, blurred vision, tachycardia, xerostomia, urinary retention, increased ocular tension, and constipation. As such, hyoscyamine is contraindicated in patients with glaucoma, obstructive uropathy, paralytic ileus, toxic megacolon, and myasthenia gravis. The drug should also be used with caution in patients with ischemic heart disease, congestive heart failure, and cardiac arrhythmias.

PEARLS AND PITFALLS

1. Hyoscyamine may be more suitable than glucagon for facilitating ERCP due to its longer half-life.
2. Caution should be used when administering hyoscyamine to nursing women, as it is excreted in human milk (Table 41-1).
3. Treatment of hyoscyamine overdose includes administration of physostigmine.

Suggested Reading

ATROPINE

Aggestrup S, Jensen SL. Effects of pirenzepine and atropine on basal lower esophageal pressure and gastric acid secretion in man: A placebo-controlled randomized study. Dig Dis Sci 1991; 9:360–364. *Atropine inhibits esophageal peristalsis and basal lower esophageal sphincter pressure.*

Cattau EL Jr, et al. Efficacy of atropine as an endoscopic premedication. Gastrointest Endosc 1983; 29:285.
Atropine, as a routine endoscopic premedication, did not improve either the ease of endoscopy or patient tolerance. The amount of oral secretions was reduced.

Gerner T, Myren J, Larsen S. Premedication in upper gastrointestinal endoscopy. Scand J Gastroenterol 1983; 18:925.
A double-blind, randomized study comparing glucagon and atropine, given in combination with diazepam and pethidine. The authors concluded that glucagon is preferable to atropine.

Ivey KJ. Are anticholinergics of use in the irritable colon syndrome? Gastroenterology 1975; 68:1300.
A thorough, critical review on the use of anticholinergics in patients with irritable bowel disease.

GLUCAGON

Anavar M, et al. The effect of glucagon on esophageal peristalsis and clearance. Gastrointest Radiol 1989; 14:100–102.
Glucagon inhibits esophageal peristalsis and decreases lower esophageal sphincter pressure.

Feczko PJ, Haggar MA, Halpert RD. A reappraisal of upper gastrointestinal response to low-dose glucagon. CRC Crit Rev Diagn Imaging 1986; 23:377.
A good summary of recent data showing that lower doses are more effective than previously thought.

Feczko PJ, et al. Gastroduodenal response to low-dose glucagon. AJR 1983; 140:935.
A prospective, double-blind clinical study.

Kahn CR, Shechter Y. Insulin, Oral Hypoglycemic Agents, and the Pharmacology of the Endocrine Pancreas. In AG Gilman et al. (eds), *Goodman and Gilman's The Pharmacologic Basis of Therapeutics* (8th ed). New York: Pergamon, 1990. Pp 1488–1489.
A concise review of the chemistry and pharmacology of glucagon.

Lin SZ, Zhang TL. Effect of glucagon on the motility of esophageal muscle. Chin Med J 1989; 102:193–199.
Glucagon caused hypomotility of the stomach and duodenum without obvious side effects in the majority of subjects.

HYOSCYAMINE

Brown JH. Atropine, Scopolamine, and Related Antimuscarinic Drugs. In AG Gilman et al. (eds), *Goodman and Gilman's The Pharmacologic Basis of Therapeutics* (8th ed). New York: Pergamon, 1990. Pp 150–165.
A concise review of the chemistry and pharmacology of antimuscarinic compounds.

Hoover DB. Muscarinic Blocking Drugs. In CR Craig, RE Stitzel (eds), *Modern Pharmacology* (3rd ed). Boston: Little, Brown, 1990. Pp 178–187.
A thorough review of antimuscarinic agents.

Hui SC, Ostroff JW. A double blinded randomized comparison of L-hyoscyamine and glucagon during endoscopic retrograde cholangiopancreatography (ERCP): Efficacy, morbidity and cost (abstract). Gastrointest Endosc 1995 (in press).
Hyoscyamine is an economical alternative to glucagon in facilitating ERCP in patients not at high risk of developing anticholinergic complications.

Moeller G, et al. Comparison of L-hyoscyamine, glucagon, and placebo for air-contrast upper gastrointestinal series. Gastrointest Radiol 1992; 17:195–198.
Hyoscyamine is as effective as glucagon in aiding the performance of hypotonic duodenography.

Iodinated Contrast Agents

Amy M. Tsuchida and Michael F. Lyons

Iodinated contrast media were introduced in the 1920s to aid in vascular and urographic imaging. They are now among the most widely used diagnostic agents, with over 17 million contrast injections given annually in the United States and Europe. These agents are extremely safe, but, with an incidence of adverse reactions occurring in 5 to 9 percent of all cases, a significant number of deaths are attributable to contrast reactions. For those with a prior history of contrast reactions, a prophylactic treatment to prevent recurrence is of proven benefit.

Standard ionic high-osmolality contrast agents are sodium, meglumine, or mixed salts of a tri-iodinated benzoic acid derivative. Newer low-osmolality contrast media approved by the Food and Drug Administration (FDA) for the US market in 1986 are nonionic and have an osmolality that results in significant reduction in toxicity with fewer than 2 percent adverse reactions for all cases. However, the cost of these agents is 20 times that of standard contrast media. While over 65 percent of the market has shifted to these newer agents, indications for general use are still being defined.

SIDE EFFECTS

Adverse reactions can be separated into three general types of side effects. These include (1) anaphylactoid (allergy-like) or idiosyncratic (independent of dose), (2) chemotoxic or dose-dependent (including molecule-specific and hyperosmolality-related), and (3) organ-specific or local reactions. Various combinations of these reactions can also be seen. The types of reactions are also classified as mild, moderate, or severe. Mild reactions require no treatment other than patient reassurance. Moderate reactions occur in 1 to 2 percent of patients, necessitating close observation and treatment but rarely hospitalization. Only 0.05 to 0.10 percent of patients receiving contrast media will have severe life-threatening reactions, which require prompt medical management and often result in hospitalization.

Anaphylactoid or idiosyncratic reactions (1–2% incidence) occur unpredictably and independently of the dose or concentration of the contrast media. Reactions are immediate, resulting in any combination of wheezing, urticaria, angioedema, laryngeal edema, pruritus, hypotension, or vascular collapse. No single pathogenic mechanism has been found to explain hypersensitivity to contrast agents. Contrast allergy mimics classic IgE-mediated responses. However, these reactions can occur on first exposure, and circulating antibodies to contrast agents are rarely found. Histamine levels are elevated in some patients after contrast exposure, but do not correlate well with allergic response. Radiocontrast agents can both activate factor XII and inhibit angiotensin-converting enzyme. These conditions favor the release and potentiation of bradykinin, which is proposed as a major mediator of anaphylactoid reactions. It is likely that several different mechanisms contribute to the allergic response.

Two groups of patients are recognized as being at increased risk for contrast hypersensitivity. Those with a history of clinical allergies are two to three times as likely to have an acute reaction. The second group consists of those with a prior history of adverse contrast reactions. The likelihood of a subsequent reaction in this group is between 35 and 60 percent. The type of previous reaction does not predict the severity of subsequent response, and at present there are no predictive tests to identify those at high risk for recurrence.

Chemotoxic reactions are due to specific physiologic effects of a contrast agent on the organs or vessels that the agent perfuses. These reactions are dose-and concentration-dependent, and, therefore, the rate and site of injection play an important role in the intensity and nature of the reaction. Reactions include pain on injection, tachypnea, vascular dilation, hypotension, alterations in glomerular permeability, and renovascular constriction. Properties of contrast agents that are responsible for these various effects include their hyperosmolality, their ability to bind calcium ions, and the nature and concentration of their cations.

Organ-specific effects are primarily categorized under central nervous system, cardiovascular, and renal effects. Contrast media do not readily cross the blood-brain barrier, but with repetitive injections over a short time, the hyperosmolality can break down the barrier, resulting in seizures, clonic spasms, and mental disturbances. Cardiovascular effects are both direct effects on the heart and peripheral circulation and indirect effects secondary to neurohumoral alterations invoked as compensatory response, which result in electrophysiologic disturbances with arrhythmias and hemodynamic compromise. The kidney is considered a target organ for contrast media, with more than 99 percent of the intravenous dose normally excreted by the kidneys. Mechanisms of nephrotoxicity are not known, but predisposing factors include chronic renal insufficiency, diabetes, dehydration, advanced age, obstructive uropathy, and contrast dose.

For the gastroenterologist involved with endoscopic retrograde cholangiopancreatography (ERCP), a concentration of 30 percent is needed for optimal visualization. At this concentration, contrast media are hyperosmolar, with an osmolality of 750 mmole/kg. In general, little contrast agent injected into the pancreatic or biliary systems is absorbed, but a dose response occurs with increasing absorption with repetitive high-volume injections.

TREATMENT OF CONTRAST-AGENT REACTIONS

Treatment of contrast-agent reactions consists of either prevention through prophylactic measures or the acute intervention of contrast reactions. When performing contrast injections in high-risk patients, the physician must ensure that there is an essential indication for the procedure, explain the risks to the patient, attempt to prevent adverse reactions with pretreatment regimen, and respond with emergency measures as needed.

Several different pretreatment regimens have been proposed. There are no randomized, controlled trials demonstrating the benefit of any one regimen for preventing recurrence, but there is convincing evidence, based on historically controlled trials, that pretreatment with steroids does provide protection. A standard regimen would include the following:

1. Prednisone, 50 mg given orally 12, 6, and 1 hour before the procedure. For emergency procedures, 200 mg hydrocortisone given a

least 4 to 6 hours prior to the procedure also appears to provide protection.
2. An antihistamine such as diphenhydramine, 50 mg given orally 1 hour before the procedure.

This protocol reduces the incidence of adverse reaction in high-risk patients to 5 to 10 percent, with most of these reactions being mild. Some radiologists would include ephedrine sulfate, 25 mg orally 1 hour before the procedure. This is reported to decrease the reaction rate to 3 percent. The use of an H_2-receptor antagonist such as cimetidine is controversial. In one trial, the incidence of anaphylactoid reaction increased after the addition of this agent. Nonionic contrast agents would be preferable in the high-risk patient.

Prophylactic treatment regimens greatly reduce the risk of reactions in a patient with previous hypersensitivity. The short-term use of high-dose steroids and antihistamines is extremely safe, and they should be used in patients with any question of previous reaction. It should be noted that there is still concern for a life-threatening reaction despite prophylactic treatment. Three of 15 deaths in a series of 912,000 patients occurred in pretreated patients.

The treatment for an anaphylactoid response to contrast is standard, consisting of intravenous fluids, SQ epinephrine (0.3 ml, 1:1000), antihistamines (intravenous diphenhydramine, 50 mg), steroids (intravenous hydrocortisone, 200 mg), and observation on a cardiac monitor.

Moderate reactions such as bronchospasms or hypotension may need symptom-directed therapy. The majority of mild reactions such as nausea/vomiting or transient urticaria require only supportive treatment.

PEARLS AND PITFALLS

1. Radiocontrast agents are extremely safe for general use, with much of their toxicity resulting from their hyperosmolarity. This is not a specific concern during ERCP because there is little absorption from the pancreatic or biliary tree.
2. The incidence of anaphylactoid reactions during intravascular procedures is 1 to 2 percent. The incidence during ERCP is significantly less than this. These reactions are idiosyncratic and can occur on exposure to minimal amounts of the agent.
3. In those with prior adverse reactions to contrast, the risk of a repeat reaction on subsequent exposure is as high as 60 percent. Pretreatment regimens that include steroids and diphenhydramine reduce the risk to 5 to 10 percent. The newer nonionic contrast media have a markedly reduced incidence of severe reactions compared with ionic agents and should be preferable in the high-risk patient.
4. Steroids should be administered at least 12 hours before elective procedures to derive benefit.
5. The use of radiocontrast agents in pregnant and breast feeding patients is summarized in Table 42-1. The paucity of data is, of course, due to the difficulty in performing clinical studies involving radiation exposure to pregnant patients.

Table 42-1. Iodinated contrast agents: Pregnancy and breast-feeding

Agent	FDA pregnancy category	Risk vs benefit (by trimester)			Breast-feeding category
		1st	2nd	3rd	
Iodinated contrast	BI	?	?	?	II

Food and Drug Administration (FDA) pregnancy categories:
A = Well-controlled studies fail to demonstrate risk to the fetus.
B1 = Animal studies fail to demonstrate risk to the fetus but no human studies are available.
B2 = Animal studies show some risk to the fetus but this is not confirmed in human studies.
C1 = Animal studies show risk to the fetus but no human studies are available.
C2 = Animal and human studies are unavailable.
D = Drug associated with birth defects but with potential benefits that may outweigh known risks.
X = Drug associated with birth defects and with potential risk that clearly outweighs potential benefit.
Risk vs benefit: R >> B = Proven or potential risk outweighs potential benefits.
B > R = Potential benefits outweigh potential risks.
R >> B? = Risks may be outweighed by benefits in some circumstances.
? = Risk-to-benefit ratio is unknown.

Breast-feeding categories:
I = Drug does not enter breast milk.
II = Drug enters breast milk but is not known to be harmful in therapeutic doses.
IIIA = Drug may or may not enter breast milk but no adverse effects are expected.
IIIB = Drug may or may not enter breast milk but drug is systemically absorbed.
IV = Drug enters breast milk and poses a potential risk to the neonate.

Suggested Reading

Bilbao MK, et al. Complications of endoscopic retrograde cholangiopancreatography (ERCP): A study of 10,000 cases. Gastroenterology 1976; 70:314–320.

Fifty-one adverse reactions were attributed to the use of drugs during ERCP. Of these, only three (0.03%) were caused by contrast.

Bush WH, et al. Acute reactions to intravascular contrast media: Types, risk factors, recognition, and specific treatment. AJR 1991; 157:1153–1161.

An overview of the various types of contrast reactions. An excellent table is included detailing the various types of reactions, with specific drugs for treating each reaction type, to include the usual dosages.

Greenberger PA. Contrast media reactions. J Allerg Clin Immunol 1984; 74:600–605.

A discussion of the various types of contrast reactions and their management.

Greenberger PA, Patterson R, Tapin CM. Prophylaxis against repeated radiocontrast media reactions in 857 cases. Arch Intern Med 1985; 145:2197–2200.

A prospective study comparing different pretreatment regimens in preventing contrast reactions. The most effective regimen included prednisone, diphenhydramine, and ephedrine, with a subsequent 3 percent reaction rate.

Greenberger PA, et al. Emergency administration of radio-contrast media in high risk patients. J Allerg Clin Immunol 1986; 77:630–634.

No reaction to contrast occurred in nine patients with a previous history of contrast allergy pretreated with intravenous hydrocortisone, given 2 to 6 hours before emergency angiographic procedures.

Lasser EC, et al. Pretreatment with corticosteroids to alleviate reactions to intravenous contrast material. N Engl J Med 1987; 317:845–849.

A randomized, placebo-controlled trial involving 6763 patients that demonstrated the efficacy in preventing allergic reactions of a regimen of prednisone given 12 hours before contrast exposure. A regimen of prednisone given 2 hours prior to exposure did not afford any protection. These patients did not have a history of prior contrast allergy.

Morris TW. X-ray contrast media: Where are we now, and where are we going? Radiology 1993; 188:11–16.

Overview of the different types of contrast media with discussion of the newer agents undergoing clinical trials.

Sabe RA, et al. Absorption of contrast medium during ERCP. Dig Dis Sci 1983; 28:801–806.

Contrast is absorbed during ERCP, as detected by measuring serum levels. The highest level of absorption was from pancreatic duct injection.

Shehadi WH. Contrast media adverse reactions: Occurrence, recurrence, and distribution patterns. Radiology 1982; 143:11–17.

A prospective evaluation of contrast reaction in over 300,000 patients. This paper describes the types of reactions that occur in patients with prior adverse reactions. The author found a general tendency against life-threatening reactions recurring in the same individuals.

Siegle RL. Rates of idiosyncratic reactions—ionic versus nonionic contrast media. Invest Radiol 1993; 28:s95–s98.

Comprehensive literature review regarding idiosyncratic reactions to iodinated contrast agents, with the rates of idiosyncratic reactions in patients receiving ionic contrast agents compared with those found in patients receiving nonionic agents. For conventional hyperosmolar agents, rates are estimated to be 5 percent, with repeat reactions greater than 20 percent. Significantly lower rates of idiosyncratic reactions were noted with the newer nonionic agents.

Stolberg HO, et al. Ionic versus nonionic contrast use. Curr Probl Diagn Radiol 1991; 20:49–88.

In-depth discussion on the types of contrast media, organ-specific toxic effects, and adverse events associated with different types of contrast agents.

Reversal Agents

Michael S. Gurney and Michael M. Van Ness

Naloxone

Naloxone is the agent of choice for narcotic-induced respiratory depression, sedation, and hypotension. It is a "pure" narcotic antagonist, devoid of known agonist activity. Because of naloxone's dramatic ability to rapidly reverse narcotic intoxication with minimal side effects, it has become a popular drug in the emergency ward and the procedure suite.

PHARMACOLOGY

Naloxone is a synthetic *N*-allyl derivative of oxymorphone. It is usually administered intravenously but can be given subcutaneously, intramuscularly, endotracheally, or intraglossally. Because of significant first-pass metabolism, an oral dose is only one-fiftieth as potent as parenteral administration (Table 43-1). Following parenteral administration, the drug is rapidly distributed throughout the body, with an estimated volume of distribution of about 200 liters. Onset of action is within 1 to 3 minutes of intravenous administration and only slightly longer after intramuscular and subcutaneous administration. Onset of action is related to how rapidly naloxone enters the brain. The brain-serum ratio of naloxone is 12 to 15 times higher than that of morphine.

Naloxone is primarily metabolized in the liver, by glucuronide conjugation, and excreted in the urine. The elimination half-life in the adult is 30 to 100 minutes (average, 60 minutes). The duration of action is from 1 to 4 hours, depending on the dose and route of administration.

MECHANISM OF ACTION

Naloxone's mechanism of action is not fully understood, but available evidence suggests that it antagonizes narcotic effects by competing for the same receptor site. Of the known, different opiate receptors, naloxone has no definite agonist effect, that is, no respiratory depression, pupillary constriction, or psychomimetic effects. It is nonaddicting and not subject to narcotics-control laws.

INDICATIONS

Naloxone is indicated for complete or partial reversal of acute narcotic intoxication and overdose. Signs of acute intoxication include hypothermia, hypotension, stupor, constricted pupils, convulsions, hypoventilation, and irregular pulse.

Untoward or exaggerated reactions to normal doses of narcotics may occur because of underlying illness or concurrent treatment with other drugs. Respiratory depression may be augmented secondary to reduced sensitivity to hypercapnia, decreased respiratory reserve, or decreased hepatic metabolism of narcotics, as seen with myxedema, chronic obstructive lung disease, asthma, obesity, severe liver disease, or concurrent cimetidine therapy.

Table 43-1. Pharmacologic properties of naloxone (intravenous)

Onset of action: 1–3 minutes
Maximum effect: 5–10 minutes
Elimination of half-life: about 1 hour
Duration of effect: 1–4 hours
Doses: 0.1–0.2 mg IV every 1–2 minutes up to 0.4–2.0 mg IV in adults and 0.01 mg/kg in children, neonates
Continuous IV infusion: 2 mg/500 ml for a concentration of 0.004 ml/ml titrated to response (0.4–0.8 mg/hr)

DOSAGE

Naloxone is supplied at a concentration of 0.4 mg/ml in 1- and 10-ml ampules. For known or suspected narcotic overdose, the initial dose should be 0.4 to 2.0 mg intravenously (one to five 1-ml ampules) repeated every 2 to 3 minutes. If there is no clinical response after 10 mg (twenty-five 1-ml ampules), acute narcotic intoxication is unlikely.

During diagnostic or therapeutic procedures, naloxone can be given in smaller doses of 0.1 to 0.2 mg intravenously every 1 to 2 minutes, titrated to the desired clinical effect. Smaller doses are preferable in patients who have been under the effects of large doses of narcotics for several hours, as they may be acutely physically dependent, and excessive doses of naloxone may precipitate withdrawal. This is clinically apparent as nausea, vomiting, tachypnea, tachycardia, mydriasis, elevated blood pressure, anxiety, and hyperalgesia.

There are no specific dosage adjustments necessary for renal insufficiency. Information is lacking on dosage adjustments for hepatic insufficiency. Investigational uses for naloxone include refractory shock, reversal of alcohol-induced coma, reversal of neurologic deficits in the setting of cerebral ischemia, and chronic idiopathic constipation.

SIDE EFFECTS AND CONTRAINDICATIONS

With rare exceptions, the use of naloxone in any dose has been demonstrated to be free of adverse effects. Doses up to 24 mg are reported to cause only slight drowsiness. There are several cases of cardiac dysrhythmias and pulmonary edema following naloxone-induced arousal after narcotic anesthesia. However, these cases may have resulted from a sympathetic discharge by the abrupt onset of postoperative pain. The use of naloxone in narcotic addicts may precipitate a withdrawal syndrome, which is not life threatening and is amenable to pharmacologic therapy. There are also case reports of naloxone-induced pulmonary edema.

The only contraindication to naloxone is a previously documented hypersensitivity. Use of naloxone in pregnant and lactating patients is summarized in Table 43-2.

PEARLS AND PITFALLS

1. While waiting for naloxone to reverse narcotic-induced respiratory depression, hypotension, and sedation, remember to always maintain a free airway, provide artificial ventilation, and provide car-

Table 43-2. Reversal agents: Pregnancy and breast-feeding

Agent	FDA pregnancy category	Risk vs benefit (by trimester)			Breast-feeding category
		1st	2nd	3rd	
Flumazenil	C1	B>R	B>R	B>R	IIIA
Naloxone	B1	B>R	B>R	B>R	IIIA

Food and Drug Administration (FDA) pregnancy categories:
A = Well-controlled studies fail to demonstrate risk to the fetus.
B1 = Animal studies fail to demonstrate risk to the fetus but no human studies are available.
B2 = Animal studies show some risk to the fetus but this is not confirmed in human studies.
C1 = Animal studies show risk to the fetus but no human studies are available.
C2 = Animal and human studies are unavailable.
D = Drug associated with birth defects but with potential benefits that may outweigh known risks.
X = Drug associated with birth defects and with potential risk that clearly outweighs potential benefit.
Risk vs benefit: R>>B = Proven or potential risk outweighs potential benefits.
B>R = Potential benefits outweigh potential risks.
R>>B? = Risks may be outweighed by benefits in some circumstances.
? = Risk-to-benefit ratio is unknown.

Breast-feeding categories:
I = Drug does not enter breast milk.
II = Drug enters breast milk but is not known to be harmful in therapeutic doses.
IIIA = Drug may or may not enter breast milk but no adverse effects are expected.
IIIB = Drug may or may not enter breast milk but drug is systemically absorbed.
IV = Drug enters breast milk and poses a potential risk to the neonate.

diopulmonary resuscitation or intravenous volume, as dictated by the patient's clinical condition.

2. If the patient is hypotensive and without intravenous access, naloxone can be injected into the venous plexus on the inferior surface of the tongue or given endotracheally.
3. During initial narcotic reversal, emesis may occur; therefore, guard against aspiration and have suction available.
4. As naloxone's duration of action is shorter than most narcotics, signs and symptoms of narcotic overdose may recur after 30 to 60 minutes. The requirement for repeat doses (given intravenously at 1- to 2-hour intervals or as a continuous intravenous infusion) is dependent on the amount, type, and route of administration of the narcotic being antagonized.

Flumazenil

Flumazenil (Romazicon) is the first commercially available benzodiazepine receptor antagonist. Although useful for emergency room treatment of suspected drug overdose, the use of flumazenil in gastroenterology appears limited more to reversal of benzodiazepine-induced sedation and treatment of the desperately ill cirrhosis patient with hepatic encephalopathy.

PHARMACOLOGY

Flumazenil is an imidazobenzodiazepine compound that antagonizes the action of benzodiazepines on the central nervous system (CNS). It does *not* reverse the effects of opiates, ethanol, or barbiturates. After intravenous administration (0.4–1.0 mg), benzodiazepine reversal is seen within 1 to 2 minutes. The drug has an effective clinical half-life of 7 to 15 minutes. The drug is cleared primarily by the liver with subsequent urinary excretion of de-ethylated metabolites for 24 to 72 hours. The half-life of flumazenil is increased to as long as 2.4 hours in patients with severe liver disease.

MECHANISM OF ACTION

Flumazenil binds competitively with central nervous system benzodiazepine receptors and closely allied CNS gamma-aminobutyric acid receptors.

INDICATIONS

In addition to reversal of benzodiazepine-induced sedation and the treatment of unknown drug overdoses, flumazenil is possibly a useful agent in temporary reversal of hepatic encephalopathy in those patients without cerebral edema.

DOSAGE

In patients who have received general anesthesia or conscious sedation, the recommended initial dosage is 0.2 mg intravenously every minute until a maximum of 1.0 mg is administered. If resedation occurs, a maximum of 3.0 mg can be given at 0.2 mg intravenously every minute.

In overdose patients, the recommended initial dosage is 0.5 mg intravenously every minute until a maximum of 5.0 mg has been given. In patients with hepatic encephalopathy, an initial 0.4-mg intravenous dose has been used, with no more than a 3.0-mg total dose.

SIDE EFFECTS AND CONTRAINDICATIONS

Flumazenil can precipitate withdrawal seizures in patients who are dependent on benzodiazepines, even in situations in which short-term, high-dose therapy (e.g., intensive care units) has been used. Flumazenil use in pregnant and lactating patients is summarized in Table 43-2.

PEARLS AND PITFALLS

1. Re-sedation after initial dosing is common, is usually seen within 20 minutes of initial therapy, and responds to repeat therapy.
2. Flumazenil has *no* benefit in opiate, ethanol, or barbiturate overdose.
3. The clearance of flumazenil is decreased significantly in patients with liver disease.

Suggested Reading

NALOXONE

Allen T. Narcotic Antagonists. In R Rosen (ed), *Emergency Medicine Concepts and Clinical Practice,* vol 2. St Louis: Mosby, 1988.
A thorough and pragmatic approach to narcotic overdose and management.

Easom JM, Lovejoy FA. Opiates. In LM Haddal, JF Winchester (eds), *Clinical Management of Poisoning and Drug Overdose.* Philadelphia: Saunders, 1983.
A comprehensive guide to the diagnosis and management of drug overdoses.

Evans LEJ, et al. Treatment of drug overdosage with naloxone, a specific narcotic antagonist. Lancet 1973; 1:452.
This paper details the physiologic changes induced by naloxone in narcotic- and nonnarcotic-induced coma.

Handal KA, Schauben JL, Salamone FR. Naloxone. Ann Emerg Med 1983; 12:438.
A comprehensive review of the biochemistry and clinical use of naloxone.

Jaffe J, Martin WR. Opioid Analgesics and Antagonists. In LS Goodman, A Gilman (eds), *The Pharmacologic Basis of Therapeutics,* vol 7. New York: Macmillan, 1985.
A concise review of opioid antagonists.

Martin WR. Naloxone. Ann Intern Med 1976; 85:765.
A concise review covering the theory and history of narcotic antagonists as well as the approved and unapproved uses of naloxone.

McNicholas LF, Martin WR. New experimental and therapeutic roles for naloxone and related opioid antagonists. Drugs 1984; 27:81
A review of endogenous opioids and their roles in the physiologic regulation of various systems and pathologic processes.

Milne B, Jramendas K. Naloxone: New therapeutic roles. Can Anaesth Soc J 1984; 31:3.
A review of naloxone use for septic shock, spinal cord injury, stroke, and nonopiate-induced respiratory depression.

Prough DS, et al. Acute pulmonary edema in healthy teenagers following conservative doses of intravenous naloxone. Anesthesiology 1984; 60:485.

Two case reports of healthy young male teenagers in whom acute pulmonary edema developed after they received naloxone, without other apparent causes.

FLUMAZENIL

Bansky G, et al. Effects of the benzodiazepine receptor antagonist flumazenil in hepatic encephalopathy in humans. Gastroenterology 1989; 97:744–750.

An intravenous dose of the benzodiazepine receptor antagonist, flumazenil (Romazicon), 0.4 mg, resulted in a transient, 1- to 2-hour reversal of stage 3 and 4 encephalopathy in a subset of patients with cirrhosis and hepatic encephalopathy. Among the responders, 7 of the 10 were ultimately discharged alive.

Birkenfeld S, et al. Double-blind controlled trial of flumazenil in patients who underwent gastrointestinal endoscopy. Gastrointest Endosc 1989; 35:519–522.

Flumazenil reverses the effects of both diazepam and midazolam given for sedation during gastrointestinal endoscopy.

Crimm G, et al. Improvement of hepatic encephalopathy treated with flumazenil. Lancet 1988; 2:1392–1394.

Since hepatic encephalopathy may result from excessive gamma-aminobutyric acid inhibitory tone, the benzodiazepine receptor antagonist flumazenil has been shown to be useful in the treatment of this condition. Failure of patients to respond to flumazenil suggests concomitant cerebral edema.

Jones EA, et al. The gamma-aminobutyric acid. A receptor complex and hepatic encephalopathy: Some recent advances. Ann Intern Med 1989; 110:532–546.

The presence of an endogenous benzodiazepine-like compound may contribute to the development of hepatic encephalopathy.

Kunert H. Benzodiazepine antagonists in ambulant colonoscopy. Gastroenterology 1993; 104:A15.

The use of flumazenil shortens patient recovery time, decreases the need for intensive postcolonoscopy observation, and does not interfere with periprocedure amnesia.

McDonald GA, et al. Benzodiazepine receptor distribution in recurrent hepatic encephalopathy. Gastroenterology 1994; 105:A936.

The authors used positron emission tomography (PET) and [^{11}C]-flumazenil to show increased benzodiazepine receptor density in severe liver disease complicated by hepatic encephalopathy.

Other Agents

Somatostatin

George Koval

Discovered in 1972, natural somatostatin is not a single molecule but rather a family of related polypeptides that includes a 14–amino acid peptide and its larger precursors. Somatostatin's name derives from its initially described physiologic effect: the inhibition of growth hormone. Since then it has been found to inhibit a long list of regulatory peptides—especially those in the gastrointestinal tract—and has earned the nickname endocrine cyanide.

Clinical use of somatostatin was limited by its extremely short half-life. In 1982, a long-acting octapeptide analogue of somatostatin, octreotide, was synthesized and marketed under the name Sandostatin. It has been applied to hormone-producing tumors of the gastrointestinal tract with remarkable success. Octreotide's further influence on intestinal functions such as secretion, motility, and absorption has now been realized, and its efficacy for a number of other gastrointestinal problems is being reported as clinical experience grows.

PHARMACOLOGY

In contrast to somatostatin's half-life of 3 minutes, octreotide has a half-life of 90 minutes. Because it is poorly absorbed from the gastrointestinal tract the drug must be given by subcutaneous or intravenous injection every 6 to 12 hours, or by continuous infusion. Approximately 10 percent of octreotide is renally excreted; the remaining 90 percent is systemically metabolized.

Somatostatin and octreotide inhibit the release of growth hormone, gastrin, insulin, secretin, cholecystokinin, vasoactive intestinal polypeptide (VIP), gastric inhibitory peptide, motilin, neurotensin, pancreatic polypeptide, and glucagon. Although octreotide has similar qualitative effects to native somatostatin, it differs in potency for certain target organs. Octreotide is 70 times, 23 times, and 3 times more potent than somatostatin in the inhibition of growth hormone, glucagon, and insulin, respectively. Octreotide does not inhibit prolactin, cortisol, or gonadotropin secretion. Its physiologic properties include inhibition of gastric acid secretion (independent of gastrin inhibition), slowing of gut motility, and inhibition of both carbohydrate absorption and pancreatic enzyme secretion.

INDICATIONS

The clearest indication for octreotide is in the treatment of hormone-producing islet cell tumors of the gastrointestinal tract. Islet cell tumors are slow growing, and patients can live for many years with metastatic disease. However, because of the release of biologically active peptides, these tumors can produce symptoms out of proportion to their size, and patients may have disabling symptoms or even die as a consequence of the secretagogue production. Thus, inhibition of these peptides is critically important in the management of patients afflicted with these syndromes. Unfortunately, despite initial reports of an antineoplastic effect of octreotide, neither Kvols nor Saltz reported any evidence of tumor regression among

56 patients with metastatic neuroendocrine tumors treated with octreotide.

The carcinoid syndrome is caused by metastatic gastrointestinal carcinoid tumor or by a bronchial carcinoid. The tumor's release of serotonin, its precursors, and other peptides into the circulation is associated with flushing, diarrhea, and abdominal pain. The carcinoid syndrome has been well studied with respect to octreotide therapy by Kvols and associates. They treated 25 patients with 150 μg 4 times a day; flushing and diarrhea were promptly relieved in 22. Three-fourths had a 50 percent or greater reduction in urinary 5-HIAA levels. Over 75 percent of the responders had continued relief of symptoms after a median therapy duration of one year. Vinik treated three such patients with lower doses (50–150 μg bid) and demonstrated relief of symptoms in all, but serotonin levels fell in only one. The effect of the analogue on long-term sequelae, such as right-sided cardiac valve stenosis and mesenteric sclerosis, has not been studied. Octreotide has also been used successfully to reverse and prevent the "carcinoid crisis" associated with anesthesia induction or surgical manipulation of the tumor. The demonstrated efficacy of octreotide in carcinoid syndrome is far greater than any medical therapy currently available.

VIPoma is also known as the Verner-Morrison syndrome, the WDHA syndrome, or pancreatic cholera. It is characterized by voluminous watery diarrhea, hypokalemia, hypochlorhydria, and, occasionally, hypocalcemia and hypophosphatemia. VIP levels have been reported to fall in the majority of patients treated with octreotide, albeit transiently in some. Symptomatic response has been more impressive, possibly because somatostatin not only inhibits VIP release, but also slows gut motility and decreases intestinal secretion at the cellular level. Over 80 percent of patients whose symptoms were resistant to other therapies have had dramatic clinical improvement. Initial treatment dosages have ranged from 50 to 100 μg twice a day to 150 μg 4 times a day. A curious feature is that in some patients the VIP suppression is prolonged, allowing a lengthening of the dosing interval to even an as-needed basis. Octreotide represents a significant therapeutic advance in the therapy of clinical manifestations in VIPoma.

Gastrinoma causes the Zollinger-Ellison syndrome of gastric acid hypersecretion, peptic ulceration, and diarrhea. It is the one islet cell tumor for which therapy is well developed; high-dose H_2-blockers, surgery, and omeprazole have drastically reduced the morbidity and mortality. Octreotide has been shown in several trials to effectively suppress both acid production and gastrin release. Gastrin levels have fallen in 93 percent of treated patients; peptic ulcers, abdominal pain, and diarrhea have been relieved in 70 to 90 percent. The effectiveness of octreotide is dose-related, with starting doses ranging from 50 μg twice a day to 150 μg 4 times a day. Dosages for chronic therapy have ranged from 50 to 1500 μg per day.

Glucagonoma, a rare malignancy of the pancreatic alpha cells, is characterized by a unique necrolytic skin rash, anemia, weight loss, glucose intolerance, and, occasionally, diarrhea. Octreotide has been reported to improve the skin rash, weight loss, anemia, and diarrhea but not the glucose intolerance of glucagonoma. Doses used ranged from 50 μg twice a day to 150 μg 4 times a day.

Insulinoma causes hypoglycemia with associated autonomic symptoms and bizarre behavioral changes. In contrast to the other islet cell tumors, the majority of insulinomas is benign and amenable to surgical removal if identified. This is fortunate since a reduction in hypoglycemic episodes has been noted only occasionally with octreotide therapy.

Somatostatin decreases splanchnic blood flow and suppresses gastric acid secretion, making it an appealing medication for management of gastrointestinal bleeding. However, clinical trials of octreotide and somatostatin in the treatment of bleeding peptic ulcers have been inconclusive. Variceal hemorrhage does seem to benefit from octreotide therapy. The mechanism of action is unclear since variable effects on portal venous gradient and intravariceal pressure have been reported. In separate studies of acute variceal bleeding, Shields and Sung compared endoscopic sclerotherapy to octreotide administered as a bolus of 50 μg intravenously followed by a 50-μg/hour infusion for 48 hours. Acute variceal bleeding was controlled in 90 percent (Shields et al.) and 84 percent (Sung et al.) of patients treated with octreotide. Outcomes were similar for patients treated with either sclerotherapy or octreotide. Shields and associates have also studied octreotide as an adjunct to endoscopic sclerotherapy in the presentation of recurrent variceal bleeding; they reported reductions in mortality and variceal rebleeding when this was compared to sclerotherapy alone.

Although octreotide reduces pancreatic exocrine secretion, it has not been shown to be beneficial in the treatment of acute pancreatitis or in the prevention of endoscopic retrograde cholangiopancreatography (ERCP)-associated pancreatitis. In the case of pancreatic fistula, octreotide has proved beneficial in reducing fistula output and in speeding closure. Dosages employed ranged from 50 μg twice a day to 200 μg three times a day. Approximately 70 percent of fistulae closed within 7 days of the start of octreotide. Response has been best in patients with fistula output of less than 200 ml per day. An efficacy similar to that of pancreatic fistula has been reported for enterocutaneous fistula.

The effects of octreotide on gastrointestinal tract motility are usually inhibitory, with slowing of gastric emptying, gallbladder emptying, and mouth-to-cecum transit. The latter property, as well as octreotide's ability to induce net water and electrolyte absorption, has led to the experimental use of octreotide in the treatment of diarrhea. Benefit has been reported in the treatment of diarrhea associated with dumping syndrome, short bowel, diabetes, and AIDS. Particular interest has been focused on AIDS-related diarrhea, since it affects up to 80 percent of AIDS patients at some time during their illness. Based on many case reports and a few studies, it appears that some patients with AIDS-related diarrhea have a diminution of stool frequency and volume at octreotide doses of 50 to 250 μg 3 three times a day.

Because of its many effects, octreotide's usefulness continues to be defined. Radiolabeled octreotide has proved effective in localizing somatostatin receptor–bearing tumors of many kinds. Octreotide may also prove useful in controlling the symptoms of irritable bowel.

CONTRAINDICATIONS AND SIDE EFFECTS

There is no absolute contraindication to somatostatin use. Hypersensitivity has not been reported, and the development of a blocking antibody has not occurred in clinical trials. The most common side effect is local irritation at the injection site. This can be minimized by warming the syringe in the palms before injection, and by injecting slowly. Cramping, bloating, and nausea are common complaints during the first week or two of therapy but usually disappear with time.

Gallstones have been reported in up to 20 percent of patients receiving octreotide for more than 30 days. Most reports of gallstone formation have been in patients treated for acromegaly. Gallstone formation may be due to increased cholesterol saturation of bile and decreased gallbladder motility.

If stool fat is analyzed before and during therapy, as many as 60 percent of patients have steatorrhea. This is rarely clinically significant. It is thought to occur from inhibition of gallbladder contraction and pancreatic secretion. The steatorrhea is partially reversible with oral pancreatic enzyme replacement and also improves on its own with time. Mild glucose intolerance has been noted in some patients, but glucose control in diabetic patients does not change significantly. About 50 percent of patients in clinical trials have had one of the mentioned side effects, but the complaints are usually minor and temporary, and they have never been severe enough to stop the medication.

DOSAGE AND ADMINISTRATION

Natural somatostatin must be given by continuous intravenous infusion due to its short half-life. It is not approved by the Food and Drug Administration (FDA) and therefore is not commercially available.

Octreotide, the synthetic analogue, is given by subcutaneous or intravenous injection. Pain with subcutaneous injection may be reduced by using the smallest possible volume of drug and by rotating the site of injection. Octreotide can also be given by intravenous push over 3 minutes. It is incompatible with total parenteral nutrition (TPN) solutions because of the formation of a glycosyl conjugate. The initial recommended dosage is 50 μg once or twice a day. Response should be apparent within a few days. The dose can be increased gradually based on patient response and tolerability. Doses of several hundred micrograms per day are usually well tolerated. A favorable response to higher doses is unlikely if no response was noted at lower doses. An oral preparation is currently in clinical trials. Somatostatin administration to pregnant or lactating patients is summarized in Table 44-1.

PEARLS AND PITFALLS

1. Steatorrhea often develops during somatostatin therapy, but it is usually mild and improves with oral pancreatic enzyme supplements.
2. Injecting the minimum volume at a slow rate and warming the syringe before injection by rolling it between the palms can reduce pain at the injection site.
3. Mild hyperglycemia may develop in nondiabetic patients; this problem often improves after a month of treatment. Paradoxically, diabetics have no decrease (and may have an improvement) in glucose control.
4. VIP can be suppressed for long periods of time with somatostatin, and injections can often be decreased to an as-needed basis.
5. Caution should be used when somatostatin is stopped. There have been several reports of dramatic rebound of tumor hormone secretion when the drug is abruptly discontinued.

Table 44-1. Somatostatin: Pregnancy and breast-feeding

Agent	FDA pregnancy category	Risk vs benefit (by trimester)			Breast-feeding category
		1st	2nd	3rd	
Somatostatin	B1	?	?	?	IIIA

Food and Drug Administration (FDA) pregnancy categories:
A = Well-controlled studies fail to demonstrate risk to the fetus.
B1 = Animal studies fail to demonstrate risk to the fetus but no human studies are available.
B2 = Animal studies show some risk to the fetus but this is not confirmed in human studies.
C1 = Animal studies show risk to the fetus but no human studies are available.
C2 = Animal and human studies are unavailable.
D = Drug associated with birth defects but with potential benefits that may outweigh known risks.
X = Drug associated with birth defects and with potential risk that clearly outweighs potential benefit.
Risk vs benefit: R>>B = Proven or potential risk outweighs potential benefits.
B>R = Potential benefits outweigh potential risks.
R>>B? = Risks may be outweighed by benefits in some circumstances.
? = Risk-to-benefit ratio is unknown.
Breast-feeding categories:
I = Drug does not enter breast milk.
II = Drug enters breast milk but is not known to be harmful in therapeutic doses.
IIIA = Drug may or may not enter breast milk but no adverse effects are expected.
IIIB = Drug may or may not enter breast milk but drug is systemically absorbed.
IV = Drug enters breast milk and poses a potential risk to the neonate.

Suggested Reading

Burroughs AK, et al. Somatostatin and octreotide in gastroenterology. Aliment Pharmacol Ther 1991; 5:331
A recent review of the use of octreotide in gastroenterology.

Creutzfeldt W, et al. Effect of somatostatin analogue on pancreatic secretion in humans. AJM 1986; 5b:49.
An excellent basic-science study of the drug's effect on pancreatic physiology. The data provide an explanation for the common side effect, steatorrhea.

Fanning M, et al. Pilot study of Sandostatin (octreotide) therapy of refractory HIV-associated diarrhea. Dig Dis Sci 1991; 36:476.
Fanning and associates' article reports on the treatment of 17 patients with AIDS-associated diarrhea.

Friedman LS, et al. Somatostatin therapy for AIDS diarrhea: Muddy waters. Gastroenterology 1991; 101:1446.
This article is a commentary on Fanning and associates' report and provides insight into the difficulty of research in this area.

Gordon P, et al. Somatostatin and somatostatin analogue (SMS 201-995) in treatment of hormone-secreting tumors of the pituitary and gastrointestinal tract and non-neoplastic diseases of the gut. Ann Intern Med 1989; 110:35–50.

The many uses of somatostatin are reviewed in this comprehensive article. Somatostatin is the drug of choice for nonresectable pituitary thyrotropin-producing tumors, for carcinoid syndrome and carcinoid crisis, and for pancreatic islet cell tumors that produce vasoactive intestinal peptide.

Hasler WC, et al. A somatostatin analogue inhibits afferent pathways modulating perception of rectal distension. Gastroenterology 1993; 104:1390.

Octreotide's effect on visceral afferent pathways may point the way for its use in the treatment of pain associated with bowel obstruction and irritable bowel.

Hurst RD, et al. The therapeutic role of octreotide in the management of surgical disorders. Am J Surg 1991; 162:499.

A review of the uses of octreotide from a surgical perspective.

Jaros W, et al. Successful treatment of idiopathic secretory diarrhea of infancy with the somatostatin analogue SMS 201–995. Gastroenterology 1988; 94:189.

A case report with a good discussion. Octreotide safely and effectively reduced stool output from 250 ml/kg/day to 80 ml/kg/day.

Krenning EP, et al. Somatostatin receptor scintigraph with [III In-DTPA-D-Phel]- and [123I-Tyr3]-octreotide: The Rotterdam experience with more than 1000 patients. J Nucl Med 1993; 20:716.

A review of the exciting new area of tumor imaging using radiolabeled peptides.

Kvols LK, et al. Treatment of the malignant carcinoid syndrome. N Engl J Med 1986; 315:663.

Octreotide was used to treat the peripheral effects of metastatic carcinoid tumors. Symptoms were relieved in 22 of 25 patients, and 5-HIAA levels fell significantly in 18.

Kvols LK, et al. Treatment of metastatic islet cell carcinoma with a somatostatin analogue (SMS 201–995). Ann Intern Med 1987; 107:162.

An excellent study of 22 patients with malignant islet cell carcinoma. These tumors are difficult to manage with conventional therapy, but good results were seen with octreotide.

McKay CJ, et al. Somatostatin and somatostatin analogues—are they indicated in the management of acute pancreatitis? Gut 1993; 34:1622

A review of the 15-year experience with the use of somatostatin in the treatment of pancreatitis.

Pedersoli P, et al. Conservative treatment of external pancreatic fistulas with parenteral nutrition alone or in combination with continuous infusion of somatostatin, glucagon, or calcitonin. Surg, Gynecol Obstet 1986; 162:428.

Somatostatin decreased the fistula closure time from 31 to 6 days, saving an estimated $2100 per patient.

Saltz L, et al. Octreotide as an antineoplastic agent in the treatment of functional and nonfunctional neuroendocrine tumors. Cancer 1993; 72:244.

A report of the Sloan-Kettering experience in the use of octreotide as the primary chemotherapeutic modality in the treatment of neuroendocrine tumors.

Shields R, et al. A prospective randomized controlled clinical trial comparing octreotide and endoscopic sclerotherapy in the control of acute variceal hemorrhage: An interim report (abstract). Gastroenterology 1993; 104:A991.

Shields R, et al. Octreotide in the long term management of portal hypertension–preliminary results of a prospective randomized controlled clinical trial (abstract). Gastroenterology 1993; 104: A991.

Two abstracts that describe the acute and chronic use of octreotide to control variceal hemorrhage.

Sung J, et al. Octreotide infusion or emergency sclerotherapy for variceal hemorrhage. Lancet 1993; 342:637.

The authors concluded that octreotide infusion and emergency sclerotherapy are equally effective in controlling variceal hemorrhage.

Van Thiel D, et al. Somatostatin in gastroenterology. Dig Dis Sci 1989; 34:15–485.

A series of papers from the American Gastroenterology Association plenary session of May 1987.

Antiserotonin Agents

Michael S. Gurney

Carcinoid tumors were first described by Lubarsch in 1888, but it was not until 1953 that Waldenström and Lundgren associated the peculiar syndrome of flushing, diarrhea, and cardiac valvular disease with elevated levels of serotonin secreted by the tumor. Pharmacotherapy was then directed against serotonin in an effort to ablate the syndrome's debilitating symptoms. Methysergide (Sansert) and various anticholinergics, particularly cyproheptadine (Periactin), were found to have antiserotonin activity and clinical benefit in such patients. The development of octreotide (Sandostatin), which has greater efficacy and fewer side effects, has relegated these drugs to lesser roles. Nevertheless, octreotide therapy is expensive and cumbersome, requiring repeated injections. The antiserotonin agents still fill a useful niche in our therapeutic armamentarium.

Cyproheptadine (Periactin)

Antihistamines competitively antagonize most of the smooth-muscle–stimulating actions of histamine on the H_1-receptors in the gastrointestinal tract. Cyproheptadine also competes with serotonin for receptor-site binding and is believed to be the most effective member of the antihistamine family for the carcinoid syndrome.

PHARMACOLOGY

Cyproheptadine is absorbed rapidly after oral administration. Symptomatic relief begins within 15 to 30 minutes, with full efficacy reached within 1 hour. Less than 5 percent of the drug is excreted unchanged in the stool. Cyproheptadine is metabolized by the liver, and the inactive glucuronide salt is renally excreted. The drug has a longer half-life than many antihistamines and can be given at 6- to 8-hour intervals.

INDICATIONS

In 1960, Brown and associates studied several antiserotonin agents in carcinoid patients and found that cyproheptadine gave the best clinical response with the fewest side effects. Since then, it has gained a reputation as the agent of first choice for relief of diarrhea and flushing. Severe flushing and diarrhea are unlikely to be completely relieved, but some improvement can be expected. Bronchospasm, on the other hand, is not well managed by this medication. There are several case reports of marked tumor regression with cyproheptadine; because of this possibility, the lower cost, and ease of administration, cyproheptadine is often recommended as first-line therapy for carcinoid syndrome, especially if flushing is not a severe problem.

Antihistamines are notorious for their lack of predictability for both clinical response and side effects in any individual patient. If cyproheptadine is not efficacious or is poorly tolerated, the entire class should not be abandoned. Good alternate choices are prochlorperazine (Compazine) or chlorpromazine (Thorazine).

CONTRAINDICATIONS AND SIDE EFFECTS

Side effects are common with all antihistamines and vary in incidence and severity with both the individual and the drug. However, serious toxicity rarely occurs.

Sedation is a common complaint with all antihistamines. Continued use of the medication or a reduction in dose often results in good tolerance. Dizziness and hypotension are also common side effects and are most common in the elderly.

Antihistamines lower the seizure threshold in patients with convulsive disorders and should be used with caution in such patients. All antihistamines also have anticholinergic activity and should be administered carefully, if at all, to patients with narrow-angle glaucoma, prostatic hypertrophy, or gastric outlet obstruction. Monoamine oxidase inhibitors intensify the anticholinergic side effects of antihistamines and inhibit the breakdown of serotonin. They should not be given to carcinoid patients, particularly those who are receiving cyproheptadine.

DOSAGE

The initial dosage of cyproheptadine is 4 mg 4 times a day, but higher doses are usually needed for relief of carcinoid symptoms; 6 to 8 mg 3 times a day is often needed for these patients. Moertal, Kvols, and Rubin found the best starting dosage to be 0.4 mg/kg in three divided doses. Total daily dosage should not exceed 500 μg/kg body weight. For acute attacks, 50 to 75 mg in 200 ml saline infused intravenously over 1 to 2 hours may be beneficial.

Methysergide (Sansert)

Methysergide is structurally related to methylergonovine maleate. Like cyproheptadine and the ergot alkaloids, it competitively inhibits serotonin binding.

PHARMACOLOGY

Methysergide is rapidly absorbed following oral administration and metabolized by the liver. As a serotonin antagonist, it has not been tested against other compounds, but in animal studies it appears to be as effective as cyproheptadine.

INDICATIONS

Methysergide was shown, in a study at the National Institutes of Health (NIH) by Brown and associates, to reduce steatorrhea and diarrhea in patients with the carcinoid syndrome. Flushing only variably responds, probably because the flush is not due to serotonin alone.

Use of methysergide has been limited because of reports that long-term use is associated with retroperitoneal fibrosis. Less commonly, fibrotic processes involving the aorta, heart, and lungs have occurred. The fibrosis may regress when the drug is withdrawn, but in some patients this regression is only partial. This complication is particularly vexing in carcinoid patients, since fibrosis in the abdomen and cardiac valves can occur late in the carcinoid syndrome and is a serious complication. Use of methysergide, therefore, should be reserved for those patients who are intolerant or unresponsive to other medications and are debilitated by their symptoms.

Table 45-1. Antiserotonin agents: Pregnancy and breast-feeding

Agent	FDA pregnancy category	Risk vs benefit (by trimester)			Breast-feeding category
		1st	2nd	3rd	
Methysergide	X	R>>B	R>>	R>>B	IV
Cyproheptadine	B1	B>R	B>R	B>R	IV

Food and Drug Administration (FDA) pregnancy categories:
A = Well-controlled studies fail to demonstrate risk to the fetus.
B1 = Animal studies fail to demonstrate risk to the fetus but no human studies are available.
B2 = Animal studies show some risk to the fetus but this is not confirmed in human studies.
C1 = Animal studies show risk to the fetus but no human studies are available.
C2 = Animal and human studies are unavailable.
D = Drug associated with birth defects but with potential benefits that may outweigh known risks.
X = Drug associated with birth defects and with potential risk that clearly outweighs potential benefit.
Risk vs benefit: R>>B = Proven or potential risk outweighs potential benefits.
B>R = Potential benefits outweigh potential risks.
R>>B? = Risks may be outweighed by benefits in some circumstances.
? = Risk-to-benefit ratio is unknown.
Breast-feeding categories:
I = Drug does not enter breast milk.
II = Drug enters breast milk but is not known to be harmful in therapeutic doses.
IIIA = Drug may or may not enter breast milk but no adverse effects are expected.
IIIB = Drug may or may not enter breast milk but drug is systemically absorbed.
IV = Drug enters breast milk and poses a potential risk to the neonate.

CONTRAINDICATIONS AND SIDE EFFECTS

Methysergide can cause vascular insufficiency and should not be used in patients with known cardiac or peripheral atherosclerotic vascular disease. It should be given with caution to patients with risk factors for coronary disease, and all patients over 40 should have their cardiac status evaluated before therapy.

Renal function must be quantified before drug administration and every 4 to 6 months during therapy. If blood urea nitrogen rises, dysuria or flank pain develops, or signs of phlebitis or venous obstruction occur, the medication should be stopped and clinical status evaluated. Patients should also be observed for pleural or cardiac friction rubs, pleural effusions, shortness of breath, and chest pain.

The drug is contraindicated during pregnancy and in patients with severe hepatic or renal disease (Table 45-1).

An estimated 30 percent of patients have side effects, and 10 to 20 percent need to discontinue the drug because of them.

DOSAGE

Methysergide is administered orally. The suggested starting dosage is 4 to 6 mg/day in divided doses, preferably with meals. The dose can be increased to 8 to 12 mg/day if tolerated. The drug should be discontinued for several weeks, and the patient reevaluated, after every 6 months of continuous therapy.

PEARLS AND PITFALLS

1. Antihistamines may prevent a positive reaction to skin-testing procedures and should be discontinued several days before such testing.
2. Gastrointestinal side effects of the antihistamines include nausea, anorexia, and epigastric distress. Administration of antihistamines with meals or milk usually alleviates these problems.
3. The incidence of peptic ulcer disease is high in the carcinoid syndrome. Not all gastrointestinal complaints should be attributed to the syndrome or the therapy, since ulcer disease may be the culprit.
4. The best study to look for retroperitoneal fibrosis is an intravenous pyelogram. Dilatation and deviation of the ureters are signs of fibrosis with obstruction.
5. Morphine is a serotonin liberator and must be avoided in carcinoid patients.
6. Alpha-adrenergic blocking agents such as methyldopa (Aldomet) or phenoxybenzamine are often helpful in control of flushing.
7. The bronchospasm of carcinoid syndrome may respond to low doses of isoproterenol aerosol or corticosteroids. Epinephrine or other adrenergic agonists must never be given to such patients since they worsen the bronchospasm and may precipitate hypotension and carcinoid crisis.
8. Carcinoid patients should be on a diet high in tryptophan and nicotinic acid; supplements may be needed.
9. Exercise, alcohol, or spicy foods may precipitate carcinoid symptoms. Patients and doctors should be aware of such associations

Suggested Reading

Brown RE, et al. Studies on several possible antiserotonin compounds in the functioning carcinoid syndrome. Clin Res 1960;

One of the few studies that compares different medications in symptomatic carcinoid syndrome. Cyproheptadine was the most effective and best tolerated.

Leitner SP, et al. Partial remission of carcinoid tumor in response to cyproheptadine. Ann Intern Med 1989; 111:760–761.

A case report of a dramatic tumor and symptom reduction due to the use of cyproheptadine. The response duration was over a year.

Maton PM The carcinoid syndrome. JAMA 1988; 260:1602–1605.

A concise and excellent discussion of the approach to the carcinoid syndrome.

Melmon KL, et al. Treatment of malabsorption and diarrhea of the carcinoid syndrome with methysergide. Gastroenterology 1965; 48:18.

A study showing good benefit and tolerance with methysergide in seven patients.

Miller R, et al. Anesthesia for the carcinoid syndrome: A report of nine cases. Can Anaesth Soc J 1978; 25:240.

A fine discussion of the perioperative management of patients with the carcinoid syndrome.

Moertal CG, Kvols LK, Rubin J. A study of cyproheptadine in the treatment of metastatic carcinoid tumor and the malignant carcinoid syndrome. Cancer 1991; 67:33–36.

Another look at the drug as initial therapy in carcinoid tumors. Patients obtained relief from diarrhea and gained weight, but flushing continued. Tumor regression was not observed in this study.

Oates JA, Butler C. Pharmacologic and endocrine aspects of the carcinoid syndrome. Adv Pharmacol 1967; 5:109.

The pathophysiology and treatment of the carcinoid syndrome are well discussed.

Warner RRP. Carcinoid Tumor. In JE Berk (ed), *Gastroenterology*, vol 3. Philadelphia: Saunders, 1985.

An excellent discussion of the carcinoid syndrome, its pathophysiology, and its therapy.

Cyclosporine and FK506

David J. Roberts

Cyclosporine

Cyclosporine is a metabolite produced by the fungus *Tolypocladium inflatum gams.* The introduction of this 11–amino acid cyclic polypeptide has revolutionized the transplantation field. In addition to its cell-mediated effects on allograft rejection in orthotopic liver transplantation, the drug is being investigated for possible use in other gastrointestinal diseases, such as ulcerative colitis, Crohn's disease, and primary biliary cirrhosis. Cyclosporine is relatively unique in its immunosuppression because its action is lymphocyte-specific, noncytotoxic, and reversible. It significantly avoids the nonspecific myelotoxic side effects of conventional immunosuppression with antimetabolites.

MECHANISM OF ACTION

The mode of action of cyclosporine involves inhibition of the early events of helper T-cell activation, thereby blocking the recruitment of cytotoxic T cells and B-cell clones. The drug is most effective if administered at the time an immune response is initiated. These properties make cyclosporine ideally suited for use in organ transplantation.

Cyclosporine exerts its major effects by inhibiting T-cell activation. The exact molecular mechanism of action is unclear, but the early T-cell signal induction pathway is repressed, leading to failure of transcription of cytokine genes. The drug binds to an intracellular receptor known as cyclophilin. The cyclosporine-cyclophilin complex interferes with the synthesis of interleukin-2 (IL-2) by activated helper T lymphocytes. Without IL-2, cytotoxic T cells do not undergo clonal expansion, and T cell–mediated rejection is inhibited. Additionally, the generation of other cytokines is affected, such as B-cell activating factor and interferon gamma. The drug spares development of suppressor T cells, which remain free to attenuate specific immune responses.

ADMINISTRATION, DOSAGE, AND MONITORING

Cyclosporine is a hydrophobic compound that must be stabilized in castor oil for intravenous infusion or olive oil for oral administration. Intramuscular administration is less effective due to inadequate absorption. Absorption following oral administration is highly variable, with peak levels occurring from 1 to 8 hours after the drug is given. Because of its lipophilic nature, cyclosporine accumulates in fat and skin; therefore, dosage requirements decrease with long-term use. Cyclosporine is metabolized and excreted mainly by the liver, with only 10 percent excreted by the kidney. Thus, patients with liver failure have decreased dosage requirements. Pediatric patients require higher doses because of more rapid metabolism.

Cyclosporine is usually administered 4 to 10 hours preoperatively and as needed intraoperatively. Postoperatively, patients should be started on intravenous cyclosporine due to the variablity of or-

absorption. Oral cyclosporine can be added to the regimen as tolerated by the patient, and drug levels should be monitored frequently. When levels begin to increase indicating oral absorption, intravenous cyclosporine can be tapered and eventually discontinued.

Since cyclosporine has significant toxicity and variable absorption, the monitoring of drug levels is critical. Radioimmunoassay (RIA) and high-pressure liquid chromatography (HPLC) are two methods available for measuring levels. Radioimmunoassay is less specific, since it measures cyclosporine as well as some inactive metabolites. Blood cyclosporine concentration is more reliable than plasma levels, which are affected by temperature, hematocrit, or plasma lipoprotein concentration. Levels should be measured before drug administration and every 2 or 3 days thereafter, until a stable clinical condition and drug level are achieved.

Each transplant center employs a slightly different protocol for administration. In general, a single oral dose of cyclosporine of 15 mg/kg/day is given 4 to 10 hours before transplantation. Postoperatively, this dose is continued daily for 1 to 2 weeks, then tapered by 5 percent per week to a maintenance level of approximately 5 to 10 mg/kg/day. Patients with variable oral absorption and those who are unable to take oral medications can be treated with the intravenous concentrate.

The intravenous dose is approximately one-third of the oral dose. The intravenous concentrate should be diluted (1 ml in 20–100 ml of 0.9% saline or 5% dextrose) and given in a slow intravenous infusion over 2 to 6 hours.

The usual dose for autoimmune disease is about 5 mg/kg/day. Currently, there is no consensus on the optimal dose for the treatment of inflammatory bowel disease (IBD), but most recent studies have used less than 5 mg/kg/day. Cyclosporine doses in the experimental treatment of primary biliary cirrhosis are also nonuniform, but are less than 5 mg/kg/day (see Gastrointestinal Indications section.)

All regimens represent only a starting point, because drug therapy must be adjusted based on the blood levels of cyclosporine, the patient's clinical status, biochemical profiles, and immunologic parameters.

SIDE EFFECTS

The most common and clinically important toxic effect of cyclosporine is kidney damage. This effect seems to be reversible with a decrease in dose; only 4 to 17 percent of patients require complete termination of the drug. Nephrotoxicity manifests as a modest increase in serum creatinine that is nonprogressive and usually occurs weeks after the start of therapy. Glomerular filtration rate usually stabilizes at 45 to 60 percent of normal despite continued drug administration. Some patients experience transient oliguria. Hypertension, hyperuricemia, and hyperkalemia, probably secondary to renal damage, are other common side effects. Renal biopsy shows vascular changes that usually do not correspond with the extent of renal failure, thus implicating a functional rather than structural mechanism.

Other, less frequent toxic effects include hepatotoxicity, gingival hyperplasia, hirsutism, and transient tremors. Rises in bilirubin, transaminases, and alkaline phosphatase occur transiently and frequently respond to dose reduction. Also reported after cyclosporine treatment are central nervous system toxicity associated with reversible white-matter changes, as well as thrombotic thrombocytopenic purpura. The central nervous system effects may be related to low serum lipid levels. See Table 46-1 for effects in pregnancy and breast feeding.

The incidence of lymphoma in cyclosporine-treated patients is about 0.3 percent, a figure not significantly different from that of conventionally treated patients. Furthermore, most patients in whom lymphoma developed were found to have previous Epstein-Barr virus infection, which has been associated in the past with B-cell tumors. Among the 2000 patients treated with cyclosporine for autoimmune disease, only three cases of lymphoma have been reported.

GASTROINTESTINAL INDICATIONS

The rapid and reversible effects of cyclosporine, predominantly modulating T-cell processes, render it ideal for use in organ transplantation. In liver transplantation treatment may be initiated simultaneously with antigen (allograft) presentation. Theoretically, cyclosporine seems less suited to affect the pathophysiologic processes in autoimmune diseases because the immunologic mediators are chronically activated, and humoral immunity appears important in pathogenesis. However, there have been a number of recent reports of the use of cyclosporine in autoimmune and other chronic inflammatory diseases. Of particular interest to the gastroenterologist is the role of the drug in treatment of primary biliary cirrhosis and inflammatory bowel disease.

Liver Transplantation

Since its discovery in 1980, cyclosporine has become the foremost agent for immunosuppression in solid-organ transplantation, including the liver. With the success of cyclosporine treatment, liver transplantation has become the treatment of choice for many liver diseases. Allograft survival rates approach 80 to 85 percent after one year and are higher in the pediatric than the adult population. Currently, morbidity and mortality more commonly result from the severity of preexisting disease or technical problems than from rejection or sepsis. In one study, 25 percent of cyclosporine-treated patients had episodes of rejection, compared with 66 percent of those treated conventionally with azathioprine and prednisone. The incidence of severe sepsis has also diminished greatly because cyclosporine suppresses the bone marrow less than agents that were previously used.

Inflammatory Bowel Disease

Several investigators have postulated that the anti-inflammatory action of cyclosporine may lend itself to the treatment of IBD. Not only does cyclosporine inhibit transcriptional activation of the gene for IL-2, but it also inhibits several other cytokines produced by different leukocyte populations. The drug may modulate tumor necrosis factor gene expression.

Use of cyclosporine in Crohn's disease is controversial. Brynskov and associates, in a multicentered randomized trial using 7.8 mg/kg/day of the drug for a follow-up period of only 12 weeks, reported mild improvement in patients randomized to a combination of cyclosporine and steroids, compared to those receiving only steroids

Table 46-1. Cyclosporine and FK506: Pregnancy and breast-feeding

Agent	FDA pregnancy category	Risk vs benefit (by trimester)			Breast-feeding category
		1st	2nd	3rd	
Cyclosporine	D	?	?	?	IV
Tacrolimus (FK506)	D	?	?	?	IV

Food and Drug Administration (FDA) pregnancy categories:
A = Well-controlled studies fail to demonstrate risk to the fetus.
B1 = Animal studies fail to demonstrate risk to the fetus but no human studies are available.
B2 = Animal studies show some risk to the fetus but this is not confirmed in human studies.
C1 = Animal studies show risk to the fetus but no human studies are available.
C2 = Animal and human studies are unavailable.
D = Drug associated with birth defects but with potential benefits that may outweigh known risks.
X = Drug associated with birth defects and with potential risk that clearly outweighs potential benefit.
Risk vs benefit: R >> B = Proven or potential risk outweighs potential benefits.
B > R = Potential benefits outweigh potential risks.
R >> B? = Risks may be outweighed by benefits in some circumstances.
? = Risk-to-benefit ratio is unknown.

Breast-feeding categories:
I = Drug does not enter breast milk.
II = Drug enters breast milk but is not known to be harmful in therapeutic doses.
IIIA = Drug may or may not enter breast milk but no adverse effects are expected.
IIIB = Drug may or may not enter breast milk but drug is systemically absorbed.
IV = Drug enters breast milk and poses a potential risk to the neonate.

However, a follow-up report on the "long-term" effect of cyclosporine in the same study population showed no sustained benefit from cyclosporine compared to steroids; further, no difference was seen in remission rates between the two groups.

The Canadian Crohn's Disease Study Group of 80 patients showed no long-term effect of cyclosporine compared to placebo. In total, the clinical outcomes of over 600 patients in four different studies do not support the early enthusiasm for use of cyclosporine in Crohn's disease. Cyclosporine appears to have a beneficial short-term anti-inflammatory effect on Crohn's disease in relatively large doses (more than 5 mg/kg/day). However, the risk of potential side effects and lack of long-term efficacy severely limit the clinical usefulness of cyclosporine in Crohn's disease.

The use of chronic, potentially harmful immunosuppressives in ulcerative colitis raises many ethical questions, and no long-term trial of cyclosporine has been attempted in this subtype of inflammatory bowel disase. A recent placebo-controlled trial of 20 patients with fulminant colitis reported over 80 percent response to cyclosporine when given intravenously (4 mg/kg/day); during limited follow-up, 60 percent of patients entered clinical remission (unpublished data). Confirmatory studies on the use of cyclosporine in fulminant ulcerative colitis must be conducted before this treatment can be recommended.

Primary Biliary Cirrhosis

Cyclosporine may attenuate the immunologic progression of primary biliary cirrhosis (PBC). A study by Routhier and associates in 1980 showed a biochemical benefit from high-dose cyclosporine (10 mg/kg/day) in six patients; however, this study was abandoned due to nephrotoxicity. Three larger trials were completed with lower doses of cyclosporine and careful monitoring of cyclosporine trough levels. The high cost of cyclosporine, hypertension, and decreased renal function have reduced enthusiasm for use of this drug in PBC.

Lombard and associates conducted the largest prospective controlled trial on PBC in 349 patients. A dose of 3 mg/kg/day cyclosporine was given initially, and the dose was adjusted to maintain safe trough levels. During a 6-year follow-up period, no beneficial effect was found on liver histology or fatigue. Effect on survival was marginal and similar to that seen with other immunosuppressants such as azothiaprine. Patients were not randomized by bilirubin levels, and advanced cirrhotics were not excluded.

A smaller study was performed at the Mayo Clinic with 29 patients using 4 mg/kg/day cyclosporine over a 2-year period. Patients with advanced cirrhosis were excluded. A significant improvement in fatigue was noted, and liver histology progressed more slowly in the cyclosporine group; however, renal toxicity or hypertension developed in 63 percent (compared to 10% in the lower-dose Lombard study). Minuk and associates reported similar results in 12 patients using doses of 5 to 6 mg/kg/day.

The value of cyclosporine in PBC remains unclear. The benefits may become more apparent when patients in earlier stages of PBC are randomized; presently, the benefits do not outweigh the clinical adverse consequences.

FK506

FK506, also known as tacrolimus, is a macrolide immunosuppressant that shares many of cyclosporine's selective anti–T-lymphocyte properties. The compound was isolated from the fungus *Streptomyces tsukubaensis* in 1984. While structurally dissimilar to cyclosporine, the drug has a similar mode of action. Like cyclosporine, FK506 binds a family of intracellular receptors (termed FK506 binding proteins), and this complex inhibits the calcium-dependent translocation of a transcription factor from the cytosol into the nucleus. In this manner FK506 blocks the transcription of the early-phase T-cell activation genes.

CLINICAL USAGE

Due to its strong hepatotrophic properties, most clinical studies of FK506 have been conducted in liver transplantation centers. In 1989, Starzl and associates reported the drug effective in salvaging chronically rejected liver allografts, with few or no untoward effects. This experience led to several randomized studies investigating the use of FK506 as primary and rescue immunosuppression in liver transplantation.

Primary Immunosuppression in Liver Transplantation

Investigators at the University of Pittsburgh reported the results of 110 patients undergoing orthotopic liver transplantation with open-label FK506 and low-dose steroids in 1991. One-year survival rates of 93 percent prompted the same group to conduct a randomized trial comparing FK506 to cyclosporine in 81 adults. The one-year survival rate for the 41 patients randomized to the FK506 arm was 12 percent better than that of the cyclosporine-treated patients. The survival rate for the allograft at one year was improved by 20 percent.

Two multicenter, prospective randomized trials are now being analyzed. If confirmatory, the use of FK506 as primary immunosuppression in liver transplantation will increase.

Salvage Immunosuppression in Liver Transplantation

The role of FK506 in salvage therapy has been actively investigated. The combination of cyclosporine and FK506 results in serious adverse effects, most notably nephrotoxicity. Most of the grafts that show either acute or early chronic rejection respond favorably when switched from cyclosporine to FK506, allowing a reduction or discontinuation of supplemental steroid therapy. Currently, salvage therapy for liver transplantation is the most common indication for FK506.

Immunosuppression in Extrahepatic Transplantation and Autoimmune Diseases

The compound has been investigated in orthotopic cardiac, kidney, and combined liver–small-bowel transplantations. Unlike its impressive record in liver transplantation, the preliminary results from these extrahepatic grafts have not been encouraging.

Currently, FK506 has no role in autoimmune disease. However, a recent report suggests a possible use of the drug in the treatment of uveitis, psoriasis, and pyoderma gangrenosum.

PEARLS AND PITFALLS

1. The clearance rate of cyclosporine in children is 40 percent higher than in adults, who require more frequent and higher doses.
2. Hepatic impairment reduces cyclosporine metabolite elimination. Since 90 percent of this elimination is bile-dependent, longer dosing intervals are necessary in the presence of elevated bilirubin or serum alanine aminotransferase.
3. Use of cyclosporine in inflammatory bowel disease remains controversial. The onset of action is rapid (approximately 2 weeks); however, relapses during therapy and after discontinuation of the drug are usual.
4. At present, cyclosporine does not appear to alter the course of Crohn's disease, reduce complications, or affect the need for surgery.
5. The role of FK506 is incompletely defined. Present data do not indicate a survival benefit over cyclosporine in renal translants. Strong hepatotrophic properties may explain the success of FK506 in liver transplantation.
6. Immunosuppressants such as cyclosporine are more likely to be beneficial in early stages of PBC. Based on currently available data, their widespread use in this disease cannot be justified.
7. The side effects of FK506 appear comparable to those of cyclosporine; nephrotoxicity is the major toxicity of both compounds.

Suggested Reading

CYCLOSPORINE: GENERAL

Anderson J, et al. FK506 and cyclosporine inhibit antigen- or nitrogen-induced monokine and lymphokine production in vitro. Transplant Proc 24: 321–325.

Recent evidence suggests that these drugs may modulate tumor necrosis factor gene expression.

Kahan BD. Medical intelligence: Cyclosporine. N Engl J Med 1989; 321:1725–1738.

A superb review of the pharmacology, toxicity, and therapeutic effects.

Schreiber SL, et al. The mechanism of action of cyclosporin A and FK506. Immunol Today 1992; 13: 136–142.

The most current synopsis of the biochemical mode of action of both of these immunosuppressants.

Van Buren CT, et al. Cyclosporine: Progress, problems, and perspectives. Surg Clin North Am 1986; 3:435–449.

This is a very good review of cyclosporine.

CYCLOSPORINE AND LIVER TRANSPLANTATION

deGroen PC, et al. Central nervous system toxicity after liver transplantation: The role of cyclosporine and cholesterol. N Engl J Med 1987; 14:861–866.

Thirteen of 48 patients receiving cyclosporine after liver transplantation had symptoms of central nervous system toxicity and radiographic evidence of diffuse white-matter changes.

Gordon R, et al. Indications for liver transplantation in the cyclosporine era. Surg Clin North Am 1986; 3:541–556.

A review of different indications for liver transplantation and their success rates.

Grant D, et al. Adverse effects of cyclosporine therapy following liver transplantation. Transplant Proc 1987; 4:3463–3465.
The side effects of cyclosporine, as observed in 62 orthotopic liver transplants.

Starzl T, et al. Liver transplantation in the cyclosporine era. Prog Allergy 1986; 38:366–394.
One of the largest transplant centers presents a general assessment of liver transplantations, including success rate, surgical techniques, tissue matching, and organ procurement.

CYCLOSPORINE AND INFLAMMATORY BOWEL DISEASE

Brynskov J, et al. A placebo-controlled, double-blind randomized trial of cyclosporine therapy in active chronic Crohn's disease. N Engl J Med 1989; 321:845–850.
A multicenter, randomized trial with limited follow-up of 12 weeks. Subsequent studies did not validate its initial enthusiasm.

Present DH. Fulminant Ulcerative Colitis, Save the Colon: Medical Management. AGA Postgraduate Course Syllabus 1994: 325–328.
Early data awaiting publication that, if confirmed, may suggest a role for cyclosporine in severe acute ulcerative colitis.

CYCLOSPORINE AND PRIMARY BILIARY CIRRHOSIS

Lombard M, et al. Cycloporin A treatment in primary biliary cirrhosis: Results of a long-term placebo-controlled trial. Gastroenterology 1993; 104:519–526.
This is the largest prospective, controlled trial with 349 patients. Only marginally prolonged survival was demonstrated by multivariate regression analysis. In a 6-year follow-up, no beneficial effect in liver histology or fatigue was seen.

Minuk GY, et al. Pilot study of cyclosporin A in patients with symptomatic primary biliary cirrhosis. Gastroenterology 1988; 95: 1356–1363.
Small randomized trial with six patients each in cyclosporine and placebo arms. A 50 percent increase in serum creatinine as observed in the cyclosporine group.

Routhier G, et al. Effects of cyclosporin A on suppressor and inducer T lymphocytes in primary biliary cirrhosis. Lancet 1980; 2:1223–1226.
Beneficial effects of the drug on serum aspartate transaminase and alkaline phosphatase levels in six patients with PBC. The study, which utilized high doses of cyclosporine, was abandoned secondary to nephrotoxicity.

Wiesner RH, et al. A controlled clinical trial of cyclosporine in the treatment of primary biliary cirrhosis. N Engl J Med 1990; 322: 1419–1424.
This Mayo Clinic group used lower doses of cyclosporine in 19 patients with PBC. Patients who received cyclosporine had less fatigue and pruritus, and reduced serum alanine transaminase, alkaline phosphatase, and bilirubin levels compared with 10 placebo-treated control subjects.

FK506

Bach JF. The new era of immunosuppressive therapy in autoimmune disease. Transplant Proc 1991; 23: 3319–3321.
The author suggests a possible role for FK506 in autoimmune processes.

Demeris AJ, et al. Conversion of allograft recipients from cyclosporin to FK506 based immunosuppression. Transplant Proc 1991; 23:14–21.

Confirmatory follow-up study to preceding report on salvage use of FK506.

Fung J, et al. Conversion from cyclosporine to FK506 in liver allograft recipients with cyclosporine related complications. Transplant Proc 1990; 22 (suppl 1): 6–12.

The authors investigate the salvage role of FK506. Interesting synergism of adverse effects with the combination of cyclosporine and FK506.

Fung J, et al. A randomized trial of primary liver transplantation under immunosuppression with FK506 vs. cyclosporine. Transplant Proc 1991; 23:2977–2988.

Starzl TE, et al. FK506 for liver, kidney, and pancreas transplantation. Lancet 1989; 2:1000–1004.

First clinical report of the success of FK506 in salvaging chronically rejected allografts.

Todo S, et al. One hundred ten consecutive primary orthotopic liver transplantations under FK506 in adults. Transplant Proc 1991; 23:1397–1402.

First primary use of the drug for immunosuppression in open-label form as phase I trial.

Index

Index